What's in this Stuff ?

The essential guide to what's really in the products you buy

PAT THOMAS

'In the absence of an effective regulatory system, it's increasingly important that we learn for ourselves what products to trust and what to avoid. Pat Thomas has made that job much easier. Every household should own a copy of this amazing book.'

Zac Goldsmith, Editor, the *Ecologist*

D0274404

This edition first published in the UK in 2006 by
Rodale International Ltd
7–10 Chandos Street
London W1G 9AD
www.rodalebooks.co.uk

The moral right of Pat Thomas to be identified as the author of this work has been
asserted in accordance with the Copyright, Designs and Patents Act of 1988.

Printed and bound in the UK by CPI Bath using acid-free paper from sustainable sources.

3 5 7 9 8 6 4 2

A CIP record for this book is available from the British Library

ISBN 10: 1-4050-9549-0
ISBN 13: 978-1-4050-9549-5

This paperback edition distributed to the book trade by Pan Macmillan Ltd

Notice
This book is intended as a reference volume only, not as a medical manual. The information
given here is designed to help you make informed decisions about your health. It is not
intended as a substitute for any treatment that you may have been prescribed by your
doctor. If you suspect that you have a medical problem, we urge you to seek competent
medical help.

Mention of specific companies, organizations or authorities in this book does not imply
endorsement by the publisher, nor does mention of specific companies, organizations or
authorities in the book imply that they endorse the book.

Addresses, websites and telephone numbers given in this book were accurate at the
time the book went to press.

Chemical names that appear in **bold italic** are listed in Chapter 10, "Chemicals: A to Z".

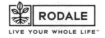

We inspire and enable people to improve their lives and the world around them

acknowledgements

I am indebted to all the usual crowd of loved ones, especially my son Alex, who has been patient and supportive while so much was put on hold during the researching and writing of this book.

My eternal gratitude goes out to my agent and partner in crime, Laura Longrigg, for more than a decade of loving care. I am also grateful to all at Rodale, especially Anne Lawrance, who understood the need for a comprehensive look at household toxins and weren't afraid of the subject matter, and to Tom Genrich, for his contributions to the pesticide section. And to Sharyn Wong my friend and favourite subeditor – another big thank you.

I am also indebted to all the authors, environmentalists, toxicologists and scientists, whose work is listed in the bibliography, for everything they have done in bringing the vital issue of toxic chemicals to the fore.

Finally, with more than mere words can express, I thank everyone at the world's best magazine, the *Ecologist* – especially Harry Ram, Tyler Moorhead and Zac Goldsmith – for reeling me into an office full of amazing, inspiring, dedicated, fearless, wildly entertaining and, above all, warmhearted people.

contents

introduction

We are what we eat. We are what we breathe. We are what we put on our skin. We are whatever we expose ourselves to. And because of all this, we are in trouble.

Today, cheap, mass-produced and poorly tested chemicals are used to make many of the products that we buy every day. The price that you pay at the checkout may seem reasonable, but there is a hidden cost – in terms of human health and the ecology of the planet – that may be higher than any of us can imagine.

The food we eat, and the products we use to clean ourselves and our homes as well as those we use in the garden and on our pets can contain carcinogens (cancer-causing substances), hormone-disrupting chemicals, central-nervous-system disrupters, reproductive toxins and psychoactive chemicals (substances that alter brain function).

While many of us have got into the habit of scanning food labels for unwanted ingredients, it can be hard to keep up to date on what is safe and what is not. What's more, intelligent consumers who scan food labels for harmful additives rarely apply the same critical faculties to the other products they buy and use.

Today, scientists have grave reservations about the witches' brew of chemicals that we are regularly exposed to. It's not just that the individual chemicals are harmful. New data are coming in all the time to show that mixtures of chemicals can often react in unexpected ways, or combine to produce entirely new compounds that are harmful to human health. Through such a combination of everyday foods and household products, we are conducting chemical warfare against our own bodies.

The bigger picture of chemical toxins and the threat they pose to health can be difficult to take in – even when all the evidence is in front of you. Nevertheless, several large studies have concluded that, because of the chemicals in the products you buy, the environment inside your home may be more seriously polluted than the air outdoors, even in the largest and most industrialised cities. Considering that we spend as much as 90 per cent of our time inside our homes, the health risks from these indoor pollutants are much greater than from those we encounter outside.

Many of us rely on the fact that the chemicals we use every day have been fully tested and found to be safe for humans. But the reality is that there are about 70,000 chemicals currently in use, with 1000 new chemicals coming on the market each year. There are no basic safety data for 43 per cent of all chemicals in use today and full safety information is only available for 7 per cent. Among the compounds commonly used in household products, there are full safety data for only a quarter of them.

While it is easy to assume the role of a 'victim' and to think of environmental toxins as things we consume involuntarily, not all toxins come from 'out there'. Many are the result of what we allow into our homes and our bodies without a second thought.

Nowadays, we ingest dozens of harmful and largely unevaluated chemicals when we eat conventionally grown produce; fertilisers, herbicides, pesticides and fungicides all combine to make so-called 'fresh' food a significant source of poisons. When we eat conventionally reared meats, we are ingesting growth hormones and a myriad of just-in-case medications given to conventionally farmed animals – not to mention the pesticides, herbicides, fertilisers and fungicides contained in their feed. As the bovine spongiform encephalopathy (BSE or 'mad-cow disease') saga has shown us, we are also sometimes ingesting deadly microorganisms.

In addition, when manufacturers try to reassure us that potentially harmful chemicals are only used in small amounts in their products, they are glossing over some relevant facts. Each day, we are exposed to many different chemicals. For example, we don't just use a shampoo once in our lives; we use it regularly, sometimes daily, and we use it in hot showers and baths so that the chemicals become vapourised and are absorbed in greater quantities into our bloodstream.

We also use a shampoo in combination with other products such as a conditioner, hair gel or mousse, hairspray, toothpaste, deodorant, washing-up liquid, air fresheners and furniture polish – each of which contains 'minute' amounts of the same harmful chemicals. Add up all these 'minute' amounts of chemicals and the potential exposure becomes disturbingly high.

Given these facts, you may wonder how we manage to stay healthy at all. The reality is, we don't. Even though we are now living longer than ever before, we are strikingly unhealthy. Chronic conditions are on the rise. Respiratory problems such as asthma and bronchitis have doubled in recent years, with young people being the most affected. Vague disorders like sinusitis and allergic rhinitis are becoming major problems, especially in inner-city areas. Heart disease, diabetes and thyroid problems are all on the rise, too. Infertility, in both men and women, is becoming more common as are other hormonally linked disorders. Cancer continues to be a persistent disease across all cultures, age groups and genders, with still no medical solution in sight.

This is not an encouraging picture. But what's worse is that we have allowed ourselves to believe that such unhealthy conditions are a normal part of being human and an inevitable result of ageing.

There is nothing 'normal' about disease. The human body is a robust and remarkable organism that is orientated towards survival and wellness. Without our even being aware of it, our body works hard every day to keep itself in balance and to eliminate the toxic byproducts of modern life. But even this most perfect automatic system can't function indefinitely without some help from its owner.

While *What's In This Stuff?* focuses on the chemical onslaught to which our bodies are subjected through the products we buy, we can't make the mistake of assuming that we buy these things in a vacuum. Often, we are coerced by high-pressure sales tactics into believing that we simply can't live without the modern conveniences of everything from bagged salad to wet wipes to anti-wrinkle creams, and that our lives would be diminished without these modern miracles.

For the purposes of this book, the supermarket has become the primary source of such beliefs. Much has already been written about the way supermarkets have changed our diets, our communities and our landscapes – and not always for the better. Because of their 'pile it high, sell it cheap' philosophy and persuasive advertising campaigns that entice us to buy and use cheaply produced products laden with chemicals, supermarkets have also become the main pushers of most of the poisons we put into our bodies and our homes.

Supermarket shopping forces us to switch off. In fact, supermarkets actively pursue the ideal of the 'switched-off consumer'. By encouraging such a mindset, the supermarket can encourage even the smartest shopper to make dumb choices over and over and over again. This book is about us switching on again, of being aware of what's on offer, of what its real value is, and of what illusions, limitations and risks are attached to all the stuff we buy, week in and week out.

Not everything you read here will be easy to take in. Not everything you read will motivate you to change. But make no mistake. The next revolution in consumer spending is an anti-chemical revolution, as more and more of us begin to realise that there may well be a darker meaning to the phrase 'shop 'til you drop' and begin to say no to products that contain harmful chemicals.

The premise behind *What's In This Stuff?* is simple. Readers will find, as they become more aware of the ingredients in the 'stuff' they buy, and of the damning evidence of harm attached to some and the unacceptable uncertainties concerning the safety of many others, that these products will rapidly lose their appeal and more of us will feel able to join this revolution.

Science may be slow to deal with issues of harm and uncertainty, but this book offers a common-sense approach that anyone can implement. When you feel uncertain as to what to believe or how best to go forward, follow what is known as the 'precautionary principle' – in other words, it's better to be safe than sorry.

Some of the alternatives included in this volume are practical and simple, whereas some require a bit of effort or a complete change of habits and lifestyle. Some may seem part of a Utopian ideal, yet other individuals are making them work – and so can you. As a first step, pick 5 or 10 – or, if you're really ambitious, 20 – of the many suggestions in this book and make a commitment to doing them. The more you are able to implement the alternatives suggested here, the more noticeable and beneficial will be the changes you'll see in your day-to-day health.

If *What's In This Stuff?* has any goal at all, it is to help you, the reader, to make more healthy choices, more conscious choices, more compassionate choices and more ecologically sound choices. In addition, the information here aims to help you feel confident about buying less and using less and, when you do decide to put something into your shopping trolley, to feel reassured that it will sustain your life rather than detract from it.

what's in store?

Y OU ARE ABOUT TO BE TAKEN on a journey … and it begins in your local supermarket.

If you are like most people, supermarket shopping has become a regular part of your weekly routine. Well stocked, competitively priced and with all the amenities laid on, these 'cathedrals of modern commerce' issue a friendly and open invitation to come on in, linger and spend.

These days, for more than 90 per cent of us, a supermarket is the main or sole place of shopping; and the weekly excursion to the supermarket is a central event in our lives. And as much as the weekly shop is a chore, it has also become a ritual – and, for some families, the only weekly outing together.

Clever advertising and marketing help to paint a picture of the supermarket as a place you can go to fulfil all your needs to excess cheaply and regularly. The supermarket has become positioned in our minds as a necessary part of life, as part of the extended family, and as able to respond to all our needs and desires.

Yet, while supermarkets promote themselves as helpful friends, the relationship is not one of equals. Supermarkets are powerful 'friends' that have become so central to our lives that we are barely aware of the power that they wield over us, how they direct and limit our shopping choices, and disconnect us from the origins of the things we buy. Many of us are completely unaware of how they shape and destroy communities by closing down local amenities, shops and post offices, how they change the physical landscape of the places where we live, and how they pollute the environment, including, for the purposes of this book, our homes and bodies.

The big weekly shop

Bringing home life's essentials has always been a challenge. Certainly, these days, we don't have to dodge tigers and bears to put food on the table, and the majority of us in the West don't have to walk miles to meet our other daily needs, such as obtaining clean water, or rely on what food we can grow ourselves. Nevertheless, providing for a family is still complicated, and sometimes just plain hard work.

In the modern world, the task is made even more difficult by the fact that we have drastically altered our idea of what is necessary. These days, most families' lists of basic requirements – most of which need to be purchased somewhere – have become unmanageably large. The larger the list gets, the more urgent the need becomes to find a way of getting the things we want quickly, easily and cheaply. The alternative – buying what we need at a succession of specialist shops such as butchers, bakers, greengrocers, shoe and clothing shops, hardware stores and off-licences – seems unthinkable and old-fashioned.

Enter the modern supermarket

While much has been made of the way supermarkets have changed how we eat, their influence stretches well beyond food consumption. Consumption of all kinds has expanded, thanks to the convenience factor of today's supermarkets, which provide an all-encompassing, one-stop solution to meeting our 'basic' needs. In addition to food and drink, most supermarkets now sell a huge variety of non-food items and, at the biggest superstores, you can kit out your entire home in one trip. Surveys show that, in a typical supermarket, you can now buy:

- Alcoholic beverages
- Baby foods and products
- Beauty products
- Breakfast cereals
- Car-care products
- Cleaning products
- Clothing and footwear
- Computer and small office goods
- Confectionery
- Dairy products
- Diet foods
- Dry-cleaning
- DVDs, CDs and videos
- Electrical items (from toasters to freezers)
- Feminine hygiene products
- Flowers
- Frozen foods
- Fruits and vegetables
- Greeting cards and stationery
- Housewares
- Lottery tickets
- Luggage
- Meat
- Medicines and first-aid items
- Mobile phones
- Newspapers, books and magazines
- Non-alcoholic beverages such as juice, mixers and water
- Personal financial products (including mortgages, credit cards and savings accounts)
- Personal hygiene and grooming products
- Pet foods and products
- Photographic processing
- Snacks
- Soft furnishings, linens and towels
- Toys and games
- Travel goods
- Video rentals
- Vitamins
- International money orders and wire transfer services

The goal of the supermarket is simple: to encourage customers to buy more of these things and more often. And several aspects of our weekly shopping experience help to accomplish this objective.

First is the clarion call of good value. In most supermarkets, there are regular announcements and product advertisements to guide shoppers to special offers. The promise of permanently low prices, bargains, buy-one-get-one-free and three-for-two offers, 'blue cross specials' and 'discount days' are all designed to give the impression that we are saving money with every item we buy.

But giant supermarket chains sell little more than the illusion of value, wrapped up in the seductive creed of convenience. Over and over again, studies have shown that – from fruit and vegetables to the Sunday roast – smaller, independent local shops can offer much better value. At the supermarket, only a few key items are sold at value prices, while the store maintains a huge profit margin on everything else, especially household goods, over-the-counter drugs and DVDs.

With so many goods in store, supermarkets make a huge effort to make us linger. As you walk down the aisles, strategically placed lighting creates an atmosphere of warmth, soothing music plays in the background, tempting scents waft through the air and brightly coloured product displays entice you to pause, reach out and put yet another item into the trolley.

In addition, the more facilities a supermarket has, the more time we spend there. Play areas for children mean mums can browse the aisles at a more leisurely pace. One-hour photo-processing counters can double the time you might otherwise spend pushing your trolley around, and cafés invite you to linger over coffee before or after you shop.

Whatever your approach to supermarket shopping – whether you go in with a list and get only what you want, or float along the aisles browsing, picking items up out of interest and inspiration – the big weekly shop is an investment of both time and effort.

Whatever we choose to believe before we enter the supermarket, and however seductive the process of cruising the aisles is, reality hits hard at the checkout where long queues and the final total make us realise that, for all the ads reassuring us that food is cheaper than ever, the weekly shop still takes a huge bite out of our monthly income.

Another persuasive factor is the illusion of control. The more a supermarket stocks, the more it invites you to spend time there, to ponder and make comparisons and choices. Thus, shopping requires decision-making ability – do you go to the fresh-foods aisle first, or get the heavy stuff like canned goods and bottles first? It also requires perseverance – for instance, to push along a trolley that has a mind of its own and to endure the long queues at the checkout – and a sense of adventure. For some, finding a parking space as near to the door as possible has become a point of principle.

The supermarket also represents freedom of choice although, in reality, the choice is limited to what the supermarket is willing to offer. Ironically, studies show that no matter how we approach the weekly shop, most of us reach the checkout with the same basic goods in our trolleys. That's because, along with the illusion of value, supermarkets can only ever offer the pretence of choice.

Witness the two-metre-wide display of toothbrushes found in most supermarkets. There is no basic difference in the way these brushes function. But by presenting them to shoppers in a range of sizes, shapes, colours and bristle strengths, supermarkets create the illusion of personal choice and control.

Once again, the reality is rather different. Most of the brands we buy are largely interchangeable. Whatever your heart may tell you, your head knows that, apart from the packaging style and occasionally the price, there are no major differences between the 10 brands of laundry detergent on the shelf, or the 12 brands of toothpaste, 20 varieties of shampoo, or 6 brands of oven chips. But, by pricing some higher than others, they can also claim to offer luxury.

This democratisation of luxury is another important aspect to the allure of the supermarket. When we shop in a supermarket, we enter a world of beautifully displayed luxury items, of shelves continually stocked to give the impression of plenty. The supermarket also flatters us that it is classless: everyone gets to spend time there, and is temporarily freed from the limitations of geography and season. Even if you live in the middle of a large city, you have access to fresh produce, and even if you live in the north Atlantic, you can still have fresh mango for breakfast.

The expanding trolley

Trolley sizes have grown exponentially over the last 30 years. The American consumer advocate Ralph Nader was the first to notice the growing-shopping-cart phenomenon, offering it as a prime example of how consumers are manipulated by the system. Bigger carts, he said, served the straightforward purpose of shaming consumers into making bigger purchases.

Other explanations have been put forward to explain the expanding-cart phenomenon – for instance, changes in women's lives. As more and more women choose to work, trips to the supermarket went from every one or two days to once a week. This led to the tendency to buy more per (less frequent) trip.

As supermarkets have grown, the width of their aisles has grown with them – and once you've got the wide aisles, you might as well have the bigger carts.

▶

Whatever the reason, today's average trolley is almost three times as large as its 1975 counterpart. It's also used for much more than just putting things in. New high-tech trolleys are being designed that will display a screen that will allow shoppers to scan items as they shop, show the purchase price of each item and keep a running tally of what they have spent.

These new 'smart' trolleys can advertise specials appropriate to whatever aisle you are in and can even remind regular customers of what they might have forgotten. And it's here that privacy issues emerge: once a shopper logs on to the trolley, it can make suggestions based on previous visits to the supermarket. So, is it a time-saver, a brain-washer or Big Brother on wheels?

How supermarket shopping changes us

Our increasingly hectic lifestyles are having a major impact on the goods we choose to buy. We want our food to be fast, our cleaners to be spray-and-wipe and our toiletries to be wash-and-go.

Many of our day-to-day decisions are made on the basis of what's convenient at the time or in the immediate future. If something is quick, easy and painless, we are far more apt to do it than if it requires forethought, the weighing of options, planning and effort.

Today, entire industries are built around the objective of making life simpler, easier and more efficient, and the convenience credo now dominates many facets of our lives – from how much sleep we get to our personal-hygiene habits, what we might eat for lunch or dinner on any given day and how we choose to raise our children.

In the name of convenience, we now buy things because we desire them, not because we need them. Retail therapy has become an increasingly common way to counter stress and dissatisfaction in our lives. Seemingly unnecessary commodities are given value by their perceived ability to make life happier and easier, to solve problems and/or change the customer into a more desirable person. Through shopping, we actively seek 'magic-bullet' solutions to the most insignificant human dilemmas – everything from the occasional upset stomach or pimple to the disinclination to peel and chop a carrot or mend a hole in a sock yourself.

The enormity of the dissatisfaction we feel with our lives has helped turn markets into supermarkets, and supermarkets into superstores. By piling it high and selling it cheap, these edifices distract us from what should be the central point of supermarket shopping – to provide healthy food for the family and safe, effective means of meeting life's other demands such as cleaning, child and pet care, and gardening.

We now buy and use – and throw away – more goods than ever before. Frivolous and highly packaged goods – like microwave popcorn or the latest cheap tee-shirt with a novelty image or slogan on it – bring short-term satisfaction and are then tossed away when they are no longer novel or fashionable, or convenient. As a result, the majority of us are buying more products than ever before, and living increasingly wasteful and over-burdened lives.

Sometimes, the price we pay is just more money but, increasingly, science is showing us that the true cost of supermarket convenience can be marked out in incremental declines in human health and well-being, and the poisoning of the environment.

Convenience at a price

When we buy into the 'convenience culture', we buy into a whole set of values and ways of life that, for the most part, remain hidden beneath the glitz, the democratised luxury and the hard sell. The convenience culture is a one-dimensional way of living, devoid of spiritual or otherworldly concerns. It encourages us to be lazy, to live beyond our means, to overindulge and spoil ourselves and our children, to ignore our past and block out all thoughts of the future.

Like the wider consumer culture of which it is a part, it celebrates the body, but is not attentive to its true needs. Thus, we can satisfy our hunger with quick-cook ready meals, and never once concern ourselves with the fact that this 'food' contains nothing that actually nourishes the body. Likewise, we can attack the 'signs of ageing' with anti-wrinkle creams, and never once think about what it is about our lives and lifestyles that is making us look and feel so old and tired.

Let's consider just some of the fallout from a convenience culture. It can, for instance:

- **skew our values.** We no longer expect excellence, we expect things to break, we expect them to fail, and we expect them to disappoint and that claims for them to be exaggerated.

- **discourage discernment,** because we take at face value all the advertising and manufacturers' claims for products.

- **disempower the individual** so that we forget how to do things for ourselves; we have lost the ability to make value judgements that go beyond price and convenience when we shop.

- **cause us to abdicate responsibility.** When things go wrong or we get sick, we blame others rather than ourselves. A litigation culture is an offshoot of a convenience culture.

- **change our social interactions.** We are more likely to talk to each other about the stuff we buy than about what we are feeling, or our thoughts or spiritual concerns. In addition, we no longer communicate with the people who make, supply or even sell the products we buy.

- **make us lose basic skills.** These days, many people don't know how to make basic repairs around the house, and can't sew or mend clothing. Some younger people don't know how to prepare or cook fresh foods.

- **waste resources.** Convenience goods are highly packaged, so you pay for and throw away packaging made from non-sustainable and often toxic materials.

- **encourage overconsumption.** We buy things in bigger 'value packs', and use more than we need to get the job done, eat more than we need to be nourished and/or throw away whatever we can't use.

- **encourage a 'live for today' attitude.** Too many consumers have stopped asking questions about goods such as where they come from, who made them and what they are made of. Living for today fails to protect us as well as our future generations.

These things impact on every individual, but there are global consequences as well. Convenience consumerism is in and of itself wasteful, and increased levels of waste and industrial pollutants in our water, air and food are the inevitable byproducts of our love affair with this increasingly unsustainable way of life.

Manufacturers are more than happy to meet our demands for cheap goods. To meet our price expectations and keep their profit margins high, these products are inevitably made or grown somewhere else – usually in developing countries – and then flown halfway across the world. The resulting air miles cause considerable environmental pollution and drain depleted petroleum reserves. They promote a system of unfair trade and low wages for workers while taking work away from local areas. When it comes to food, intensive-farming practices to speed up the journey from farm to table means an increased use of pesticides, flirtations with unsafe technologies to create GM (genetically modified) foods, increased productivity at a cost to animal health, and unsafe eggs, meat and fish.

The human cost

There are many ways in which we humans are hoist by our own petard by the convenience culture. For instance, according to Harvard researchers in 2004, cheap convenience foods are the driving force behind the rising rates of obesity in the West. Partly based on food diaries kept by the study's participants, a surprising picture emerged of American eating habits. In the US, people are not consuming any more calories at mealtimes than they did 20 years ago, but they have nearly doubled their consumption of calories from snacks and sodas between meals.

Food companies, seeking an outlet for the glut of cereals and other raw foodstuffs in the 1980s and 1990s, developed literally hundreds of new products that increased the demand for food beyond previously imagined levels. The industry took advantage of the burgeoning science of chemical flavouring, and new technologies for processing and preserving foods, to create high-fat, high-sugar and high-taste foods. In just a few years, processed foods grew cheaper, more convenient and, more important, tastier.

At the same time, snacking was legitimised as American culture celebrated the practice of 'grazing' as a supposedly healthful alternative to heavy meals at mealtime.

Some could reason that the convenience and pleasure of snack foods is worth carrying a few extra pounds but, of course, obesity carries with it a high risk of developing type 2 (non-insulin-dependent) diabetes, hypertension, heart disease and other serious illnesses.

The results from this Harvard study could easily have come from Britain or Australia or anywhere else that the free market rules the food industry, where regulatory systems are lax and allow almost any amount of additives to be put into foods, and where snacking and, as a result, obesity are on the rise.

While changes in agricultural and manufacturing processes, and in consumer habits are the most obvious example of the problems of a convenience-obsessed society, examples abound from all sectors of the marketplace.

Fifty years ago, most of us wrapped our sandwiches in waxed paper, poured our milk from glass bottles, wore rubberised coats when it rained, drove cars made from steel and reheated dinner in an old pie tin in the oven. Nowadays, our sandwiches come in plastic boxes or aluminium-plastic pockets that can be popped in the microwave. Pizza boxes and containers for french fries keep the grease off us with high-tech Teflon coatings. When it rains, we wear Gore-Tex – a relative of Teflon – which keeps the water out, but lets our skin breathe.

The common thread running through all these things is man-made chemicals. Most convenience goods are mass-produced, and the ability of manufacturers to make vast amounts of identical goods at dirt-cheap prices has increased enormously since the end of World War II. Since that time, manufacturers have created, overproduced and then looked for new uses for a glut of waste chemicals, including organochlorines, and plastics and other petroleum-derived substances.

Many of these chemicals were the result of wartime research and development. When the war ended, the dovetailing of excess production of these substances with the spirit of enterprise and a desire to expand our personal horizons created an unprecedented appetite for the selling and consuming of 'stuff'.

The advantage of the chemical society is that these cheap industrial chemicals can be used to produce cheap everyday goods. Added to food, they give us ready meals that can be made a long time in advance and stocked on the shelves for ages. In cosmetics, they promise professional results without ever stepping inside a salon or spa. And why call an exterminator when you can buy a spray can of powerful insecticide at the supermarket that will make the bugs go away? Our cars are now lighter, cheaper and more energy-efficient because they are made from an astonishing array of metals and plastics. At night, we can pull dinner out of the refrigerator in plastic containers that can go straight from freezer to microwave without cracking or burning.

The chemical advances that have made these things possible may, on the one hand, seem miraculous. But every one of these products has a knock-on effect on our health since their use increases our exposure to potentially toxic chemicals. For instance:

- Around 90 per cent of us are carrying trace amounts of a chemical called 'perfluorinated acid' (PFOA) in our blood. That's because PFOA or its byproducts are used in the making of Teflon and Gore-Tex, and can be released from products with stain-proof coatings such as Scotchguard and Stainmaster. PFOA is an industrial chemical and, in 2006, the US Environmental Protection Agency (EPA) recommended that it be classified as a potential human carcinogen. PFOA has also been shown to be toxic to the kidneys while, in animals, it causes reproductive problems and growth retardation.

- Numerous studies have shown that a commonly used ingredient in plastic called 'bisphenol A' causes abnormal pregnancy in mice and could cause reproductive problems in people, too.

- Likewise, studies have found that polybrominated diphenyl ether (PBDE), a flame retardant used in TV sets, computer circuit boards and casings, foams and fabrics is rapidly accumulating in the breastmilk of women in Sweden and the US. The chemical has been shown to cause thyroid cancer and neurodevelopmental problems in test animals.

These are by no means the first examples of innovative new technologies we've taken and run with, only to find out years later that we've unwittingly been endangering ourselves as well as our planet.

The pesticide **DDT** was touted as revolutionary in the 1940s before it became apparent that it caused the eggshells of predatory birds such as the bald eagle to become too thin, lowering their numbers dramatically. Soon after, DDT was found to cause cancer in humans and is now banned in most developed countries. ***Chlorofluorocarbons***, or CFCs, were prized for their chemical stability until scientists discovered they eroded the ozone layer. ***Polychlorinated biphenyls***, or PCBs, were the darling of manufacturers until their toxicity to people and wildlife became evident.

At the dawn of the 21st century, the question many are asking is whether the short-term convenience we gain from all these new materials is worth the trouble they cause us in the long run. We also need to ask whether there should be more stringent testing rules to avert both human and environmental catastrophes.

Quick fixes

The wide availability of convenient prepackaged foods and other quick fixes is something that most of us believe makes our lives a little easier. Science is only too happy to oblige us in our pursuit of such things. So if you want to get a jump on your day, you can now use soap with caffeine in it that is absorbed into your skin as you wash. Soon, it may even be possible to fix sugar cravings with a shampoo that sends chemicals to your brain to mimic the effects of a sugar rush. It's only a matter of time before cigarette companies start putting vitamin C or calcium in cigarettes so that you can get your vitamins while destroying your – and other people's – lungs.

Buying convenience goods has become such an ingrained habit for most of us that we can't imagine life without them. Most of us never really question whether such goods are good for us, whether they actually save us significant amounts of time or what impact they may have on our health or our planet over the longer term.

Some innovations such as vacuum cleaners and washing machines do genuinely save us hours of backbreaking work. Imagining life without them is almost impossible. But along with these devices are thousands of false conveniences that we buy into every day without thinking. Thanks to clever marketing, we have genuinely come to believe that the mere seconds we save by buying prepackaged lettuce or pregrated cheese buy us even more extra time to live better, fuller lives.

In your heart of hearts, you know this isn't true and, what's more, every convenience item you buy or use has a hidden cost. Sometimes you are simply paying more, but often the cost is to your own health and well-being, and to the environment. Consider the true cost of some well-known convenience and 'quick-fix' items and, whenever you can, try to get out of the quick-fix habit.

Item/Quick fix	True cost	Try this instead
Air fresheners *Cover up bad smells*	• Effect is temporary • Made from neurotoxic solvents and synthetic fragrances that can cause headaches, mood swings, memory loss and depression • Strong perfumes trigger asthma and allergies • Spray varieties contain ozone-depleting propellants	• Open a window • Don't smoke in the house (in fact, don't smoke at all!) • Use a ventilator when cooking • Keep bathroom surfaces clean and dry
Aspartame *Allows you to consume sweet foods without consuming calories*	• Breaks down into carcinogenic formaldehyde during storage and in the body • Other breakdown products – such as phenylalanine and aspartic acid – damage and destroy brain cells • Women, children and those with poor immune function are particularly vulnerable to its effects • According to the US FDA, common adverse effects from regular use of aspartame include headaches, memory loss, skin rashes, seizures, heart palpitations, disorientation, dizziness, hives, joint pain, sore throat and impaired vision	• Use the real thing, but use it less often – sugar only contains 15 calories per teaspoon

Dryer sheets/fabric softeners *Soften clothes and eliminate static cling*	• Surfactants in dryer sheets can irritate skin
	• Contain more synthetic fragrance chemicals than any other household item, including:
	  – *benzyl acetate*, linked to pancreatic cancer
	  – *benzyl alcohol*, an upper respiratory tract irritant
		• Add baking soda to your wash cycle *or*
		• Add vinegar to your wash cycle (don't add both)

Item/Quick fix	True cost	Try this instead
Dryer sheets/fabric softeners (continued)	– *ethanol*, linked to central nervous system disorders – *limonene*, a known carcinogen – *alpha-terpineol*, can cause respiratory problems, and central nervous system damage – *ethyl acetate*, a narcotic – *camphor*, causes central nervous system disorders – *chloroform*, a neurotoxin, anaesthetic and carcinogen – *linalool*, a narcotic that causes central nervous system disorders. • Heated in the dryer, they release toxic vapours onto clothes and into the air • Scents used in fabric softeners are designed to stay in your clothing for long periods of time; when you wear 'softened' clothes, your body heat helps to release chemicals into the air for you to inhale and onto your skin for you to absorb	
Microwave popcorn *Tasty popcorn in a jiffy*	• Artificial butter flavouring is made from a caustic chemical, diacetyl, a relative of paint stripper • Heating diacetyl produces vapours that irritate the skin, eyes, mucous membranes and respiratory tract • Long-term exposure to diacetyl can permanently damage your airways • Packaging is lined with Teflon, which releases lung-damaging and cancer-causing micro-particles into the air when heated • Many brands of microwave popcorn contain tartrazine (FD&C Yellow No. 5), a synthetic dye linked to hyperactivity, asthma and other health problems	• Use an air popper and add real butter

Item/Quick fix	True cost	Try this instead
Prepackaged lettuce *You don't have to cut the lettuce yourself*	• More expensive than a regular head of lettuce • Washed in a chlorine solution 20 times more concentrated than in the average swimming pool – to prevent deterioration • Ingesting chlorine raises the risk of liver, kidney, heart and neurological damage, is harmful to unborn children and a trigger for cancer • Chlorine destroys the taste of the leaf • Bacteria on lettuce become resistant to chlorine so 'washed' lettuce can still contain virulent strains of *Listeria* and *E. coli* • Packed in modified-atmosphere packaging (MAP) in which normal levels of oxygen and carbon dioxide are altered to maintain the appearance of freshness • MAP destroys many vital nutrients such as vitamins C and E, polyphenols and other micronutrients	• Buy a fresh head of lettuce and cut it up yourself
Standby electronics *Your computer, TV, DVD player are ready to use at any time*	• Pump millions of tons of carbon into the atmosphere each year • Electrical goods on standby in all the G8 nations waste the equivalent of the electricity generated by 20 power stations each year • Many appliances use as much power on standby as when turned on • Accelerate climate change • Can add as much as £200 a year to your energy bills	• Unplug electrical items when not in use • Buy products that allow you to choose whether or not you will use a standby function
Wet wipes *A quick wash without water*	• Once opened, they are a breeding ground for bacteria • Contain lots of preservatives and antibacterial ingredients which can cause skin rashes and encourage bacterial resistance	• Use soap and water • Carry a face cloth in a plastic bag for a quick wipe when with kids

Item/Quick fix	True cost	Try this instead
Wet wipes (continued)	• Detergents and perfumes can also irritate the skin, especially as they are not washed off • Made from plastic, cellulose and polyester fibres, so are not biodegradable • Highly perfumed, so can cause neurotoxic effects such as headaches, agitation, forgetfulness, mood swings, depression • Chemicals can be transferred to food during cooking and eating	

Supermarkets as sources of mass poisonings

Most of us are so busy with the challenge of 'getting the shopping done' that we never stop to analyse what's actually in the trolley. And because we buy so much from the supermarket, it has become the most significant source of pollutants in our homes. This may seem an incredible statement, yet, as subsequent chapters will show, almost all the toxic chemicals that we are exposed to on a daily basis – solvents, aerosols, food additives, plastics, pesticides, heavy metals, GM organisms and antibiotics – are brought home from the supermarket.

The Sudan 1 red dye crisis of 2004 – which reached international proportions, with products withdrawn in Europe, the US and Canada – was a good illustration of how supermarkets really are the best way to poison large numbers of people within the shortest period of time. Sudan 1, an illegal toxic dye found in a range of ready-prepared foods, was just one of the many chemicals used in everyday products such as convenience foods, cosmetics, household cleaners, and pet and garden supplies that go unnoticed and untested.

As this book will reveal, the true extent to which our bodies have become polluted by these man-made chemicals is shocking, and the effects of living with a polluted body are wide-ranging.

Many of us are so used to feeling below par that we no longer even question why we suffer from regular headaches, stomachaches, skin rashes, pain, fatigue, breathing problems or poor memories. 'That's life', we say, as we pop another pill or eat something or turn up the automatic air freshener a notch and carry on regardless.

Throughout the world, supermarket shoppers have become part of an unregulated experiment that involves the buying and consumption of a whole range of toxic and contaminated products.

Supermarkets may have revolutionised certain aspects of our lives. But most people, when encouraged to dig deeper and to ask questions about the direction this revolution has taken, find that they cannot shop in supermarkets with the same level of enthusiasm and blind faith they once did. There are just too many unanswered questions related to the pollution of our bodies and our planet, the destruction of genuine communities, and the poor quality of food and other goods purchased in supermarkets to feel as easy as you once did, pushing your super-sized trolley up and down the aisles.

Is there a way out?

Our life may have been made somewhat more convenient by the chemical revolution, but it has also been made inexorably more complicated, too. The more goods we buy, the more government controls are necessary to regulate those goods. Agencies are established and regulated by the government to regulate and supervise economic activity, and to protect us the consumer from exploitation and health damage, from other sources, but also ourselves.

The more government agencies there are involved in the regulation of commercial goods, the more manufacturers spend on lobbying and influencing regulators to keep their goods on the shelf. The more lobbying that goes on, the more corruption there is, and the more corruption there is, the greater the need for consumer groups and whistle-blowers to guard the guards.

Historically, in the West, a risk–benefit analysis – that is, assessing whether the potential benefits of a new technology outweigh the potential risks – has been the yardstick, and most businesses still evaluate their products on this basis.

But consumer advocates are increasingly turning towards a theory which is, at the same time, more sophisticated and more simple. It's known as the 'precautionary principle'. This is based on the notion of the *Vorsorgeprinzip*, literally the 'forecaring principle', which emerged in Germany when laws were enacted to save forests by reducing the power-plant emissions causing acid rain. It was considered an act of forecaring, or precaution, because, at the time, there wasn't 100 per cent scientific certainty that power-plant emissions were in fact the cause of acid rain.

The concept was defined at a major conference in 1998 as: '*When an activity raises threats of harm to human health or the environment, precautionary measures should be taken even if some cause-and-effect relationships are not fully established scientifically.*'

In ordinary language: better safe than sorry.

The precautionary principle doesn't mean that we have to go back to living in the Stone Age, but it does provide regulators – and ordinary people – with a framework that encourages them to act *before* disaster strikes and so avoid what could be called the 'ooops! factor' – which we so often experience when a product that has been on sale for years is suddenly found to cause widespread and irreversible damage to human health.

By applying the precautionary principle to your own life, you can also avoid the 'ooops! factor', linked to so many of the products that we buy and use on a regular basis.

▶ NEW WAYS TO SHOP

If you believe that supermarket shopping is just 'the way things are', then you have been seduced into believing in a world where maximising the production and consumption of goods is the only worthy goal. We all have the power to do something different. We can rethink the weekly shop, and rethink what we buy and why we buy it. We can begin to change the way we shop to reduce our exposure to toxic chemicals, to make an investment in our local area, to ensure we are getting more nutrients per mouthful and even to spend less.

It's all too easy to point the finger of blame at supermarkets for their misleading advertising and abuse of power, and at industry for polluting the planet. Such things are a given. But as consumers, we are also part of the problem. Our thoughtless demands for more throwaway stuff – plastic containers, aerosol sprays, wet wipes and ready-made everything – are damaging the planet and adding to the pollution. If we stopped buying unnecessary 'stuff', there would be no reason for manufacturers to produce it, and without public demand, the convenience culture would die away. You have the power to change things. If you are ready to apply the brakes on a toxic modern lifestyle that is accelerating out of control, consider taking these first simple steps.

Buy less. We buy and eat too much food; we buy and often only half-use too many toiletries and cosmetics; we buy too much stuff for babies in the belief that the investment in wipes and plastic toys makes us good parents. Get off the treadmill; ignore all those '3 for 2' offers that supermarkets use to offload products they have a surfeit of. Think about what you really need, about what is essential to your life, and stick to that.

Reuse, repair, recycle. Sometime after World War II, the concept of doing without, making do, sticking to the necessities became practically unpatriotic, and somewhere along the way, the personal freedom that had been fought for got confused with the freedom to buy things, to have things, to show off the things to others and be envied for them. As a result, many of the skills that sustained our forefathers fell out of fashion. It's not just that we don't know how to build our own barns or grow our own food any more. Many of us don't know how to repair clothing or make a meal from scratch or fix a blocked drain. Frugality, too, has gone out of fashion but, in a world rapidly running out of resources, it's time to resurrect it.

Shop local. It can be hard to shop if you have no local retailers or a car but, remember, supermarkets are the reason for this, and the way most of us shop these days has fostered the demise of the local shopkeeper. There are plenty of online stores you can now order quality food from. Farmers' markets are popping up in more places, and organic farms make weekly deliveries. Now's the time to ask yourself: 'How well do I know my local area? Are there people who offer goods and services that I can and should be taking advantage of?' And if there are, then use them.

Forget brand loyalty. When you are buying food or toiletries, brand loyalty may mean that you are getting poor value for money, and you may even be exposing yourself to more chemicals than you have to. By learning to read labels and make comparisons, you will find that there is often little between brands, that cheaper brands are just as good and that there are low-chemical options for almost everything you buy.

Voluntary simplicity. Many of the toxins we encounter every day are the result of our unbridled consumerism, so choose not to buy into this unhealthy addiction. The fact is, the less stuff you have in your life, the less likely you are to come into contact with environmental toxins.

If you only use the microwave to heat up coffee or bake potatoes, perhaps the time has come to get rid of this significant source of radiation in your home altogether. If you declutter your home, chances are you will not need so many plastic boxes to store things, thereby reducing the amount of formaldehyde gas in the air. Likewise, if you use fewer cosmetics, toiletries, air fresheners and harsh household cleaners, you will be lowering your exposure to solvents and other volatile organic chemicals (VOCs) as well as environmental hormone mimics.

Cultivating simplicity in your life is not some vague hippie ideal. These days, it requires an iron will to resist advertising pressure to buy more stuff and consume more than you need. Dig down deep and see if you can find that will in yourself.

not everything gives you cancer ... but lots of things do

IT WOULD BE EASY, WHILE READING THIS BOOK, to believe that it's simply not safe for any of us to live in the modern world. Conclusive evidence that our chemicalised society is damaging our health is accumulating rapidly, and if we don't take action to protect ourselves, the prospect of living long and healthy lives gets slimmer with each and every compromise we make in the name of convenience and quick-fixes.

Even in the face of all the evidence, those who shine a light on the problems associated with environmental chemical exposure and who advise caution are often derided or portrayed as 'scaremongers' or 'killjoys'. They are continually challenged with objections along the lines of 'Well, everything gives you cancer these days, doesn't it?' or 'Why worry when I could get hit by a bus tomorrow'.

Yes, you could get hit by a bus tomorrow. But would you deliberately throw yourself in front of that bus? Not making the effort to understand which toxins you are exposing yourself to every day is very much like throwing yourself in the path of an oncoming vehicle. You know that it's coming, you know that it will harm you and that doing nothing to get out of the way is an act of profound irresponsibility to yourself, your family and all those whom you love and who love you.

Not everything gives you cancer, but a great many things do. Indeed, according to the US National Toxicology Program, around 200 chemicals encountered every day are either known or potential human carcinogens. There is no established 'safe' dose for any carcinogen, so why are we continually surprised when cancer rates soar? In the same vein, not everything causes infertility or birth defects or dementia or migraines or allergies, but many hundreds of chemicals that we encounter every day do – and again, it is hardly surprising to see rates of these conditions rising rapidly amongst the general population. Why invite these risks into your home if you have the power to keep them out?

How polluted are you?

It is impossible to say how many different chemicals we each carry in our bodies. This is because beyond the chemicals that are added to food or used as drugs, there is no requirement for manufacturers to disclose how their chemicals are used or to keep track of the various routes through which people may be exposed. Neither are they required to understand the fate of their chemicals in the environment, to measure concentrations of their products in either the environment or people, or develop and share methods of analysis that would allow other scientists to gather this kind of information independently.

In the largest study of chemical exposure ever conducted on humans, the US Centers for Disease Control and Prevention (CDC) showed that most American children and adults are carrying in their bodies more than 100 substances that aren't supposed to be there, including pesticides and the toxic compounds used in everyday consumer products, many of them linked to potential health hazards.

Many toxicologists and environmental scientists reviewing the report expressed grave concerns that in studies of animals and, in some cases, of people, most of these compounds could affect the brain, hormonal balance, reproductive system or immune system, or were linked to cancer.

The report documented the fact that many children are carrying much higher levels of these chemicals than adults. These include pyrethroids, which are found in virtually every household pesticide, and phthalates, plasticisers that are found in nail polish and other beauty products as well as in soft plastics.

Throughout the world, the phenomenon of polluted people is becoming more commonplace. For instance, to reveal more about how much toxic material we carry around in our bodies, the World Wildlife Foundation environmental group conducted a series of blood tests on people from all walks of life in the UK. In 2003, they tested the blood of individuals across the country and found an average of 27 chemicals in every one of them. These compounds included long-banned chemicals such as the organochlorine pesticide **DDT** (dichloro-diphenyl-trichloro-ethane), and PCBs from old electrical equipment and building materials, as well as more common chemicals found in everyday materials such as paints, glues, toys, electrical goods, furniture, carpets and clothing.

The following year, they tested the blood of environment ministers from 13 European Union countries and found a total of 55 different chemicals in the ministers' blood. The lowest number of chemicals found in any one minister's body was 33 and the highest was 43. These chemicals were pollutants commonly found in sofas, pizza boxes and pesticides.

Most recently, in 2005, the WWF tested the blood of a handful of British celebrities and found, on average, 24 chemicals in each one. The chemicals they found included DDT and PCBs, brominated flameretardants found in furniture and electrical equipment, phthalates found in perfumes, cosmetics and flexible plastics, perfluorinated chemicals found in the Teflon used on non-stick pans and Scotchguard used for stainproofing.

In 2005, a Canada-wide study by the group Environmental Defence tested for a broad range of chemicals in average Canadians, and found toxic chemicals such as DDT, PCBs, stain repellents, flame retardants, mercury and lead in every person sampled.

What these unique surveys show is that no matter where you live, you are unlikely to be able to avoid the kind of chemical exposure that can lead to chemical overload.

Total body load

As research in the field of chemical exposure has advanced, two pivotal concepts have emerged: the 'total body load' and 'the low-dose effect'. Essentially, these measures allow scientists to study and determine how much we carry in our bodies, and the level at which this is likely to be harmful.

Many of the chemicals we are exposed to each day are 'persistent' – that is, instead of breaking down, they remain intact, and dangerous, in the environment and in our bodies for years, even decades. Small regular doses can and do build up to health-harming levels over time.

Scientists refer to the accumulation of such chemicals as an individual's 'body burden' or 'total body load' – the consequence of lifelong exposure to industrial chemicals used in thousands of consumer products and which linger on as contaminants in our air, water, food and soil.

These chemicals come from household products like detergents, cosmetics, fabric treatments and paints as well as upholstery, computers and TVs. They accumulate in the fat, blood and organs, or are passed out of the body via breast milk, urine, faeces, sweat, semen, hair and nails. Over time, if the total body load is high, the likelihood of the body breaking down under the weight of it becomes higher.

Quiz

Your total body load

It's not always easy to gauge what your daily exposure to toxic chemicals is. Take this simple quiz to help you get an idea of how much you might be carrying in your body.

About you

☐ Do you have children?

☐ Are you a woman?

☐ Are you of retirement age?

☐ Do you work with chemicals?

☐ Do you have pets?

About the products you buy

☐ Do you read and understand the ingredients labels on the products you buy?

☐ Is the greater proportion of your diet made up of preprepared or convenience foods?

☐ Do you buy your cleaning products at the supermarket, hardware stores or other mainstream outlets?

☐ Do you regularly use air fresheners?

☐ Do you use bleach in your laundry?

☐ Do you use fragranced household cleaners and cosmetics?

☐ Do you use disinfectants or antibacterial products?

☐ Do you use a commercial oven cleaner?

☐ Do you use commercial carpet cleaners?

☐ Do you use mainstream commercial bath, tile and toilet cleaners?

☐ Do you store a number of partially used cleaning products from commercial sources under your kitchen sink?

☐ Does your furniture polish say 'flammable'? Do you spray a commercial dusting product?

☐ For all-purpose cleaning, do you use a mainstream commercial product?

About your health

☐ Are you sensitive to chemicals, car fumes, odours, perfumes or fragrances?

☐ As you get older, are you becoming increasingly sensitive to caffeine, alcohol or medications?

☐ Do you have bad reactions to monosodium glutamate (MSG); foods containing sulphites such as wine and dried fruit; salad-bar food; or beverages that contain caffeine; or diet sodas?

☐ Do you suffer from fibromyalgia (widespread musculoskeletal pain and fatigue), chronic fatigue syndrome (ME), cancer or an autoimmune disease?

☐ Do you have acne, eczema, hives or unexplained itching?

☐ Do you suffer from fatigue, lethargy, joint pain, muscle ache or weakness?

☐ Are you subject to irritability, mood swings, anxiety, depression, poor concentration, a 'spaced-out' feeling or restlessness?

☐ Do you get headaches, a stuffy nose, frequent sinus infections or allergies?

☐ Do you suffer from nausea, bad breath, foul-smelling stools, a bloated feeling, or intolerance to fatty or starchy foods?

☐ Do you keep getting sick 'for no reason'?

☐ Do you drink more than two alcoholic beverages a day?

☐ Do you use over-the-counter, prescription or recreational drugs on a regular basis?

If you answered yes to five or more of these questions, you may be exposing yourself to harmful chemicals on a regular basis, and these may be building up in your body. Follow the advice in this book to help you decrease your total body load.

Small doses, big effects

The 'low-dose effect' suggests that even small doses of certain chemicals can have big repercussions on health in both the short- and long-term. What constitutes a 'low dose' is not always clear, although it's generally defined as a dose much lower than would normally be expected to have an effect.

The idea that small doses can have big effects is beginning to receive a great deal of serious attention from scientists throughout the world, some of whom have found that chemicals in amounts as diluted as only a few parts per trillion (ppt) can have profound biological effects. Worryingly, these low-dose effects are often seen at levels well below those that have been deemed safe by regulatory authorities.

This phenomenon has been particularly well researched in the field of hormone disruption, where even minute quantities of different oestrogen mimics present in the environment can produce an effect on the body that is many times greater than would be expected.

For instance:

- **Phthalates.** Extremely low levels of these oestrogen-like chemicals, found in toys, building materials, drug capsules, cosmetics and perfumes, have been linked to sperm damage in men, and genital changes, asthma and allergies in children.

- **Bisphenol A.** Minuscule doses of this compound, which is used in polycarbonate plastic baby bottles, in resins that line food cans and in dental sealants, have been found to cause health effects at levels 2500 times lower than the US EPA's 'lowest observed effect' dose. Exposure to low levels of bisphenol A can alter brain structure, neurochemistry, behaviour, reproduction and immune responses in animals.

- **Atrazine.** This weedkiller unbalances a number of hormones necessary for the normal development and functioning of the reproductive system, including oestrogen, prolactin, luteinising hormone and follicle-stimulating hormone. It has been linked to gross sexual malformations in frogs that were exposed to water containing just 1/30th of the concentrations that the US EPA regards as safe for use in drinking water.

There are several reasons why low doses can be dangerous. One is that some people are simply more sensitive to it than others. Allergy specialists understand this problem well. If a person becomes sensitised to an allergen – for example, peanuts or cat dander – then exposure to even the tiniest amounts can set off a dramatic reaction. In chemically sensitive individuals, exposure to even small amounts of certain chemicals may be all that is required to start their health spiralling downwards.

The timing of an exposure is also influential. With many chemicals, a low dose to a baby in the womb or during childhood can produce potentially much more serious toxic effects than similar exposures as an adult. Good examples of this can be seen with the heavy metals lead and mercury, where low-dose exposures *in utero* and during infancy cause permanent brain and nervous-system damage, while the same doses appear to have no observable effects in adults. Similar problems have been found with exposure to certain pesticides in babies and infants.

The cocktail effect

Another way that low doses of chemicals can become dangerous is through what is known variously as 'synergy', 'the cocktail effect' or 'the additive effect'.

This happens when two toxic, or potentially toxic, chemicals are combined either in a product or in the human body, and produce a toxic effect much greater than would be predicted by the sum of their individual effects.

As with low-dose effects, most of the research into synergy has so far centred on the cocktail effect of hormone-disrupting chemicals. British research published in the journal *Environmental Health Perspectives* in 2002 found that combinations of minute levels of 11 environmental oestrogens, including genistein (one of the main oestrogens in soya), resorcinol monobenzoate (a protective coating commonly found on plastic items such as computer mice, sunglasses, hearing aids and ballpoint pens), phenyl salicylate (a sunscreen agent) and bisphenol A had more than double the oestrogenic effect on living cells that would have otherwise been predicted.

While the number of oestrogen mimics – 'xenoestrogens', or oestrogens produced outside the body – used in this study may seem high, it's worth remembering that most of us are exposed to many more than this number each day simply through household products, cosmetics and toiletries. It's also worth bearing in mind that oestrogen in amounts higher than those naturally produced by the body can cause cancer.

The authors concluded: 'Considered in isolation, the contribution of individual environmental oestrogens, at the concentrations found in wildlife and human tissues, will always be small. However, such reasoning cannot be used to support claims of negligible health risks from weak xenoestrogens, because the number of xenoestrogens present in wildlife and humans is unknown but likely to be very large ... by not taking combination effects into account, significant underestimations of the effects associated with exposure to xenoestrogens are likely.'

This kind of synergy occurs with many different classes of chemicals and, in the real world, we are exposed to multiple chemicals every day. Yet, chemicals such as food additives, pesticides and cosmetic ingredients are still tested for safety in the laboratory one at a time, with no allowance being made for cocktail effects.

The effects of synergistic interactions are not widely reported in the press, so many consumers remain unaware of the dangers of exposure to more than one chemical at a time. The notion is hardly new, however. In the 1960s and early 1970s, Dr Samuel Epstein, then with The Children's Cancer Research Foundation in Boston, and Dr Keiji Fujii, with the National Institute of Hygienic Sciences in Tokyo, published a series of papers highlighting the increased carcinogenicity of everyday pesticides used in combination, even at very low levels, or when applied as far apart as 200 days. Epstein has since gone on to become the chairman of the Cancer Prevention Coalition in the US, and is a recognised expert in the way chemicals in everyday products can harm health.

Most of us, however, only became aware of the idea of the cocktail effect after the Gulf War, when soldiers who returned from their tours of duty complained of numerous chronic illnesses. Gulf War soldiers were given an extraordinary mixture of drugs in preparation for life in the region, and the interactions among these compounds was the suspected cause of a range of health problems, especially the abnormal neurological function experienced by so many veterans.

Animal research has suggested that this suspicion is correct. Researchers at Duke University Medical Center and Texas Southwestern Medical School reported in 1996 that the simultaneous exposure to the topical insecticides **DEET** (N,N-diethyl-meta-toluamide) and permethrin, and pyridostigmine bromide, a drug taken as a prophylaxis (just in case) against toxic gas-warfare agents, can cause nervous-system damage in chickens.

The researchers found that the many symptoms experienced by Gulf War veterans, including headaches, fatigue, muscle aches, decreased attention and rashes, were similar to the symptoms seen in exposed chickens.

Chickens given any two chemicals became lethargic, unable to fly, lost weight and their coordination, and demonstrated tremors. For those administered all three chemicals, paralysis and death was a common outcome.

Because of the inadequacies of chemical testing, we have little concrete knowledge of the way the cocktail of chemicals we are exposed to each day will impact on our bodies and/or minds. The failure of regulatory authorities to acknowledge and allow for the synergism that occurs within just a single product, or in the human body due to exposure to several chemicals at once, is one the greatest failures of modern health regulation.

how your body reacts

OUR BODIES ARE MIRACULOUS. In spite of all the man-made pollutants we are exposed to each day, we seem to stay healthy – at least in the short term. This is because our bodies are equipped with numerous biological mechanisms that aid the process of defending and repairing our cells, tissues and organs.

These mechanisms work quietly in the background minute by minute and day by day. Skin, for example, is the largest excretory organ in the body. It helps to rid the body of toxins through sweat. It also protects us from dehydration and from external temperature variations. The immune system protects us from foreign bodies such as bacteria, which can make us ill. The kidneys eliminate waste products; the liver detoxifies the blood; the respiratory system enriches the blood with oxygen as well as filters out irritants and toxins.

There are, however, limits to what the body can do without support, and certain lifestyle factors can make it considerably harder for the body to provide 24/7 protection. For example, a person may be eating foods laced with pesticides or to which they are sensitive; exposing themselves daily to chemical toxins in the home or office; allowing emotional and psychological stress to build up; not taking regular exercise; not getting enough sleep; not allowing themselves to recover fully from illness before starting back at work; taking too many painkillers; drinking too much; and smoking cigarettes. This person's body is overloaded and will eventually break down.

Who is vulnerable?

Each of us has some vulnerability or weakness that makes exposure to toxic chemicals risky. Some of these weaknesses are mediated by gender or age. Women, the very young and the elderly are, for instance, much more likely to experience health problems from daily exposure to toxic chemicals and pollutants. Other types of vulnerability are genetic; if you have symptoms of illnesses that run in your family, you may have this kind of constitutional weakness.

Where you fall on the socioeconomic ladder is another factor. Lack of education and a very low income can often dovetail with lifestyle risk factors such as excess alcohol intake, broken families, inadequate diet, older housing with lead paint and ageing water pipes, drug abuse, smoking and exposure to industrial pollution as well as inadequate prenatal healthcare and high rates of bottle-feeding babies with artificial milk. This means that the poorest urban populations are already at the highest risk of health and behavioural problems. Adding exposure to toxic chemicals to the mix can often quickly tip these people over into ill health.

However, the relatively affluent should not consider themselves immune to toxic effects. Our consumer-orientated society encourages us to buy and use a wide range of products that contain toxic chemicals, endocrine disrupters and heavy metals, all of which can cause similar health problems in the longer term.

We are all of us vulnerable to a greater or lesser extent. The unique vulnerability of children is discussed in Chapter 4. Nevertheless, there are some things that make women and the elderly more likely to be harmed by exposure to toxic chemicals.

It's different for girls

Women are more likely to use a greater number of toxic products while carrying out everyday grooming and household cleaning. Many women also work in jobs that expose them to toxic substances. This higher rate of exposure is one significant reason why women are more likely to suffer health problems from chemical exposures.

As is the case with children, women tend to have smaller body frames, so their exposure per kilogramme of body weight will also be greater than men's. In addition, women naturally carry more body fat than men and, as many toxic substances are stored in fat, this means that women carry potentially more toxins in their bodies.

Once again, trends in health and behaviour tell us something about how women are likely to be affected by these toxins. Rates of disorders such as diabetes, arthritis and systemic lupus erythematosus (SLE or lupus) are rising, as are reproductive disorders such as endometriosis, polycystic ovarian syndrome (PCOS) and infertility.

Many cancers, including those of the breast, endometrium (lining of the womb), lungs and skin are becoming more common in women, too. Because cancer is a multifactorial disease, it can be difficult to pinpoint its origins. But an examination into the rise in once-rare cancers such as non-Hodgkin's lymphoma (NHL) may shed an entirely different light on the subject.

The term 'non-Hodgkin's lymphoma' is a catchall phrase used to cover several different cancers that develop from the lymphatic system, a complex network of tissues and organs that runs throughout the entire body. Scientists admit that they are baffled by the steady rise of this immune-system cancer, which now accounts for around 3 per cent of all cancers. Yet, in the last 20 years, the incidence of NHL has increased by about 73 per cent. A large proportion of that increase occurred between 1973 and 1987, when the incidence of NHL rose by a massive 51 per cent. Most victims are women.

To understand how important the link is between toxins and immune-system cancer, it is helpful to know that the primary function of the lymphatic system is to clear debris and help defend the body. A cornerstone of the immune system, the lymphatic system is made up of fine vessels that branch out like veins into all parts of the body and carry lymph, a watery colourless fluid, to the lymph nodes – small bean-shaped nodules found in clusters in the neck, armpits, pelvis and abdomen. The lymph nodes produce infection-fighting cells such as lymphocytes and antibodies, and also act like a filter and drain, sifting out foreign matter into the lymph fluid.

A number of significant associations between NHL and solvent exposure have been reported in the medical literature. In 1976, the accidental release of large quantities of poisonous industrial byproducts called *dioxins* in

Seveso, Italy, resulted in the exposure of more than 5000 local residents. Follow-up studies revealed elevated rates of NHL and soft-tissue sarcomas – cancers of the muscle, fat, blood vessels or any of the other tissues that support, surround and protect the organs – among exposed individuals.

But chemicals such as those used in everyday pesticides are also implicated in raising the risk of NHL by 50 per cent or more. One investigation by the US National Cancer Institute (NCI) in 1986 found that farmers who used the pesticide **2,4-D** – a common ingredient in garden 'weed and feed' products – on more than 20 days a year were six times more likely to develop NHL compared with unexposed persons. Another found that people who frequently mixed or used herbicides themselves were eight times more likely to develop this type of cancer.

Increased exposure to PCBs (*polychlorinated biphenyls*; found in flame retardants, plastics and insulation materials as well as in some detergents, hairspray and other personal-care items) has also been linked to the continuing rise in NHL. Similarly, those exposed to the flame retardant tetra-BDE (bromodiphenyl ether) such as professional car, bus and truck drivers are also at an increased risk (and women should note that this same flame retardant is used in all vehicles, even 'mum's taxi').

NHL, however, is not just an occupational hazard. Women who use hair dye (particularly dark brown, black and red) may be increasing their risk of rare cancers, including NHL and multiple myeloma (a progressive blood disease), by anywhere from two to four times over non-users.

Rare cancers, of course, are not the only effect of toxic exposures. Women are also at greater risk of menstrual disorders, mood swings, headaches, allergies and chronic fatigue. Women, of course, also have the responsibility of bearing children, and decades of research show that a woman's fertility can be affected by pollution. Should she conceive, her child's level of health will be largely dependent on her own. Many of the environmental illnesses that children suffer from have their roots in toxic exposures in prenatal life – in other words, in the womb.

The elderly at risk

There are a number of reasons why older people may be at an increased risk from environmental toxins. Natural ageing, for instance, involves decreases in bone mass and blood flow through the heart, and diminished pancreatic, thyroid and lymphatic functioning. These changes make the body less effective at clearing toxins. Other factors that can add to the risk include:

- A lifetime of environmental stress, which can lead to increased stress hormones such as corticosteroids that, in turn, can lead to immune suppression and a diminished healing capacity.

- The accumulation of free-radical damage, cellular 'garbage' and DNA damage due to environmental toxins, which can result in mutations that make cells less resilient and more prone to disease.

- The development of diseases such as atherosclerosis (clogged arteries) that prevent the elderly from taking regular exercise and staying active, which then has the knock-on effect of exacerbating any other health problems they may have.

It is also widely acknowledged that the elderly are generally overmedicated. Doctors who prescribe unnecessary drugs to the elderly are not only compromising these patients' health, but also adding to the toxic burden of their bodies. Even more worrying, some medications and environmental toxins interact with each other, making their individual effects on the body even more powerful (see 'The Cocktail Effect', page 28).

What to look for

Because everyone is different, the first symptoms of toxic exposure in some may be in the digestive system whereas, for others, it may be the skin or immune system. Others may get headaches, mood swings or symptoms of depression when exposed to certain chemicals.

Certain conditions – such as pregnancy or breastfeeding, or if you're trying to conceive – and particular illnesses can also make you more susceptible to the adverse effects of toxic chemicals than others. If any of the following conditions apply to you, you may find that lowering the total toxic load on your body may be beneficial for your health in both the short and long term.

- Constant tiredness, chronic fatigue syndrome

- Autoimmune diseases such as osteoarthritis, diabetes, multiple sclerosis

- A family history of cancers

- Respiratory problems such as asthma or chronic bronchitis

- Sinusitis or hayfever

- Frequent colds or susceptibility to flu

- Watery, itchy eyes or eyes that produce excess mucus

- Skin problems such as dermatitis or eczema

- Regular headaches or migraines

- Mental symptoms such as depression

- Menstrual problems such as PMS, irregular periods and anovulatory cycles

- Parasitic infestations

- Overweight or underweight

Most of us would not automatically look for chemical causes of these conditions and, while no one is suggesting that chemical overload is the sole cause of such problems, it cannot be ruled out as a contributing factor. What's more, diseases that do not appear to respond to conventional treatment often do respond once your environment and your body are cleared of toxins.

Taking a look at some of these conditions in greater depth may help to clarify the role of chemical exposure in your day-to-day health.

Stress

Feeling stressed is a common experience of modern life. Most of us equate stress with the physical and emotional experiences of everyday life. But, as humans have evolved, so have our sources of stress. Today, we can come under physical, chemical, electromagnetic, nutritional, traumatic and even psychospiritual stress – and, in all cases, the body's reaction is the same.

The body does not differentiate between emotional and environmental stress. Anything that threatens to unbalance or harm the body can trigger our primitive fight-or-flight responses and trigger the release of a flood of stress hormones.

In the right proportions, stress hormones help to keep our bodies healthy. But too much or too little of them, and they become a form of slow poison, depressing your immune system and leading to a staggering list of stress-related disorders, including:

- Allergies
- Anorexia nervosa
- Arthritis
- Asthma
- Atherosclerosis
- Cancer
- Constipation
- Depression
- Diabetes
- Diarrhoea
- Eczema
- Fatigue
- Headaches
- High blood pressure
- Indigestion
- Infections
- Insomnia
- Irritability
- Irritable bowel syndrome
- Loss of appetite
- Muscle tension
- Neck and back pain
- Nutritional deficiencies
- Peptic ulcer
- Premenstrual symptoms
- Psoriasis
- Psychological problems
- Sexual problems
- Weight changes

Stress, whatever its origin, can also follow a circular pathway. For instance, physical stress can lead to emotional stress and vice versa. Whatever the origin, a stressed-out body is simply less able to deal with poisons in the environment and, therefore, one that may be more likely to become overwhelmed and less efficient at defending and repairing itself.

Chronic fatigue syndrome

When a person has chronic fatigue syndrome (CFS), several body systems are affected. These include the immune, the endocrine, the haematological (responsible for the formation of new red blood cells) and the nervous systems.

Severe fatigue is the most common symptom of CFS. In some cases, it can be so overwhelming that just minor exertion, such as a short walk or light housework, can be debilitating. While many sufferers try to curtail their normal daily activities and rest more, this doesn't appear to help.

CFS produces other symptoms as well, including headaches, low-grade fever, swollen lymph nodes, sore throat, depression, poor concentration and decreased mental acuity, muscle and joint aches and pains, allergies, digestive complaints, weight loss and skin rashes.

Mental and emotional symptoms are also common. CFS sufferers often have trouble remembering specific names or places, or doing complex mental work such as bookkeeping, administrative tasks or teaching.

Many CFS sufferers have a history of extreme and prolonged emotional stress, anxiety and depression, and a history of poor nutritional habits, which are thought to contribute to the disease. But environmental pollutants and contaminants are also thought to play a significant role. Having run the body down, it becomes much more susceptible to the viruses known to trigger CFS.

Perhaps not surprisingly, given their higher rate of chemical exposure and increased vulnerability, 70 per cent of CFS sufferers are women.

Autoimmune diseases

Chemical overload and autoimmune diseases often go hand in hand. A good example of this is the role that toxic exposures and allergic reactions often play in the development of arthritis. Studies where arthritis patients have been exposed to various pollutants such as natural gas, car exhausts, perfume, hairspray, insecticides and tobacco smoke have shown a clear link between such exposure and worsening of symptoms.

Likewise, there is good evidence to show that the autoimmune disease systemic lupus erythematosus (SLE) can be made worse by fluoride. Lupus is a connective tissue disorder, and connective tissue is around 30 per cent collagen. *Fluoride*, which is added to water supplies in many places and to most commercial toothpastes, disrupts the synthesis of collagen and leads to its breakdown in skin, muscle, tendons, ligaments, bone, lungs, kidneys, cartilage and elsewhere.

While we have always assumed that diabetes, another common autoimmune disorder, is linked solely to diet, this may not be the case. There is evidence that exposure to pesticides during pregnancy may raise a child's risk of developing juvenile diabetes. Such findings have opened the door to the possibility that other types of chemical exposure may also be contributing factors to both juvenile and late-onset diabetes.

Most recently, exposure to small amounts of **bisphenol A** have been shown to increase the risk of diabetes. This synthetic plasticiser is used to make dental sealants, sturdy microwavable plastics, linings for metal food and beverage containers, and baby bottles – to name but a few. Bisphenol A can leach into food and water from these products and, not surprisingly, it's widely found in human blood. In animals, repeated exposure over several days provoked insulin resistance, a prediabetic state in which tissues lose their sensitivity to normal levels of insulin.

Cancer

Cancer rates are on the rise. In the UK, the number of cases diagnosed each year has increased by a massive 50 per cent in the last 25 years. Researchers say it's not just because the population is getting older, or because we are getting better at detecting the disease in its early stages. So why is this happening?

Cancer doesn't just suddenly appear. It is generated in two steps: initiation and promotion. The initiation process is what triggers the development of cancer. This is the factor(s) that interacts with cellular DNA to start the process of producing abnormal cells. Initiators can be carcinogens (cancer-causing agents), viruses, radiation, oxygen, cell-destroying free radicals and hormones, particularly oestrogens.

While none of your daily exposures to these toxins may be significant on their own, added together, their action is cumulative, challenging the immune system and damaging cells over a long period of time until, eventually, cancer develops.

Many of the ingredients in consumer products – volatile organic compounds (VOCs) and solvents, surfactants, **formaldehyde**, nitrosamines, plastics and preservatives – can act as initiators either because they are directly cancer-causing or because they disrupt hormonal or other normal bodily functions.

Several lifestyle factors can also become disease-causing agents, working away silently for years and damaging body cells. For instance, a low-fibre diet means that waste products remain in the gut longer than they should, giving the body ample time to absorb more toxins. Toxins in the body can interrupt the process of cellular repair and cause cells to replicate too quickly or to mutate.

After initiation, the disease may lie dormant for many years until something comes along which signals it to grow. Promoters, which cause the disease to develop, are factors that damage the body's defence mechanisms. Promoters may also alter body tissues, predisposing them to cancer growth. A diet that is high in fat can make toxic chemicals much more efficient promoters. This is because chemicals can accumulate in fatty tissues, from where they can leach back into the body, causing continual damage and, eventually, the development of disease.

Because cancer can lie dormant for many years before it begins to grow and spread, it can be difficult to link it conclusively with toxic exposures. Nevertheless, when cancer clusters (large numbers of people in one area with the same type of cancer) appear, environmental factors such as toxic exposure are always the leading suspects. It is estimated that between 10 and 30 per cent of cancers are the result of regular exposure to toxic chemicals.

Asthma and allergies

An allergy is a response to something the body identifies as foreign or toxic. Around 15 to 20 per cent of the population experience significant allergic reactions to consumer products.

Asthma is an extreme allergic response. It can be triggered by a variety of stimuli, the nature of which varies from individual to individual. Upper respiratory tract infections, either viral or bacterial, can often trigger an asthmatic attack. Changes in weather or temperature, exposure to moulds, animal dander, grass or tree pollens may all be triggers for asthmatics, and so are the preservatives, fragrances and colourings used in prepackaged foods, cosmetics, toiletries and household cleaners.

Fragrances in particular are major triggers for asthma attacks, with around 70 per cent of asthmatics reporting that exposure to perfumes can worsen their condition. Other chemical triggers include the *formaldehyde* used in products such as medicated shampoos, germicidal soaps, mouthwashes and toothpastes. The solvents commonly found in toiletries and household cleaners can also cause respiratory problems.

Often, the triggers for such reactions can remain undetected for years, only revealing themselves as toxins when they are taken out of the diet or environment, and the body is given a chance to recover and repair itself.

Skin disorders

Rashes and other disorders of the skin now constitute a frequent complaint in the GP's surgery. Commonly reported problems range from simple hives to more complicated conditions such as eczema and psoriasis.

The skin is the largest organ in the body and performs many life-sustaining functions. It is a physical barrier that protects us from harmful organisms in our environment, but it is also a major organ of excretion. Skin reactions are commonly localised reactions to something that has come into contact with the skin. But they can also be the result of the body trying to rid itself of circulating toxins deep within the body.

The fragrance portion of toiletries and cleaning products is responsible for a large percentage of skin reactions. However, other chemicals are also implicated. These include preservatives, detergents and antibacterial agents.

While the skin does act as a barrier, it can be easily breached by harsh chemicals that dissolve the protective oils lying on the surface of the skin, thereby allowing toxins to be more easily absorbed into the bloodstream. Many substances such as solvents, perfumes, preservatives, fatty acids, and other emollients and nanoparticles actually aid the absorption of other, more harmful chemicals into the body. These agents are known as 'penetration enhancers' (see Chapter 6). Skin permeability is also increased by heat, such as when taking a hot bath or shower.

Headaches

If you get headaches regularly, it is likely to be because your body is under some kind of stress. In fact, the most common type of headache is the tension headache. While we often dismiss such headaches as the result of emotional stress, they are also likely to be the result of biological stress – due to food allergies, or exposure to pollutants and toxins. Migraines are more complex, but also respond remarkably well to the removal of allergens and synthetic chemicals from the environment.

Research into migraine shows that fragrances are a common trigger. This is because scents can breach the blood–brain barrier and gain direct access to the central nervous system. Many other chemicals such as solvents and propellants, which are so prevalent in toiletries and household products, also affect the central nervous and vascular systems, and are implicated in chronic headaches.

Research shows that pregnant women who frequently use aerosol products such as air fresheners, deodorants, furniture polishes and hairsprays have significantly higher rates of headaches and post-natal depression compared with those who use these products less than once a week.

Depression

There is some evidence that environmental pollutants can both cause depression and other emotional problems as well as make them worse. The chemicals known to trigger depression include solvents, VOCs and endocrine-disrupting chemicals. The fragrances used in perfumes, toiletries and household cleaners contain many of these substances and, not surprisingly, are often implicated in mood swings and emotional problems.

Many environmental practitioners have had good results in relieving depression by putting mild-to-moderately depressed patients on chemical-free regimes. Once patients begin to limit their exposure to compounds like fragrances, they often then find it easier to recognise when a particular chemical ingredient or fragrance has triggered a depressive episode.

Depression also has a circular link with immunity. Depressed immune function – often a result of toxic overload – can affect mood. Likewise, a depressed mood can lead to impaired immune function, resulting in a vicious circle of poor mental and emotional health. Similarly, hormone disruption can also be a factor in depression.

Infertility and reproductive problems

Many of the chemicals in everyday products are hormone-disrupting. Often, they mimic the effects of oestrogen in the body. While women (and men) need oestrogen to remain healthy, too much of this hormone has profound effects on our well-being, and our sexual and reproductive health, as well as being a known risk factor for oestrogen-dependent cancers of the breast, ovary, endometrium and prostate.

Much of what we know about the influence of everyday toxins on fertility comes from research into those who work with these chemicals every day. A recent Canadian study, published in the *Journal of the American*

Medical Association, showed that women who work with organic solvents – such as artists, graphic designers, laboratory technicians, veterinary technicians, cleaners, factory workers, office workers and chemists – have a greatly increased risk of both miscarriage and of giving birth to premature, low birth-weight or damaged babies compared with women who aren't so exposed.

Hairdressers and others who work in the beauty industry are also exposed to these kinds of organic solvents. And again, they have much higher rates of infertility, miscarriage and babies with birth defects than women who are not exposed to these chemicals every day.

These kinds of solvents are not restricted to the workplace. They are also commonly used in cleaning products, toiletries and paints. Pregnant women who live near petrochemical factories also experience more threatened abortions, toxaemia (toxic spread of an infection via the bloodstream), anaemia, nausea and vomiting.

A man's fertility can also be affected by chemical exposures. Men who work in jobs that bring them into regular contact with pesticides and toxic chemicals are more likely to father children with birth defects. Such men often bring residues from their work home with them on their clothes and hair, and in their semen, increasing their partners' exposure to these toxins as well.

Hormone-disrupting chemicals that find their way into the food chain are now believed to be responsible for the global decline in sperm counts. Some 20 different toxic chemicals with the potential to harm sperm quality and production have been found in studies of sperm quality. In contrast, there is evidence from the US suggesting that men who eat organic foods have sperm counts that are twice as high as those who don't.

Finally, studies show that more than 350 man-made toxic chemicals are being passed on to babies in increasing amounts through pathways such as the placenta. Unlike adults, a developing baby is very sensitive to changes in the supply of nutrients and the presence of poisons.

Eating disorders

Both obesity and slimming disorders have been linked to toxins in the body. Continual ingestion of toxins can, for instance, produce nutritional deficiencies, particularly in zinc. Several studies show that zinc deficiency is a contributing factor to slimming disorders such as anorexia. Hormone disruption may also cause slimming disorders.

One German review concluded that distorted hormonal patterns are often found in young women before the onset of anorexia. Other researchers have found that one reason why bulimics report feeling uncomfortably full after eating may be irregularities in the hormonal process that regulates fluid volume in the body. Where this hormonal disruption comes from, and whether it begins at a young age with exposure to everyday toxins, may be useful avenues of research in coming years.

Similarly, some experts believe that obesity can be a response to accumulated toxins in the body. This may be due to the way toxins can alter thyroid function, making it more sluggish and unable to respond to the energy intake of the body.

However, it may also be because some of the most harmful toxins are absorbed by the body and stored in fat. As a rule, the body doesn't like to allow the concentration of potentially harmful substances to rise too high, and will excrete them if it can. However, if for some reason the body cannot excrete them, or cannot excrete them quickly enough, the body's other option is to 'dilute' the toxins by storing them in fat cells. Under these circumstances, fat becomes the body's way of controlling and preventing high levels of toxins from circulating around the body.

During weight loss, as we lose fat, we release toxins into the body. This may be why some dieters feel so unwell when they begin a slimming regime. To protect your body from the release of toxins while dieting, you need to ensure a greater intake of water and fibre, and of the antioxidant nutrients such as vitamins C and E, beta-carotene, selenium and zinc.

Another way in which the body attempts to dilute toxins is through the accumulation of water. Those who feel that their extra weight is the result of water retention may also benefit from a sensible detoxification programme.

▶ MAKING CHANGES

Few of us have the choice of living in an unpolluted environment. City dwellers are often obliged to travel and live in places where pollution from cars and factories is a fact of life. In fact, many of us work and live in buildings so full of chemicals that they have come to be known as 'sick buildings'. Good evidence shows that many of the substances that we come into contact with each day are causing a health crisis in our bodies, and it behoves us to do what we can to reduce our exposure whenever and wherever we can.

Because they tend to bypass our conscious awareness, environmental and other stressors that are not emotional or psychological in nature are arguably the most harmful to our health. But, in a body overwhelmed by environmental poisons, the usual recommendations such as relaxation and exercise may no longer be enough to completely counteract the effects of stress.

To cope with environmental stress, you need to be aware of the environment and to understand how it affects you even when you are not immediately aware of these effects. Once you know the particular sources of your environmental stress, you can begin to make positive changes in your home and in your regular routines. The first step is to remove as many chemical pollutants as you can from your everyday activities.

Other supportive steps include:

Improve your diet. Little changes can make a big difference. Switch to organic foods when you can, and make sure your diet includes lots of fresh fruit and vegetables. Fresh produce contains those important nutrients called 'antioxidants', which help to correct the damage caused by pollutants. In addition, the water-soluble fibre in these foods can help eliminate accumulated toxins. A diet that is low in saturated fat will also keep toxins from accumulating in the body. Try to choose oily fish over red meat whenever possible as the essential fatty acids in mackerel, trout, salmon, herring and sardines can also help fight the effects of chemical exposure in the body.

Exercise regularly. Our bodies are designed to be used. When we don't use them to their optimal extent, muscles deteriorate, metabolism becomes sluggish and breathing becomes shallow. For these reasons, it is desirable to develop good, sensible habits of exercise – whether they are aerobic routines, an active lifestyle or weight-training – that you can easily incorporate into your life for the rest of your life.

Studies also show that regular aerobic exercise can help detoxify the body, so choose two or three activities that you really enjoy and work these into your schedule each week. Aerobic exercise – or anything that makes you sweat (such as a regular sauna) – is particularly useful for boosting metabolism and aiding the release of toxins through the skin.

Investigate stress relief. The state of your body often reflects the state of your mind. Too much stress depletes the body of nutrients needed to fight the effects of pollution. Any activity that absorbs you completely and allows you to switch off can be useful in lowering stress levels. However, activities that involve deep breathing such as yoga or meditation can be very relaxing as well as promote the release of toxins via the lungs. Any activity that relaxes you will also have a knock-on effect on your immune system, helping it to function more efficiently.

Have regular massage. Consider booking an appointment for regular massage. It's relaxing, and can improve the movement of blood and lymph through the body, encouraging the removal of toxins, cell regeneration and better all-round circulation.

Try hydrotherapy. Water in all its states helps to purify the body. Try a relaxing bath with cider vinegar; add Epsom or sea salts to stimulate the skin to release toxins. Invest in a home whirlpool for your bath. Or, if you belong to a health club with a steam sauna, make regular use of it.

Use plant power. A two-year study by NASA scientists suggests that the most sophisticated pollution-absorbing device in your home is a potted plant. Living, green and flowering plants have an amazing ability to remove several toxic chemicals, including formaldehyde, benzene and carbon monoxide from the air. You can use plants in your home or office to improve the quality of the air as well as to make it a more pleasant place to live and work, where people feel better, perform better and enjoy life more.

The 15 most effective houseplants for this job are: English ivy, spider plant, golden pothos, peace lily, Chinese evergreen, bamboo or reed palm, snake plant, heartleaf philodendron, selloum or elephant-ear philodendron, red-edged *Dracaena*, cornstalk *Dracaena*, Janet Craig *Dracaena*, Warneck *Dracaena* and weeping fig.

Use food therapy. There are some simple kitchen cupboard solutions to help you combat everyday toxins. For instance, all leafy, dark-green vegetables, but especially cruciferous vegetables (belonging to the cabbage family), can inhibit the carcinogenic effects of chemicals. So, include plenty of kale, spinach, broccoli and brussels sprouts in your diet. Other foods are helpful, too:

- The pectin found in apple and pear seeds can protect your body from damage by toxic metals. These work by blocking the absorption of toxins while aiding detoxification. Try making apples or pears, stewed with their seeds, a regular feature of your diet.

- Garlic and onions contain powerful antioxidants that aid the body's natural day-to-day efforts to detox. Use these liberally in cooking.

- Peas, beans and lentils also contain special antioxidants. They are also high in fibre that can bind to toxins and aid their excretion from the body. Pulses are a good alternative source of protein, so why not substitute a couple of meat meals each week for one based on (organic) pulses.

- Bananas have been shown to have antioxidant qualities.

- Eggs protect against lead and mercury contamination.

- A high-fibre diet in general is useful for trapping toxins and assisting in the elimination of heavy metals. Consider adding water-soluble, mucilaginous fibres such as psyllium seeds and flaxseeds to your diet. These can be ground up and added to cereals, soups and baked foods.

- Seaweeds and alginates can also bind to heavy metals. There is evidence, for instance, that the freshwater green algae *Chlorella* can draw persistent chemicals, such as PCBs, out of the system.

Learn to breathe properly. (and preferably in a clean environment). Most of us breathe in a shallow, inefficient way high into the chest. This reduces oxygen consumption and denies the benefits of breathing. When the breath is shallow, we not only don't take in enough oxygen, but we also don't get rid of enough carbon dioxide. As a result, our bodies become oxygen-starved, allowing toxins to build up. In addition, shallow breathing fails to exercise the lungs and so reduces their ability to function optimally, creating a vicious circle of lost vitality.

The kind of deep-breathing practices found in yoga, for example, draw air into the very bottom of the lungs, helping to clear the lungs and bloodstream of toxic buildup. Studies also show that breathing deeply is more relaxing, and so lowers levels of stress hormones and encourages the immune system to work more efficiently. Getting more oxygen into the lungs is reputed to have the knock-on effect of improving the function of your eliminatory organs, such as the liver and kidneys, as well as your digestive tract. Oxygen-rich blood also feeds the nervous system, in particular, the brain, which requires three times more oxygen to work properly than other organs in the body.

Kick the habit. Excess use of tobacco products, alcohol and caffeine wreak havoc on your body. They also encourage toxic damage. Smoking exposes you to cadmium and carcinogenic polycyclic aromatic hydrocarbons (PAHs). Alcohol can alter immune and endocrine functions, and is poisonous to your internal organs – specifically, your liver. In this day and age, no one needs to justify advice to cut down. Too much caffeine dehydrates the body, and a dehydrated body is less able to function properly, to fight off infection and the effects of toxic exposures.

especially for parents

MOST PARENTS KNOW that the greatest gift they can give their children is good health. Once upon a time, this may have seemed like a simple matter of putting a roof over their heads, making sure they had a good winter coat and giving them decent food. The rest, parents may have reasoned, was up to chance, genetics or Divine intervention.

Today, life is more complex. We live in a polluted world surrounded daily by hundreds of man-made toxins that we can't see, taste or even smell, but which nevertheless have the potential to damage human health. When we go to the supermarket, we buy 'fresh' foods which are covered with pesticides and not really fresh at all. Instead, they have been stored for long periods of time, during which time they have been sprayed with even more chemicals to maintain the appearance of freshness. As our schedules get busier, we rely more and more on convenience foods laced with additives, flavourings, colours and aromas, all of which can cause a variety of health problems.

While it may appear that, in spite of all this, our children are being born alive and well, a closer look at infant health trends says otherwise.

Children are more vulnerable

Children are uniquely vulnerable to environmental pollution in part because their response to toxic exposure is often very different from that of adults. Good examples of this are the paradoxical responses to phenobarbital and methylphenidate (Ritalin) in children compared with adults. Phenobarbital acts like a sedative in adults, but produces hyperactivity in children; Ritalin, a cocaine-like drug, is used as an anti-hyperactivity drug in children, but has a stimulant effect in grown-ups.

There are many reasons for this paradoxical response. But perhaps the most influential is that, in the womb and during the first two years after birth, children undergo extraordinary cell growth in every part of their bodies, from brain neurons to immune cells, so there are more disruptive opportunities for toxic compounds. During childhood, different systems and organs develop at different rates and in different phases. Growing tissue is also much more sensitive to toxic exposure than other tissues, and remains sensitive right through to the teen years. Indeed, studies of exposure to cigarette smoke have shown that the risk of dying of breast cancer is greater for those who started smoking before the age of 16 than for those who started smoking after the age of 20.

In addition to growing and developing, children differ from adults in a number of other ways that can increase their susceptibility to toxins. For example:

- Their systems have a less-developed ability to break down toxic substances and their bodies may also have less capacity to repair any damage as well.

- They eat, drink and breathe in more for their weight than adults, which means they take in more toxins per kilogramme than grown-ups – in fact, even at rest, an infant breathes in twice the volume of air as an adult does.

- They crawl around on the floor near dust and other potentially toxic particles.

- They are more likely to put things in their mouths and eat things that they shouldn't.

The developing foetus reacts strongly to toxic chemicals. This is because the developing body is extremely sensitive to the signals and complex interactions of hormones. Disruption of these signals and interactions can permanently skew the body's development.

Many studies show that hypertension, coronary heart disease, thyroid dysfunction, cancer, diabetes, asthma, arthritis and even Alzheimer's disease – things which can't be picked up on a prenatal scan – are all programmed into a baby while still in the womb. What determines the programming is maternal nutrition and exposure to environmental toxins.

More cancer

The worst effects of environmental poisons on children can clearly be seen in the increasing rate of childhood cancers.

According to medical scientists, the reason for the rise in childhood cancers is something of a mystery. Indeed, some experts continue to promote the idea that childhood cancer is rare. Yet, statistics show that, after accidents, childhood cancer is the second biggest killer of children.

Just like adults, children can develop cancer at any site in the body, but two sites – the bones and the brain – are now particularly common. Figures from the US National Cancer Institute show that most childhood cancers are on the rise. Rates for acute lymphocytic leukaemia (ALL) have risen 10 per cent in the last 15 years, and the incidence of central-nervous-system tumours are up by more than 30 per cent.

Cancer is, of course, a multifactorial disease – many things can trigger it. But while scientists continue to focus their research on the genetic links to childhood cancer, important environmental triggers – in the form of mercury-containing vaccines, pesticides, food additives and electromagnetic radiation – are being ignored.

In addition to obvious birth defects and cancer, more subtle trends have emerged. Population studies tell us that the rate of birth defects has actually gone up in recent years. In the US, one report showed that 18 of the 20 most common birth defects were on the rise – some by as much as 1700 per cent. Reports from the UK show a similar trend. But this fact has been successfully obscured by an increase in medical terminations – as long as the baby is not born at term, the fact that it had an abnormality does not count in the 'official' records. Also, in the West, some problems, such as undescended testicles, have become so commonplace that they are no longer recorded as malformations.

Furthermore, rates of asthma and other respiratory problems among children are on the rise, as are skin conditions, learning and behavioural difficulties, and serious conditions such as attention-deficit/hyperactivity disorder (ADHD).

Life in the womb

Many parents-to-be believe that, as long as the baby is inside its mother, it is safe from environmental toxins. This belief stems from a long-standing view that the placenta – the baby's life-support system – acts like a filter, letting only the nutrients and immune-protective agents like antibodies into the baby's system. In reality, the placenta acts more like a sponge.

The placenta consists of a complex mass of blood vessels (if laid out flat, enough to completely cover more than half a tennis court) that carry nutrients and oxygen to the baby, and remove waste products and carbon dioxide. While the placenta can protect your baby to some degree, it is not a total barrier; studies show that, nowadays, more than 350 man-made toxic chemicals are being passed on to babies in increasing amounts through pathways such as the placenta.

Absolutely *everything* that enters the mother's system also enters the baby's system via the placenta. So, along with all those vitamins, minerals, amino acids and antibodies, there are also heavy metals, car fumes, pesticides, cigarette smoke, drugs, and the chemicals from household cleaners and cosmetics.

The World Wildlife Fund (WWF) in the UK has stated, in its report *Chemical Trespass: a Toxic Legacy*, that: 'It is now recognised that the foetus can be damaged by relatively low levels of contaminants which do not affect the adult ... Exposure in the womb can cause birth defects and can affect our children's future ability to reproduce and their susceptibility to diseases such as cancer. Functional deficits may also be caused, such that some children may not reach their full potential. Put simply, the integrity of the next generation is at stake.'

There is a huge body of evidence to show that a combination of inadequate nutrition and exposure to environmental toxins can have a profound effect on the developing child. Consider the following:

- According to the US-based National Birth Defects Prevention Network, a 50 per cent reduction in birth defects could be achieved if parents simply improved their diets and limited their exposure to toxic substances.

- The UK's preconceptual care group Foresight has published figures showing that a prepregnancy health programme that includes dietary correction and reduction of toxins can lead to an overall birth-defect rate of less than 1 per cent – compared with the 5–7 per cent that is the national average.

- Everyday toxins such as food additives and those in unfiltered, contaminated tap water raise the risk of your baby having a birth defect. Pesticide exposure during pregnancy has also been linked to an increase in birth defects along with a greater risk of cancer later in life.

- Hormone disrupters, which can be found in large amounts in pesticide residues, but also in everyday household detergents and toiletries, and even in disposable nappies, may alter a child's thyroid function and sexual characteristics. These types of chemicals have already been implicated as responsible for low sperm counts in young men, and there is fear that exposure to too many of these synthetic oestrogens may predispose young girls to oestrogen-dependent cancers of the breast, ovary and endometrium later in life.

Cutting down on toxic toiletries

Certain everyday toiletries may also pose a threat to your unborn child's health. There is a substantial body of evidence to show that hairdressers are at greater risk of having babies with malformations than other women, and that they are more prone to miscarriages as well. This is because hairdressers are exposed daily to the poisonous chemicals in hair preparations such as shampoo, conditioners, hairsprays, gels, mousses and hair dyes. The average

▶

woman is not exposed to these chemicals in the same concentrations, but a quick look through your bathroom cupboard may give you pause for thought. If it is filled with lots of different types of haircare products, you may wish to consider cutting down.

Similarly, a study of 14,000 women from the University of Bristol revealed that pregnant women who constantly use aerosol products such as air fresheners, deodorants, furniture polishes and hairsprays have significantly higher rates of headaches and post-natal depression than those who use these products less than once a week. The high-users' babies had higher rates of ear infections and diarrhoea (see 'Air Fresheners', page 192).

Cutting down on unnecessary toiletries is a good habit to get into now as it may help you to resist the temptation to smother your baby with the unnecessary and harsh chemicals contained in many baby products.

The toxic baby

Human babies are unlike any other young animals in that they are born completely helpless and with many of their bodily functions, such as their digestion and immune system, still not fully functioning. This is why extra consideration is worthwhile when making choices about feeding, and when looking around for potential sources of exposure to toxic chemicals and fumes in the home.

Babies also indulge in lots of hand-to-mouth activity, making it easy to transfer more foreign substances into their bodies. Young children are also more likely to have close encounters with the pesticides on lawns or in pet collars, and toxins in carpets, as they spend a lot of time playing or crawling on the ground.

There are other, less obvious threats to health as well. The average newborn, with his faster metabolism, and immature immune and detoxification systems, may:

- Spend his first year of life in a new crib with a mattress that's been treated with pesticides and fire-retardant chemicals. The foam inside the mattress can give off toxic *formaldehyde* gas, and the dyes used in the sheets and covers are usually carcinogenic. The typical crib headboard or bed frame is constructed from particleboard – wood shavings pressed and glued together with a urea-formaldehyde resin that also gives off toxic gases.

- Wear disposable nappies made of bleached paper that emits a slow, steady dose of cancer-causing *dioxins*. These nappies also contain a 'chemical sponge' that emits hormone-disrupting chemicals.

- Obtain some or all of his nourishment from plastic bottles that give off *phthalates* (plasticisers) in amounts that can be measured in the bloodstream.

- Travel in brand-new, moulded, plastic baby carriers and car seats that have been treated with toxic flame-retardants, and which off-gasses toluene and more plasticisers.

The average parent may simply shrug and reason that none of these things on their own could possibly expose their child to enough toxins to cause

---

Household cleaners raise asthma risk

Household chemicals, such as *bleach*, disinfectant and cleaning fluid, have been blamed for the huge surge in childhood asthma, and the data suggest that the chemical formaldehyde present in many household products could be the reason. A 2004 British study of more than 7000 children found that those born into households that are high users of such products are twice as likely to suffer persistent wheezing, often a precursor to asthma. The results, published in the journal *Thorax*, came from an ongoing study at Bristol University dubbed 'Children of the 90s', as it has been following children born in the Avon area in the early 1990s and tracking their health in relation to chemical exposure in the home.

▶

Their findings echoed those of an Australian study published earlier in 2004 that linked volatile chemicals in household products with asthma.

According to these two studies, the following household products were the ones most likely to trigger an asthma attack:

- Disinfectant
- Bleach
- Aerosols
- Air freshener
- Window cleaner
- Carpet cleaner

- Paint or varnish
- White spirit
- Pesticide
- Paint stripper
- Dry-cleaning fluid

illness. In a sense, that is correct. None of these things *individually* is likely to cause harm. But collectively, they create a powerful combination of harmful chemicals from which a baby has no escape.

Toddler to child

Children grow quickly and, watching their remarkable progress from helpless babies to walking/talking individuals, it is easy to believe that they are no longer as vulnerable as they were as newborns. To some extent, this is true. Your child's immune system has matured – but not fully.

As a child grows, so does the potential for greater exposure to environmental toxins. Starting playgroup or nursery can expose a child to more bacteria, viruses and allergens than are normally encountered at home. To combat this, parents may start giving their children conventional medicines. Time constraints and 'faddy' eating habits may mean resorting more and more to convenience foods. More time out of the house also means more exposure to pollutants and, if it is sunny, more chemicals in the form of sunscreens.

Scientists are only just beginning to make the connection between toxic exposure in childhood and developmental disorders. For instance, researchers at Johns Hopkins University School of Hygiene and Public Health in the US recently went on record saying that childhood exposure to lead, mercury, pesticides and ***polychlorinated biphenyls*** (PCBs) can affect brain development, and may be linked to eventual ADHD, autism, Parkinson's disease and other developmental disorders.

Children's brain development and behaviour are vitally important to their health and to their ability to contribute to society throughout life. Yet, there is currently no system for testing pesticides and other chemicals to see what impact their ingestion has on the brain and neurological system of growing children. This research is desperately needed but, in the meantime, some parents may feel it's prudent to live by the axiom: 'Look before you leap'.

▶ WHAT YOU CAN DO

Overexposure to chemical toxins is not inevitable for your children at any stage, nor is it out of your control. There are many simple ways to protect your developing baby and your child, and to keep everyday chemical exposures to a minimum.

If you are pregnant or trying for a baby

Change your lifestyle before you become pregnant. As little as six months of effort can make all the difference, and many parents might reason that this effort is nothing compared to the emotional, physical, mental and financial drain it may be to look after a handicapped child.

Don't forget dad. While the mother's health plays a major role in the state of her child, fathers do have some influence as well. Men who smoke are more likely to father children of low birth weights. Those who work in jobs that bring them into contact with pesticides and toxic chemicals are more likely to have children with birth defects. Such men often bring residues from their work home with them, raising their partner's exposure to toxins through contact with clothing and semen.

Some 20 different toxic chemicals with the potential to harm sperm quality and production have been found in random male samples. Contrast this with evidence from America suggesting that men who eat organic foods have sperm counts that are twice as high as those who don't.

Eat organic foods, which are free from pesticide residues, food additives and GM (genetically modified) additives. Organic foods are also significantly higher in nutrients. One American study found that organic tomatoes had 500 per cent more calcium than the convention-ally grown variety. You'll also get more iron, potassium, magnesium, manganese and copper in every bite as well, which is good for you and your baby.

If you're thinking of making the switch to organic, but budgeting is an issue, then consider buying organic for those foods you eat the most of. Even a small switch to organic teas and coffee (preferably decaffeinated) can substantially reduce your intake of pesticides. Or you may wish to replace the most contaminated types of conventional foods with organic alternatives. This means dairy products and meats (especially beef and offal). Watch out also for orchard fruits such as strawberries, cherries, apricots and apples. Research into pesticide residues on such produce shows that these types of fruits are among the most heavily contaminated.

Cut out caffeine. You probably don't think of caffeine as a toxin but, in large quantities and especially when you're pregnant, it is. Caffeine, which is found in coffee, tea, sodas and chocolate, leaches essential nutrients out of your system, leaving little for your baby to grow on.

The most recent medical evidence also suggests that consuming large amounts of coffee daily – five to six cups – can encourage miscarriage. What isn't known is whether this risk is higher in some women than in others. Caffeine also dehydrates the body. This means that the relative concentration of toxins in your blood will be higher than in a woman who limits caffeine. Instead of caffeinated beverages, try drinking herbal teas, or grain coffees such as dandelion and chicory.

Limit or avoid cured meats such as hot dogs, salami, bacon and smoked fish. These are treated with known carcinogens called 'nitrites'. Prenatal exposure to nitrites raises the risk of your child developing cancer. For example, it has been found that men who regularly consume hot dogs run the risk of fathering children at an increased risk of leukaemia. Women who eat cured meats during pregnancy appear to increase their child's chances of developing brain cancer. Read the labels on organic cured meats carefully because organic standards in most countries allow the use of nitrites in cured meats.

Use non-fluoride toothpaste. and check with your local water authority to see if your water is fluoridated. If it is, switch to filtered water. Fluoride is a toxic substance that arrives at the toothpaste manufacturer in a barrel marked with a skull and crossbones. Pregnant women who consume large amounts of fluoride increase their child's risk of birth defects and cancer.

Limit alcohol, especially in the crucial preconceptual stage and during the first few months of life in the womb. Binge-drinking and chronic alcoholism can deplete your body of nutrients such as vitamin B6, iron and zinc, and interfere with normal hormonal function. It also interferes with the proper formation of organs such as the kidneys, and raises the risk of congenital malformations.

There is also evidence to show that consuming alcohol can interfere with a woman's ability to conceive. Once pregnant, it can stop your baby developing properly. There are no official rules for preconceptual and prenatal drinking, but government guidelines suggest that pregnant women should not drink more than one or two units of alcohol (one unit equals one small glass of wine) once or twice a week. Nevertheless, many women still prefer to avoid alcohol while trying to conceive and during the first trimester, when the foetus is developing.

Rethink soft drinks. Fizzy drinks like colas, lemonade and squashes provide empty calories and have the potential to cause harm. They contain caffeine as well as sugar, which can significantly depress immune function and leach nutrients from the body. They can also contain artificial sweeteners such as aspartame and other harmful ingredients such as phosphoric acid.

Artificial sweeteners have been shown to harm the developing brain of young animals, and scientists now believe they are likely to do the same in developing human babies (see Chapter 5). They have also been shown to increase your sweet tooth so, ultimately, these calorie-sparing drinks may defeat their purpose.

Recently, American researchers have made the connection between soft-drink consumption and brittle bones in teenagers. They are now turning their attention to what happens when mothers consume large quantities of phosphoric acid during the developmentally sensitive time in the womb. Phosphoric acid blocks the absorption of calcium and magnesium by the intestines, which means less is available for your developing baby's bones.

Quit smoking. Smoking can poison your body with carcinogenic nicotine and the toxic metal cadmium. Once pregnant, smoking decreases the flow of blood and oxygen to the placenta, and reduces the availability of essential amino acids necessary for proper growth. Smokers are also twice as likely as non-smokers to miscarry or have an ectopic pregnancy (when the egg gets implanted outside of the womb). According to recent data, women who smoke also have a 78 per cent higher risk of giving birth to a baby with a cleft palate or lip.

In addition, babies of smokers are also more likely to have chronic breathing problems. Studies have shown that the lungs of babies whose parents smoke are 10 per cent smaller than those of non-smokers, and their risk of cancer is 50 per cent greater. Babies of smokers are born with fewer natural reserves to fight off infection, and have a 43-per-cent higher risk of blood disorders, neurological and sensory disorders, bladder and kidney problems and skin disorders than children of non-smokers.

Follow a stress-relief programme. Stress depletes the body of essential nutrients – especially the B vitamins. Mothers who are under lots of stress tend to have babies that are smaller and less active in the womb. Stress also depresses the immune system – making you less able to fight off the effects of any toxins that are ingested and inhaled.

In a recent US study, women who had strenuous jobs, such as those which require repetitive tasks, had a higher rate of problems during pregnancy, including pre-eclampsia, premature delivery and low birth-weight babies. Not all stresses can be dealt with easily, but try to do what you can. A large study in Sweden has recently found that the kinds of stress most likely to affect a baby's growth are a lack of emotional and practical support, social isolation and an unstable home life.

Anything that relaxes you – whether it is yoga, swimming or just 'vegging out' in front of the TV – should become a regular part of your routine.

After your child is born

Serve organic foods. It may be the most important step you take. In spite of what appears to be a junk-food culture, children still eat fruit and vegetables at a much higher rate than adults do, thus consuming up to 12 times as much pesticide residues. In the US, it is estimated that three to four million children now have toxic lead levels in their bodies. So-called 'safe' levels of lead and pesticides as defined by government agencies are only applicable to adults. No safe levels have been established for children and, indeed, many argue that there is no such thing as a safe level of these toxins.

In addition, make sure that your child gets plenty of variety in their diet. Many children's day-to-day diets are made up of the same types of foods over and over again. This can lead to food allergies and nutritional deficiencies, which can alter appetite and weaken the immune system (see page 66).

Use a non-fluoride toothpaste. Fluoride is only slightly less toxic than lead and more toxic than arsenic, yet we continue to add it to toothpaste and to our water supplies. As we can take in fluoride from other sources – such as produce grown in soil with a high fluoride content or sprayed with fluoride as a pesticide, Teflon cooking utensils, and car exhausts and other industrial pollution – our children may be getting between 4 and 12 times the 'safe' limit of 1 mg/day. Mounting evidence shows that fluoride overdose can cause health problems such as fatigue, skin rashes, visual disturbances, stomach problems, headaches and dizziness. In the long term, it is also considered to be a carcinogen.

Avoid exposure to passive smoke. There is nothing passive about passive smoke. It actively destroys health. Children breathing in second-hand smoke have higher rates of respiratory illness than those who do not. Remember: healthy lungs are necessary to excrete accumulated toxins. Passive smoke depletes levels of the antioxidant vitamin C by as much as 20 per cent, and increases the risk of cancer over the short and long term, and the risk of heart disease by 25 per cent.

Rethink storage. Brightly coloured plastics in a child's room such as storage crates, plastic toys or vinyl wallpaper give off poisonous gases such as formaldehyde. We may not always be able to smell these gases, but they are entering our bodies and have the potential to cause harm. Consider untreated wood boxes or traditional wooden toy chests for toy storage.

Go fragrance-free. Fragrances, used in room fresheners, soaps, deodorants, baby wipes and lotions and cleaning agents all contain highly volatile fragrance compounds that have been shown to be both carcinogenic and allergenic. If that's not bad enough, fragrance also alters central-nervous-system function and lowers immunity. Using fragrance-free products goes part of the way towards reducing your child's risk of such toxic exposure.

Consider supplements. It would be nice to think that our children could get all the nutrients they need from their diets, but this is just not possible. As our world becomes more and more polluted, it is even more important to give your child a daily multivitamin and mineral supplement, as a well-nourished body is better able to cope with environmental insults. Many popular brands of children's vitamins only contain a few essentials such as vitamins A, B, C, D and E. These are not enough. You may need to make a trip to the healthfood shop to find a supplement designed for children with a full range of nutrients.

Teach your children to drink water. Sodas, fruit juices and milk top the list of favourite drinks for many children. Equally, some parents feel that they are somehow depriving their children of a 'good' drink if they only offer water. But water is necessary for life and is more thirst-quenching than any other drink. Adequate amounts of water can also help the body to flush out toxins, and is necessary to maintain the efficiency of many other bodily functions.

Breast or bottle?

Your baby is born with an immature immune system. Just as she relied upon you for protection in the womb, she will rely upon you for some time to come for protection outside the womb. The first and most important step in providing this protection is by breastfeeding your baby for as long as possible.

No matter what formula manufacturers claim, no matter how healthy the baby in the magazine advert looks and no matter how much some would like to believe it, artificial milk cannot provide anywhere near the full range of short- and long- term advantages that breastmilk does.

Breastmilk is economical, always the right temperature and always 'on tap'. While you are breastfeeding your baby, you are providing, among other things:

- Good bacteria that guard against intestinal infection and aid digestion.

- Essential fatty acids, necessary for brain function and to help kill off parasites such as *Giardia lamblia*, a common cause of diarrhoea in infants.

- Antioxidants, to help your baby fight off infection and the effects of pollution.

- Immune-boosters such as antibodies, immunoglobulins and interferon.

- Active protection from disease, as mothers pass on their own immunity to several diseases against which babies are routinely vaccinated.

TOXIC BREASTMILK?

There has been a great deal of attention in the press recently regarding toxins in breastmilk. Women who are considering breastfeeding their children have expressed concerns that the

▶

benefits of breastmilk may be negated by the presence of harmful chemicals such as *dioxins* and PCBs (*polychlorinated biphenyls*).

According to a World Health Organization (WHO) survey, published in the *British Medical Journal*, the daily estimated intake of dioxins and PCBs by breastfed infants is around 170 pg/kg of body weight at two months and 39 pg/kg at 10 months. The tolerated daily intake is around 10 pg/kg of body weight.

So, how can we know whether or not breastmilk is safe? This is an area that has been extensively studied, and the overwhelming conclusion is that, while prenatal exposure to these levels of toxins has a definite negative effect on neurological development, exposure via breastmilk did not have the same dramatic effect.

This does not mean that the issue of contaminated breastmilk is not serious. It is. But along with any contaminants, breastmilk also has constituents that fight against toxic overload. The overwhelming opinion among paediatricians and child-health experts is that the benefits of breastfeeding still far outweigh the potential risk of ingesting chemicals. What's more, according to child-health experts like Dr Michel Odent, of the Primal Research Centre in London, if a woman is following an organic regime, the longer a woman breastfeeds, the less contaminated her milk can become. Breastfeeding uses up calories (it burns up fat), and as toxic fat is burned up, this is replaced by non-toxic fat.

Remember also that a baby formula made with conventional tap water is likely to contain many harmful chemicals and heavy metals, but without conferring even a whisper of the benefits that breastmilk has.

food and drink

THE FOOD WE EAT is inexorably linked with our well-being. It is the bedrock on which a healthy life is based. It is the body's ready store of nutrients and energy – the thing that holds us up, bolsters our immunity, fights free-radical damage and maintains our energy cycles in the face of an increasingly polluted world.

We have to eat and drink to live, and yet, increasingly, eating and drinking has become an act of faith as most of what we consume today does not resemble 'food' in any reasonable sense of the word.

Indeed, much of what we call food today would only have existed in the realms of science fiction a hundred years ago: exotic items grown without soil, flown in daily from far away, made from ingredients synthesised in test-tubes and preserved long beyond their natural shelf life using a variety of industrial chemicals derived from petroleum byproducts.

We eat meat byproducts enhanced with artificial meat flavours to make them palatable. We eat processed, quick-cook microwave and oven meals. Even the so-called healthy cereals we eat for breakfast are so highly processed and nutritionally poor that the manufacturers have to add vitamins to them simply so that they can be classified as foods.

These foods also contain a myriad of additives – occasionally at higher levels than any actual nutrients in them – and contaminants such as pesticides. These days, it is estimated that every one of us ingests a gallon of pesticides and herbicides a year from our daily diet.

Every day, we put this nutritionally poor, adulterated, unbalanced stuff into our bodies, and when our bodies eventually stop functioning properly, we wonder why. The fact is, our daily diets are the most influential aspect of our day-to-day health. What we eat is reflected in the strength of our immune and hormonal systems, the way our minds function, our muscle coordination, the health of our bones, the quality of our skin and hair, and the short- and long-term health of the children we produce. The health problems associated with a poor diet – heart disease, obesity, cancer, arthritis and diabetes – are real and tangible.

Eat, drink and be worried

Food can be 'bad' for you in lots of ways. You can eat too much of it and become obese (a major risk factor for heart disease, stroke and diabetes, among other things). It can contain pesticides, contaminants and 'anti-nutrients' (substances such as soya flour that prevent the body from absorbing essential nutrients). Or it can contain so few nutrients that you 'starve' even when you appear to be eating plenty.

Each of these problems is linked. For instance, when you eat nutrient-poor food, your body doesn't get all it needs to stay healthy. The body instinctively knows this, and craves more and more food to get what it needs. When you give in to these cravings and continue to eat calorie-rich but nutritionally poor foods, you gain weight. The more excess weight you carry, the more capacity you have for storing compounds such as pesticides and other synthetic chemicals in your body. And the more chemicals in your body, the greater the risk of declining health.

Food fads have also drastically altered the way we eat. Most of us have a list of 'good' and 'bad' foods compiled by the cult of food 'experts' who offer advice in newspapers, books and magazines, and subtly inform our food choices. Much of the constantly changing advice of dietitians and government bodies – reduce fat, eat raw foods, follow a 'Mediterranean diet' – has never been researched in detail, with the result that some of it can be downright damaging to our health. In fact, it has been said that you have a better chance of winning the lottery than you have of hitting on clear and accurate advice as to what you should be eating.

Humans thrive on variety, yet diet faddists encourage us to cut out specific types of foods, even entire food groups, from our daily diet for the sake of being 'healthy'. At the same time, market forces encourage us to consume a whole range of new and novel convenience foods – often in great quantity – that may not be good for us.

Anyone interested in long-term good health would certainly benefit from a healthy daily dose of scepticism about food fads that questions whom all this ever-changing dietary advice really serves. Chances are, you will find that, ultimately, it benefits multinational food manufacturers.

These companies have massive influence worldwide and have no interest in our eating fresh, unprocessed food. A steak is a steak is a steak, for instance. But a prepared meat product, seasoned and formed from 'select cuts of beef' is a patented recipe, and patented recipes (which, with a bit of clever marketing, can be sold to the public as healthy, nutritious, quick and easy) are where the profits are. Fresh food is not high on the priority lists because there is considerably less profit in it.

It is the lack of variety, toxic additives, long storage times and highly processed foods that have led us to where, nutritionally, we are today – a place where the food we eat detracts from, rather than adds to, our ongoing sense of well-being.

Synthetic additives

There are thousands of food additives approved for use in our foods. If your diet is high in processed or convenience foods, you will be consuming a staggering amount of these additives and artificial ingredients each year.

Sugar, corn sweeteners, salt, *citric acid*, pepper, vegetable colours, mustard, yeast and baking soda account for the vast majority – some 98 per cent – of the total amount of food additives we consume. But, even though the rest are used in very small amounts, it has been estimated that the average American, for example, consumes 2.4 kg (5 lb) of additives per year. If you include refined sugar – the food-processing industry's most used and abused additive – the total skyrockets to 61 kg (135 lb) a year.

Additives are placed in foods for a number of reasons. They facilitate the preparation of processed foods or lengthen shelf life. They can make food more appealing. With the use of chemical additives, food technicians are able to mimic natural flavours and to colour foods that are well past their nutritional best to make them look more 'natural' or 'fresh'. They are used to preserve foods for increasingly longer periods of time and allow the creation of highly manipulated forms of bread, biscuits, fruits, vegetables, meats and dairy products.

Chemicals can also be used to make the product more marketable in some way – for example, by adding a sugar substitute, a manufacturer can advertise its product as 'sugar-free'. Some 'foods' such as coffee creamers, chewing gum and sweets consist almost entirely of artificial ingredients derived from synthetic chemicals.

Are all additives harmful?

Although we eat them every day, food additives are not subject to the same scrutiny by the regulatory authorities as drugs are, and the history of food additives includes a number of products that were once deemed safe, but were later banned or allowed to be used only if accompanied by warnings. Certain food colourings, the artificial sweeteners *cyclamate* and *saccharin*, and the flavour-enhancer *monosodium glutamate* (MSG) are examples of such products.

At their best, additives add little or no nutritional value to a food product. At their worst, they can detract from your health and your day-to-day well-being. Moreover, some food additives provoke powerful adverse effects in some people while appearing to cause no problems for others. For instance, *sulphites*, a group of preservatives/antioxidants used in dried fruits and wines, are known to cause sensitive individuals (such as those suffering from asthma) to experience severe reactions. People with the genetic disorder phenylketonuria (PKU) are unable to fully metabolise the artificial sweetener *aspartame*, which can lead to a buildup of its break-down products in their body that can potentially result in serious brain damage. The flavour-enhancer MSG, a relative of aspartame and also a neurotoxin, can cause sensitive individuals to have headaches, nausea, weakness and breathing difficulties.

While food additives and preservatives undergo a required series of premarketing tests, often involving laboratory animals being given huge doses of individual additives, no one can ever test for what really happens when all the different additives in a food break down and interact with each other in your body.

The problem of mixtures

When we eat processed foods, we ingest a mixture of different chemicals and, yet, until recently, scant studies have been conducted to enlighten us as to what risks there might be attached to this.

Recent reports have shown that we should be paying more attention to the problem of mixtures. In 2005, British researchers at the University of Liverpool examined the toxic effects on nerve cells in the laboratory using a combination of four common food additives: aspartame, MSG, and the artificial colourings Brilliant Blue and Quinoline Yellow. The findings, published in the journal *Toxicological Sciences*, revealed that, when nerve cells were exposed to MSG and Brilliant Blue or to aspartame and Quinoline Yellow, in concentrations that are easily found in the bloodstream after a typical children's snack and drink, the paired additives stopped the nerve cells from growing and interfered with proper signalling processes. Mixing the additives had a much more potent effect on the nerve cells than each additive had on its own.

Not long after this report, in the US, the Environmental Working Group (EWG) sampled a range of popular juices and sodas, and presented evidence showing that two ingredients – ascorbic acid (vitamin C) and either sodium **benzoate** or **potassium benzoate** – found in many popular children's drinks, when mixed together can form the potent cancer-causing chemical **benzene**. After this was revealed, consumer groups elsewhere in the world began testing for and finding benzene in a range of popular soft drinks.

The EWG found that the US regulatory authority, the Food and Drug Administration (FDA), had known about this interaction since 1990, but instead of notifying the public and acting to ban the use of the combination, the FDA left it to the beverage industry to voluntarily reformulate its products while keeping quiet about the problem.

As more data like these emerge, it becomes clear that our ability to formulate foods from chemical mixtures has far outstripped our ability to ensure that these mixtures are safe. The next time you buy yourself a chemical meal, ask yourself a simple question: just because it is on sale, does it mean that it is safe to eat?

A lesson in labels

Food labels are the inevitable result of our reliance on prepackaged, highly processed convenience foods. Most of us have become so accustomed to buying food with labels that we can hardly imagine purchasing a food that doesn't come with an ingredients list, and cooking, heating and storage instructions. Totally natural foods need no cooking instructions, no statements about nutritional content (or lack of it), no cautions about containing traces of nuts or other allergens, no disclaimers about how this information affects your statutory rights and no hype about how much better this product is for you than a dozen other similar products on the supermarket shelves.

Given how ubiquitous processed food is in our diets, some label information is useful. Statements about fat, protein, carbohydrate, sodium and calorie content can be helpful. But the truth is, most labels are designed for a less worthy purpose. Food companies use packaging and labels as mini-

Food for thought

We tend to think of food as being fuel for the body. Government campaigns on health often focus on the importance of a good diet to combat conditions like heart disease, diabetes and cancer, and most of us accept that poor-quality food can produce poor physical health. Less often publicised is the role that good-quality food plays in shaping our minds.

Your brain is the most metabolically active organ in your body. It uses up 20 per cent of the body's energy stores. It is extremely sensitive to changes in its chemical environment. In fact, one of the first reactions to a poor diet, or to ingesting toxins, will be mental and behavioural rather than physical.

In the last 100 years or so, we have drastically altered the number and kinds of chemicals we take into our bodies – and at a rate much faster than any human organ could evolve to cope with. When people complain about the 'dumbing-down' of society, or about the seeming rise in senseless violence, aggression and crime, few

▶

make the connection between not feeding the brain with necessary nutrients and a brain-dead society.

Yet, consider studies done among prison populations, where prisoners were given food and supplements that met all the body's and brain's requirements. In these populations, aggressive behaviour and re-offending were cut by an average of 40 per cent. Furthermore, these individuals were not given mega-doses of expensive supplements, but just basic, recommended daily allowance (RDA) levels of what each of us needs to not fall ill.

In addition, there are now over 500 studies linking diet to a range of mental-health conditions, including depression, schizophrenia, Alzheimer's and other types of dementia, as well as attention-deficit/hyperactivity disorder (ADHD).

No one is suggesting that a poor diet is the only cause of these problems, but it can make a substantial contribution. In many cases, making some simple dietary adjustments can significantly improve symptoms and modify problem behaviour. Ensuring that both children and adults get adequate nutrition each day, then, seems a simple, safe, inexpensive, effective and humane step in the direction of turning the world into a more peaceful and more thoughtful place.

advertisements for their products. Sometimes, the two functions of a label – to provide accurate information and to entice someone to buy the product – are in conflict. When this happens, the manufacturer will do everything possible to distract you from the truth about their product. For this reason, food labels can be misleading, especially if you don't learn how to read between the lines and examine the fine print. Knowing what the words on the label really mean is a big step in learning to make better choices at the supermarket.

Getting beyond the hype

Smart shoppers ignore the hype on the front of the package. This part of the label is designed by the company's marketing and advertising departments, and contains whatever pleasing images and fashionable words will best sell the product.

While the meanings of many of the terms found on food packages are regulated by law, it's still easy to be deceived by them. The food may not be as good for you as its large and colourful claims would have you believe and, while manufacturers cannot legally lie on a food label, they are allowed, within reason, to stretch the truth. Be wary of these tricky terms:

- **'Pure'** Everyone wants to eat food that's pure. You would not want to put contaminated food into your body. But the word 'pure' has no regulated, agreed-upon meaning in food-labelling. It tells you nothing about what's in the product that perhaps should not be there. Even pure foods can contain unwanted processing aids and contaminants. The packaging of most ready-made foods can leach chemicals such as adhesives, polyvinyls and hormone-disrupting **bisphenol A** and **phthalates** into food. This is especially true of canned goods and foods that go from freezer to oven.

- **'Natural'** is probably the least trustworthy of all label terms. Once again, there is no agreed-upon legal definition of 'natural' in the food business. While it sounds appealing, the word says little about the nutritional quality of the food, or even its safety. 'Natural', for example, is not the same as nutritious. The 'natural flavours' included in many processed foods are, almost without exception, synthesised in the lab to be 'natural-identical'. They contain nothing that the average consumer would equate with a product that is truly natural. Instead, they're derived from a range of neurotoxic and carcinogenic chemicals that are best avoided in any diet.

- **'Made from …'** simply refers to a starting material. For example, the claim 'made from 100 per cent vegetable oil' may be technically correct, but it is misleading. A lot can happen to a simple vegetable oil before it gets into our food, or ends up as a margarine or spread. Along the way, it may have been diluted or hydrogenated, changing it from a healthy fat to an artery-clogging trans fat. Another common label lie is 'made from natural …' This simply means that the manufacturer started with a natural source. But, by the time the food was processed, it may be anything but 'natural'. The chicken nuggets you feed your child may be made from chicken, but ask yourself: which part of the chicken? In many cheap products, every part of the chicken, including organs, feet, beaks and other non-nutritious parts, are included to support the 'made from ...' claim.

- **'Made with real fruit'** This boast is particularly prevalent in snacks for children. Sadly, there is no law requiring labels to say how much real fruit is in the product. Often 'real fruit' snacks contain more sugar, preservatives and colours than fruit.

- **'Made with whole grains'** is a similar labelling 'white lie' that leads the consumer to believe they are buying and eating a healthy wholegrain cereal or bread. But the package label is not legally required to say how much 'whole grain' is in the product. Its main ingredient could be refined flour with just a small amount of whole wheat (and brown colouring) added. This means that the food won't contain all the fibre and other nutrients associated with wholegrains.

- **'Fat free'** Fat content provides the pleasing 'mouth feel' in natural foods and removing it alters the consistency of food as well as the way it tastes. As a result, fat-free foods are often full of emulsifiers, modified starches, sugar (or worse, poisonous sweeteners), salt and artificial flavourings. Sugary foods may not contain fat, but when you eat more sugar than your body can effectively process, not only will it increase your risk of diabetes, but it will also eventually result in your body storing this extra sugar as fat.

  Some intake of fat is necessary for health, and we need a combination of both saturated and unsaturated fats in our diet each day. A good example of why this is so can be seen in salads. The dominant nutrients in fresh vegetables are mostly fat-soluble ones known as 'carotenes'. These are powerful antioxidant and disease-fighting substances. Adding a drizzle of oily dressing to your salad aids your absorption of these nutrients, whereas studies show that a fat-free dressing or no dressing at all effectively stops your body absorbing any of these beneficial nutrients from fresh vegetables.

- **'Enriched'** is a tip-off that this food may have been rendered so nutritionally poor through processing that the manufacturers had to put some of the good stuff back in to call it 'food'. Enriched flour, enriched white bread and enriched cereals are all good examples of foods that have been processed to such a degree that all the beneficial nutrients have been removed. Enriched foods are not as healthy as their whole-food counterparts because they are often missing important cofactors found in unprocessed foods.

- **'Smoked'** legally describes the flavour of the food, not how it was smoked. The consumer imagines the food is smoked in a backyard bar-becue or in an old-fashioned smokehouse. In truth, the food could be artificially or chemically smoked and/or just use smoked flavouring and still be legally labelled 'smoked'.

- **'Fruit drink'.** When the word 'drink' appears on the label, it tells you that this is not 100 per cent juice. Indeed, a fruit drink may contain little or no real fruit juice. Look at the ingredients to find out what's really in there. It may, in fact, be mostly sugar and water, with added vitamin C. This enables the manufacturer to add another buyer incentive – 'high in vitamin C' – even if the product is a long way from being real orange juice.

Experienced label-readers look right past the banners and marketing hype on the front of the package and, instead, look for the facts in the small print ingredients list on the back.

What to avoid

While many of us are now used to checking labels for salt and sugar content, and even for artificial colourings or artificial flavourings, it can be difficult to get into the habit of searching for other undesirable ingredients, too. Of course, the way to get out of reading labels altogether is to buy fresh food and prepare your own meals. However, if you are not willing to give up the convenience food habit, then there are a number of additives you and your family could do without.

To find them, you have to get into the habit of reading food labels as you shop. Don't be fooled into thinking that a high price tag guarantees quality. Some very high-priced name-brand convenience foods are full of the worst kinds of additives, while some of the more moderately priced, non-name brands may be perfectly acceptable. Equally, some organic foods, especially cakes and biscuits, can contain more sugar and fat than conventional brands.

With more than 10,000 chemicals added to our foods nowadays, it can be a daunting task to decipher labels and decide which products you should and should not be buying. The best way to avoid synthetic chemicals in your food is to buy fresh ingredients and make it yourself. But on those occasions when you do resort to second-best, consider avoiding foods that use certain ingredients (see table, below). In Europe, these additives will usually be listed by their 'E number'. In Australia, they tend to use the same numbers, but without the E prefix – a system that is due to be adopted internationally in the next few years.

When shopping for food, try to avoid products that contain the following additives (also, see the A–Z, page 289, for health effects).

Additive	E number	Found in
Allura Red AC	E129	Food colouring in snacks, sauces, preserves, soups, wine, cider, etc
Amaranth	E123	Food colouring in wine, spirits, fish roe
Aspartame	E951	Sweetener in snacks, sweets, alcohol, desserts, 'diet' foods
Benzoic acid	E210	Preservative in many foods, including drinks, low-sugar products, cereals, meat products
Brilliant Black BN	E151	Colouring in drinks, sauces, snacks, wines, cheese, etc
Butylated hydroxyanisole (BHA)	E320	Preservative, particularly in fat-containing foods, confectionery, meats
Calcium benzoate	E213	Preservative in many foods, including drinks, low-sugar products, cereals, meat products
Calcium sulphite	E226	Preservative in a vast array of foods – from burgers to biscuits, frozen mushrooms to horseradish; used to make old produce look fresh
Carboxymethyl cellulose sodium salt	E466	Bulking agent found in ice creams, beverages and other foods
Carrageenan (seaweed extract)	E407	Thickener used in a wide variety of foods including dressings, ice cream, jams and custards

Additive	E number	Found in
Monosodium glutamate (MSG)	E621	Ubiquitous flavour enhancer found in almost every pre-prepared food
Nitrite chemicals	E249–252	Curing agents commonly found in cured or preserved meats
Polyoxyethylene sorbitan chemicals	E432–E436	Emulsifiers found in spreads, cake mixes, dressings, desserts and beverages
Ponceau 4R, cochineal Red A	E124	Food colouring found in sweets, desserts and beverages
Potassium benzoate	E212	See calcium benzoate
Potassium nitrate	E249	Preservative in cured meats and canned meat products
Propyl p-hydroxybenzoate, propylparaben, parabens	E216	Preservative in cereals, snacks, paté, meat products, confectionery
Saccharin and its sodium, potassium and calcium salts	E954	Sweetener in diet and no-sugar products
Sodium metabisulphite	E223	Preservative and antioxidant used in dried and frozen fruits and fruit fillings
Sodium sulphite	E221	Preservative used in winemaking and other processed foods
Soya protein isolates	–	Protein source widely used in ready meals and breads
Stannous chloride (tin)	E512	Antioxidant and colour-retention agent in canned and bottled foods, fruit juices
Sulphur dioxide	E220	Preservative found in dried fruits and condiments
Sunset Yellow FCF, Orange Yellow S	E110	Food colouring found in sweets, desserts and beverages
Tartrazine	E102	Yellow food colouring found in sweets, desserts and beverages
Tri- and polyphosphate chemicals	E450(b)	Added to meat to make it take up water to increase weight (and so the price) at no extra cost to the manufacturer

Hidden additives

Apart from the known additives that are listed on the label, modern processed foods also contain a number of unintentional contaminants such as pesticides, genetically modified (GM) ingredients, chemicals that have leached from the packaging and, most recently, nanoparticles. Many of these 'hidden additives' can have a profound effect on health and, what's more, as they are generally industrial chemicals, food will not be your only source of exposure to them. That's why choosing to cut your exposure to them whenever and wherever you can makes good sense.

Pesticides

Health professionals recommend that you eat at least five servings of fruit and vegetables every day as part of a varied diet. Unfortunately, if you eat conventionally grown produce, you may also unknowingly be ingesting a mixture of harmful pesticides, including:

- insecticides to control insects
- rodenticides to control rodents
- herbicides to control weeds
- fungicides to control mould and fungus
- antimicrobials to control bacteria.

Just because you can't see or taste them doesn't mean they aren't there. The most comprehensive testing for the presence of unwanted chemicals in food is the ongoing US Total Diet Study (TDS), conducted by the FDA and updated yearly. The TDS looks for the presence of many different chemicals in food, but its findings on levels of chlorinated pesticides have been particularly distressing. In its 1988 report, **DDE** (dichlorodiphenyldichloroethylene), a close relative of **DDT** (dichlorodiphenyltrichloroethane), was found in every single sample of raisins, spinach (fresh and frozen), chilli con carne (beef and beans) and beef.

DDE was also present in 93 per cent of processed cheeses, mince, hot dogs, collards (spring greens), chicken, turkey and ice-cream sandwiches sampled. It was also present in 87 per cent of lamb chops, salami, canned spinach, meatloaf and butter, and in 81 per cent of sauces and creamed spinach.

Since DDT and DDE have been banned in the US since 1972, it is likely that some of this contamination is from produce imported from other countries that still use these chemicals. But some of it is also due to the persistence of these chemicals in the soil. Growing crops or rearing animals on land contaminated with DDT and DDE means that we 'recycle' these toxins back into the food chain.

In the intervening years, things didn't get much better. The 1999 TDS report showed that, among the foods sampled, 17 different pesticides were found in butter, 32 different ones in cherries, 29 in strawberries and 27 in apples. The baked potato samples contained 23 pesticides, and hamburger, 22. Milk chocolate samples contained 18 different pesticides. Once again, DDE/DDT was the residue most often found, with *chlorpyrifos-methyl*, *malathion*, *endosulfan*, *dieldrin* and *chlorpyrifos* also being very common (see also Chapter 8, page 239, on pesticides).

In the UK, the 1999 Annual Report by the Working Party on Pesticide Residues (WPPR) found that 27 per cent of the full range of foods tested showed pesticide residues. Among them, DDT (which is banned in the UK) was found in beef slices, corned beef and lamb's kidney, and *2,4-D* (also banned in the UK) was found in over half the oranges tested. Oranges, pears, lettuces, chocolate and apples contained the highest numbers and levels of residues. Three-quarters of the chocolate samples contained *lindane* (a relative of DDT), and one in eight jars of baby food were also contaminated. Surveys in Australia and New Zealand have found similarly high levels of pesticides in foods.

Government surveys around the world continue to show that many everyday foods can increase our exposure to this cocktail of chemicals exponentially. For instance, in the UK:

- **Apples:** in 2003, 71 per cent contained residues and 39 per cent had residues of more than one chemical.

- **Beer:** in 1999, 35 per cent contained pesticide residues. Growing non-organic hops involves 12 to 14 annual sprays using an average of around 15 chemical products.

- **Bread:** in 2003, residues were found in 61 per cent of the ordinary bread sampled, and 12 per cent contained multiple residues.

- **Cereal bars:** two surveys were carried out in 2001. The first found that

64 per cent contained detectable residues, with 22 per cent of these containing multiple residues; the second found that 71 per cent had detectable residues, with 14 per cent containing more than one chemical. There is currently no maximum residue limit for cereal bars.

- **Feta cheese:** in 1999, 67 per cent of samples contained residues of DDT.
- **Cucumber:** in 2003, 24 per cent contained residues, and 4 per cent had multiple residues.
- **Grapes:** in 2003, 63 per cent contained residues and 32 per cent had multiple residues.
- **Lemons:** in two surveys carried out in 2001, one found that 100 per cent contained detectable residues, with 90 per cent of them containing multiple residues, while the other found 93 per cent with detectable residues, 81 per cent containing multiple residues.
- **Pears:** in 2003, 58 per cent of those tested contained residues, and 22 per cent had multiple residues.
- **Potatoes:** in 2003, 35 per cent contained residues, with 9 per cent containing multiple residues.
- **Raspberries:** in 2003, 57 per cent contained residues, 31 per cent with multiple residues.
- **Rice:** in 2003, 54 per cent of samples contained residues, with 10 per cent containing multiple residues.
- **Spinach:** in 2003, 24 per cent of samples contained residues.
- **Wine:** in 2003, 10 per cent contained residues.

Pesticides are harmful to people – no one would dispute that. We can't always detect the immediate health effects from eating pesticide-laden food, but that doesn't mean that they are safe. The World Health Organization (WHO) estimates that between 3.5 and 5 million people globally suffer acute pesticide poisoning every year.

Studies of people regularly exposed to pesticides show that these poisons can cause nerve damage, cancer, diabetes and other effects that can take a long time to manifest.

These ill-effects depend on how toxic the pesticide is and how much of it is taken in. Also, when researchers test the amount of pesticide in a single carrot or apple and declare that it is too low to be harmful, they are missing an important point. In the real world, we do not eat foods singly. We eat them in quantity and in combination, day in and day out.

As with food additives, little is known of the effects of multiple residues – the 'cocktail effect' (see Chapter 2, page 28). Very little research has been done, but the current knowledge points to the distinct possibility that these chemicals would react with each other to form even more potent toxins.

Officials continue to argue that levels of pesticide residues in food are within legal limits, but until those limits are proven safe beyond all reasonable doubt, we should not allow ourselves to be lulled into a false sense of security – 'legal' does not necessarily mean 'safe'.

▶ HOW TO AVOID PESTICIDES IN YOUR FOOD

Once they are on or in food, pesticides are very difficult to avoid. Some authorities recommend that we wash and scrub all fresh fruit and vegetables thoroughly under running water. Running water has an abrasive effect that soaking doesn't have, so this may help to remove traces of chemicals from the surface of these foods as well as dirt from crevices. But not all pesticide residues can be removed just by washing because many are designed to be water-resistant so they won't wash off crops when it rains.

Peeling the skin off fruit and vegetables whenever possible and discarding the outer leaves of leafy vegetables can reduce your exposure. Trimming the fat from meat, and the skin from poultry and fish will also help as most pesticide residues collect in fat.

Eating a variety of foods is sometimes recommended to help reduce your exposure to any one pesticide. However, it is uncertain how effective this is as most pesticides work in similar ways, whatever the produce. Also, on the journey from farm to table, many foods are coated with multiple pesticides and fungicides. From a nutritional-health standpoint, however, eating food from a variety of sources will give you a more comprehensive mix of nutrients, which may have a protective effect.

In fact, the best, and probably the only, way to avoid pesticides in your food is to include as much organic food in your diet as possible (see page 94).

You are what they eat

In recent decades, our consumption of meat products has grown dramatically. In the West, the average person eats around 62 kg (137 lb) of beef, chicken, fish and shellfish per year. But, if you're a meat-eater, then you are also eating whatever the animal ate before it was slaughtered.

There was a time when animals reared for food ate what grew naturally – cows and chickens ate grass and grain, and big fish ate small fish or other sea creatures. In industrialised meat production – often a 30,000-cow feedlot or a 60,000-chicken coop – things are very different. The artificial conditions the animals are kept in – often without light or regular exercise – and the requirement for the animals to grow to a saleable weight quickly means that the animals require special 'scientific' diets.

Such facilities thus require huge quantities of high-protein rations, and this has coincided with the need for slaughterhouses to find a cheap, safe way to dispose of more and more waste. Both industries have now entered into a marriage of convenience, which means that a number of animal byproducts are now included in animal feeds – even for those animals that are not normally carnivores.

Cattle and chickens are still given plant-based feed: corn (for carbohydrates) and soya bean meal (for amino acids) make up 70 to 90 per cent of most commercial animal feeds. But the remaining 10 to 30 per cent of feeds can differ radically from what cows and poultry would normally eat in their natural habitats.

Processed feathers, for instance, are an acceptable source of protein in cattle feed, as is chicken faeces. Plastic pellets are permitted as roughage. Chickens can be fed meat and bone meal. And, in addition to their main diet of fishmeal and fish oil, farmed fish may be given rendered meat, bone and feather meal. These animal byproducts can be contaminated with bacteria such as *Salmonella*, and the recycling of animal byproducts into animal feed is an acknowledged risk for mad-cow disease.

Other animal-feed additives contain worrying industrial toxins. Every year in the US, 11 billion pounds of animal fat are recycled into animal feed – a serious cause for concern as many toxins and pesticides, such as *dioxins* and *PCB*s, concentrate naturally in animal fat. Dioxins are also found in the clays that occasionally get mixed into animal feeds.

Also included in the food of intensively reared animals are medications such as growth promoters and antibiotics, given routinely even to healthy cattle and chickens to hasten growth and keep infections at bay. There is growing concern over the high use of antibiotics and its possible effects on human health. Antimicrobial drug residues in food (including antibiotics) are suspected to cause allergies, cancer, paralysis and respiratory failure, anaphylactic shock and aplastic anaemia in both humans and animals. In particular, every time we ingest antibiotics via our meat, we are contributing to the worldwide problem of antibiotic resistance. Nevertheless, the default position of many official government committees is that these residues pose no risk to consumers.

Stress affects meat quality

Animals are, of course, subject to the same stresses that we humans are. Like us, extremes in temperature, humidity, light, sound and confinement, as well as excitement, fatigue, pain, hunger and thirst, can stress animals out – and so can environmental toxins such as sheep dip and pesticides in their food. Dairy cows and sheep living near sources of electromagnetic radiation, such as power lines, also exhibit signs of greater stress and lowered immunity.

When an animal is under severe stress due to fear or pain, increased levels of stress-related hormones such as epinephrine (adrenaline) and cortisone are found not only in the blood, but also in body tissues. The stress experienced before slaughter is not only cruel, but can cause undesirable effects on the quality of the meat, resulting in PSE (pale, soft, exudative) meat which, as the name suggests, is colourless and overly liquid, or DFD (dark, firm, dry) meat, which lies at the other end of the scale.

The quality of the meat may also be compromised in other, more important ways. As stress levels in animals go up, immunity goes down, making them more prone to bacterial and viral infections (and more likely to be given antibiotics and other medicines as prevention and treatment). These microbes and chemicals as well as all the other toxins, such as pesticides, remain in the fat and muscle of the animal and are passed on to humans when we consume conventionally reared meats. The health effects of this have not yet been properly evaluated. However, it may be an early and persuasive argument against eating commercially reared meats, reducing your overall meat intake or, for some, switching to a vegetarian diet.

Genetically modified ingredients

Increasingly, news headlines about genetic modification leave many of us anxious and confused about the food we eat. We now have the technology to alter the most basic building blocks of life. Sadly, we have not conducted the studies necessary to prove or disprove the safety of GM foods over either the long or short term. It is still not clear whether GM foods can, for instance, cause damage to a vulnerable foetus at certain stages of its development.

GM foods don't taste better and are not cheaper to buy; they have, however, been implicated in increased resistance to antibiotics and the creation of 'superbugs'. They have also been linked to an increased incidence of allergies, unpredictable rises of toxins in the body, increased cancer rates and a decline in the nutritional quality of foods. Ironically, studies show that, contrary to most industry reports, US farmers growing GM crops are using just as many toxic pesticides and herbicides as conventional farmers – and, in some cases, are using more.

Indeed, one of the 'benefits' of these herbicide-resistant crops is that farmers can spray as much of a particular herbicide on their crops as they want, thereby killing the weeds without damaging their crop. Scientists estimate that herbicide-resistant crops planted around the globe will triple the amount of toxic, broad-spectrum herbicides used in agriculture.

Although it is claimed by the biotechnology companies that there have been no ill-effects seen in people consuming GM food in the US, there have been no large or in-depth studies to support this statement. Observations in the medical press, however, suggest that negative effects are becoming more apparent. For instance:

- **In the UK:** a 50 per cent rise in soya allergies has been reported since imports of GM food started.

- **In Ireland:** doctors have reported an increase in child soya allergies since the start of GM soya imports.

- **In the US:** coinciding with the introduction of GM ingredients, food-derived illnesses are believed to have doubled over the last seven years.

Food can either be genetically modified itself or contain genetically modified ingredients. The issues are complex but, if you are concerned, you might want to consider avoiding or limiting:

- **Tomatoes (and tomato purée),** the first GM foods to be sold. In the US, you can buy fresh tomatoes that have been genetically modified; in the UK, you can only buy puree made from these tomatoes. Watch out for ready-made foods such as pizza that may use GM tomato purée.

- **Soya,** modified to resist weedkiller. In the US, supplier of most of the world's soya, GM and unmodified soya are not kept separate, and processed foods may contain both. Soya is present in most baked and prepackaged foods in several forms: oil (often just labelled as 'vegetable oil'), vegetable fat, flour, lecithin and vegetable protein.

- **Maize,** which has been modified to contain bacteria toxic to a common crop pest. Maize is used as a grain, as corn (or maize) flour, corn meal, corn starch, corn syrup, dextrose, glucose, fructose, xanthan gum and maltodextrin, and as corn oil. Be aware of things like chocolate bars and sweet drinks that contain sugars derived from maize.

- **Cheese,** which can be made with a GM enzyme called chymosin instead of traditional rennet. Chymosin is used in many vegetarian cheeses and increasingly in hard cheeses for general consumption.

- **Enzymes,** used in a large number of products, including drinks, bakery goods and dairy products. Manufacturers are not obliged to include these on the product information.

- **Canola, or rapeseed,** mainly used as oil. Some crops now contain human genes.

- **Yeast,** which has been genetically modified and approved for making bread; it is difficult to know the extent to which it is used in bakery products.

- **Vitamin B2,** known as riboflavin, and now widely produced from genetically modified microorganisms. It is generally added to breakfast cereals, soft drinks, baby foods and diet foods.

- **E numbers,** which indicate preservatives, flavourings and colourings. Watch out for E101, E101a, E150, E153, E161c, E322, E471 and E621, all of which may be GM derivatives.

To spot GM foods, you will have to read the labels. But even this will not guarantee that your diet will be GM-free. Labelling laws can be very confusing, and seem to exist mostly to protect the manufacturer rather than the consumer. Certain GM ingredients, such as flavourings and additives, do not need to be listed on the label, and very few manufacturers volunteer this information. For the moment, the best way to avoid GM foods is to eat as much organic and freshly prepared (by you in your home) food as possible, and to avoid prepackaged foods when you can.

In addition to GM organisms in our food, concerns have recently been expressed that some excipients (inert ingredients) in nutritional supplements may also include genetically modified ingredients. Most health supplements that are not licensed medicines are classed as foods and, as such, are obliged to warn the consumer on the label if they are known to contain GM ingredients. Supplements that are licensed medicines (for instance, some folic acid and cod liver oil supplements) are not required to alert consumers to the presence of GM ingredients or derivatives, and so could contain these ingredients without any indication on the label.

According to Genetic Food Alert (GFA) in the UK, unless expressly denied by the manufacturer, the following excipients may be genetically modified:

- Derivatives of soya, maize (corn), cotton or rapeseed, including oils which are used as carriers for vitamins (A, D and E) in supplements; lecithin and vitamin E, which are used as antioxidants; and sweeteners such as dextrose, glucose, dextrins, maltodextrins and sorbitol.

- GM microorganisms or their products, including some bacteria, brewer's yeast and baker's yeast. Products of GM bacteria can include aspartame and enzymes used as processing aids (which may not be listed on the label) such as alpha-acetolactate decarboxylase, alpha-amylase, catalase, chymosin a, chymosin b, cyclodextrin-glucosyltransferase, beta-glucanase, glucose isomerase, glucose oxidase, hemicellulase (xylanase), lipase, tria-cylglycerol, maltogenic amylase, pectinesterase, protease and pullulanase.

● Products of GM-fed or treated animals, including gelatine, bonemeal and albumen from animals raised on GM ingredients or injected with GM growth hormones such as BST (bovine somatotropin).

Packaging

A wide range of materials come into contact with food during its production, processing, packaging, storage and preparation. All of these have the potential to leach chemicals into the product.

If your intake of packaged foods is high, then your potential exposure to the chemicals that migrate from packaging into the foodstuffs is also high. In the EU, the 'safe' exposure of migrants from food-contact materials (FCMs) is an estimated intake of 1 kg of packaged food per 60 kg (130 lb) person per day. But this figure applies only to adults. Children tend to consume more food than adults per kilogram of body weight. Worse, food products that are targeted specifically at children are often packaged in small single portions, so the potential for greater migration into the food is higher. There is no reliable 'safe' limit of food-contact materials for children.

Examples of the kinds of chemicals that can migrate from package to food include:

● **Harmful chemicals from plastic or Styrofoam packaging** which can penetrate into foods, and may cause health problems such as cancer. The chemical of concern is 1,3-butadiene but, because of the varying amounts of this chemical that are used in plastics and Styrofoam, it is impossible to make an accurate estimate of how much gets into your food from any one container.

● **Aseptic or Tetra Paks** have recently been shown to leach *isopropil-ThioXantone* (ITX). ITX can get into any fatty product like milk when it is exposed to sunlight's ultraviolet rays. Little information is available as to the safety of ITX, which is a chemical produced in relatively small quantities globally. The US Environmental Protection Agency (EPA) considers it a potentially high hazard in the environment based on studies showing that it is toxic to aquatic species. A 1999 American report noted a case in which six workers exposed to ITX developed skin rashes on the head and neck following exposure to the sun. Industry has not yet provided clear, verifiable information on the health effects of ITX, especially if consumed as a contaminant in foodstuffs.

- **Teflon,** widely used in the paper wrapping of fast and microwaveable foods such as french fries, popcorn and pizza, as well as sweet wrappers and other products. It helps to prevent grease stains from coming through the wrapper. You don't see it, you don't feel it and you can't taste it, but when you open that bag and start removing your french fries from there, you are extracting and eating a fluorochemical called Zonyl, which can further break down into perfluorooctanoic acid (PFOA). According to the EPA, PFOA stays in the bloodstream and is a suspected carcinogen. The US government says this chemical is now believed to be in the blood of nearly every American.

- **Aluminium,** found in the packaging of freezer-to-oven ready-meals and in soda cans, and implicated in a range of neurological disorders. The more acidic the food product is, the greater the chances that aluminium will migrate into it.

- **Plastics,** used for microwaveable packaging and as liners in tins. They contain several chemicals that mimic the action of oestrogen, including **phthalates** and **bisphenol A.** The latter has recently been found to provoke insulin resistance, a prediabetic condition in which tissues lose their normal sensitivity to insulin. Plastic wrapping on microwaveable foods can also transmit the chemicals during heating.

Less obvious packaging materials that can pose health risks include **isocyanates**, adhesive components in laminates and can coatings; **semicarbazide**, used in the plastic sealing gaskets on jars of food, especially baby food; volatile substances, such as those present in adhesives and in the printing inks used for packaging; and microwave susceptors, usually a mixture of metals and minerals incorporated into a plastic film to make certain microwaved foods crisp during cooking.

Even if your food isn't in something that you recognise as packaging, it may have been 'packaged' in some way to make it more appealing on the supermarket shelf. Fresh fruit is a good example. Many 'fresh' foods are coated in petroleum-derived waxes to help maintain freshness. The waxes on fruit and vegetables are based on petrochemicals and may trigger allergies. They may also contain **morpholine** which, according to World Health Organization reports, turns into the carcinogen N-nitrosomorpholine.

Foods that are regularly waxed include thin-skinned produce such as cucumbers, peppers and apples. In addition, all fruit and vegetables are repeatedly sprayed with a multitude of pesticides and fungicides while in storage. Unwanted additives can also seep in from packaging. For example, if the plastic packaging is derived from vinyl chloride – a known carcinogen and endocrine disrupter – this can easily migrate into foods, especially those that are acidic or fatty.

Nano-additives

Nanotechnology deals with particles so small – a million of them would fit on a pinhead – that the laws of physics no longer apply. After experiencing widespread rejection of genetically modified foods, the food industry is somewhat skittish about owning up to its research into 'atomically modified' food products. But this research is ongoing and nanofood products are already on the shelves.

In 2005, a UK-based study revealed that 200 food-manufacturing companies are already working on ways to insert nanotechnology into foods. These companies are already celebrating the future profits of their endeavours. The food industry calculates that the nanofood market is already worth around $7 billion in 2006 and that this figure will grow to $20 billion by 2010.

But no research at all has been done to investigate how these particles might affect human health (in this, there is a disturbing parallel with GM). Worse, no one knows how to regulate these technologies as they span the regulatory boundaries between pharmaceuticals, medical devices and biological agents. The US Food and Drug Administration considers that particle size is not the issue in regulation. But this is clearly not the case since the defining characteristic of nanoparticles is that, because of their size, they behave in ways that defy physics and, thus, may interact with the body on entirely new levels. None of the current crop of safety tests is designed to investigate the effects of nanoparticles, and none can prove them to be entirely safe for human consumption.

Where does your food come from?

One of the inevitable consequences of advanced preservation systems for food is our new-found ability to ship food over long distances and store it for long periods of time, without provoking spoilage. Thus, people in the middle of a dark winter morning by the North Sea can have papayas or lychees for breakfast, if they so desire.

There is a price to pay, however, for the luxury of eating long-haul foods. A recent survey in the UK showed that an alarming number of children have no real understanding of how, where or why their food is produced. Indeed, many don't know that eggs came from chickens or hamburgers from cows.

Some of the 100 youngsters, aged between 10 and 14 and living in England and Wales, who took part in the survey for the Country Landowners Association thought that a ewe was a bird, that mutton came from rabbits, that free range means 'not genetic' and that cows produce milk because they eat grass. If this survey had been carried out 20 or 30 years ago, it would have produced a very different set of answers.

Nevertheless, grown-ups shouldn't feel too superior either. Many know little more than the basics as to the origins of their food or the consequences of the overuse of certain ingredients. Few can claim to understand, for instance, how the overuse of palm oil in junk foods is killing off orang-utans in far-flung corners of the world such as Borneo and Sumatra by destroying their natural habitats. And few know just how significantly our love of long-haul food contributes to the destruction of our natural environment.

Yet, according to the Soil Association, which is the UK's main organic-certification board, the number of food miles accumulated by many of the foods we take for granted every day is staggering. Indeed, the carbon-dioxide emissions from moving food around the planet is a direct contributor to the catastrophic problem of global warming. For instance:

- Through the food consumed, the average person is responsible for 9.63 tonnes of carbon-dioxide emissions.

- A weekly basket of imported food for a family of four could add 1.1 tonnes to per capita emissions.

- A typical Sunday meal could travel 49,000 miles – equivalent to two journeys around the world and releasing 37 kg (82 lb) of carbon dioxide.

- Distributing products by plane results in 50 times more carbon dioxide than sea freight.
- For every 1000 fruit products bought in the UK, only six will be grown here.
- The food system accounts for up to 40 per cent of all UK road freight.

What is missing from your food?

Apart from the things that are added intentionally or otherwise to our food supply, there is a whole host of things that we have lost due to modern intensive agricultural practices. These also have important implications for our long-term health.

While fruit, vegetables and whole grains are commonly thought to be high in essential nutrients, the majority of today's produce and grains are grown in depleted soil, doused with pesticides and stored for long periods of time (all the while being sprayed with more insecticides and fungicides) before being sold. They may be stored for an even longer time after purchase, before being eaten or used in cooking.

Because of this, some modern nutritionists believe that, in the midst of all this plenty, many people in the West are starving – for the basic nutrients that were once in our everyday food.

Conventional farmers are caught in a vicious circle of production. They add chemical fertilisers to the soil in the hope of increasing crop yields, but doing this ultimately increases many plants' susceptibility to pests. So more pesticides are used. But the pesticides they use can also affect the soil's capacity to sustain and generate fertility.

Using synthetic fertilisers to make plants grow in otherwise depleted soils has other disturbing consequences. For instance, while the fertiliser will stimulate the plant to grow in the absence of any of the usual protective nutrients they should contain, the plants will also take up more of the heavy metals in the soil such as aluminium, mercury and lead, and these, in turn, are passed on up through the food chain.

All the while, the nutritional value of our food is plummeting.

Nutrient deficits

In 1940, British chemists Robert McCance and Elsie Widdowson published the first of what would be their periodical examinations of the nutrient content of food. When the fifth edition of this tome – which has over the years become a standard reference work on the subject – was published in 1991, British geologist-turned-nutritionist David Thomas undertook the work of comparing the values as published in the first and latest editions of the book.

He examined the data for 28 raw vegetables and 44 cooked vegetables, 17 fruits and 10 types of meat, poultry and game. His findings make frightening reading. What he found was that, among today's foods:

- **Potatoes** have 30 per cent less magnesium, 35 per cent less calcium, 45 per cent less iron and 47 per cent less copper.

- **Carrots** have 75 per cent less magnesium, 48 per cent less calcium, 46 per cent less iron and 75 per cent less copper.

- **Broccoli** (boiled) has 75 per cent less calcium.

- **Spinach** (boiled) has 60 per cent less iron and 96 per cent less copper.

- **Swedes** have 71 per cent less iron.

- **Spring onions** have 74 per cent less calcium.

- **Watercress** has 93 per cent less copper.

- **All meats** contain 41 per cent less calcium and 54 per cent less iron.

- **All fruits** contain 27 per cent less zinc.

- **Apples and oranges** have 67 per cent less iron.

Among the other worrying findings was that the practice of seeding the soil with only certain minerals (sodium, phosphorus and potassium) has greatly altered the natural mineral profile of our foods. Thus, swedes now contain 110 per cent of the phosphorus they once did. Humans who eat this nutritionally altered food cannot help but experience an alteration in the natural mineral profiles of their own body tissues and bones as well, which can affect their health.

A similar exercise was carried out in the US in 1999, when nutritionist Alex Jack compared nutrient values in that year's US Department of Agriculture (USDA) handbook with those published in 1975. He discovered a number of mineral deficits as well as the fact that cauliflower had 40 per cent less vitamin C than it did in 1975.

Many classes of herbicide can alter plant metabolism and, thus, nutrient composition. For example, herbicides that inhibit photosynthesis (such as triazine or phenoyacetics) produce effects similar to growing a plant in low-light conditions. Under such conditions, the carbohydrate, alpha-tocopherol (vitamin E) and beta-carotene (a precursor of vitamin A) content of a plant is reduced, and protein, free amino acid and nitrate levels are increased. Equally, bleaching herbicides can reduce beta-carotene levels, and sulphonylurea herbicides are known to reduce levels of branched-chain amino acids (which people need to maintain muscle tissue).

▶ MAKING CHANGES

When you begin to realise the health risks associated with processed foods and food additives, it makes good sense to start eating less of them or, better yet, cutting them out altogether. The problem is that the widespread use of additives has greatly changed our perception of what food is and should be. Food riddled with additives is convenient. It can be bought in bulk and stored for long periods of time. It's always on tap. It is highly flavoured and brightly coloured, appealing to our senses.

If giving up all the foods you like seems too big a task, then start slowly. If there are special treats that you just can't imagine living without, have them on occasion. But be aware of what those special treats contain. Where possible, look for wholesome alternatives that taste just as good and which don't put your health at risk.

Also, consider changing your buying habits. Are there farmers' markets in the area where you could shop frequently? If you don't know, use the Internet or the local press to find out. Is there a natural-foods market with organic produce nearby that you've never bothered to patronise? If so, now is the time to investigate it.

Eating local

When it comes to eating good food, most of us would automatically think organic. Organic food has undoubted advantages but, in the big picture of food production, locally produced food has a much more important role to play in keeping our bodies and communities healthy.

Consider the conclusions of a 2005 study by British researchers, published in the journal *Food Policy*. The team calculated a shopping basket's hidden costs, which mount up as produce is transported over large distances. The study found that 'road miles' account for proportionately more environmental damage than 'air miles'. While organic farming is valuable, the distance that organic food often travels to reach our plates creates environmental damage that outweighs the benefit of buying organic.

Instead, these scientists argued that people can help the environment even more by buying food from within a 20-km (12-mile) radius. By their calculations, if all foods were sourced from within 20 km of where they were consumed, environmental and congestion costs would fall from more than £2.3 billion to under £230 million – an 'environmental saving' of £2.1 billion annually.

Buying locally produced food might seem impossible if you live in a big city. But by patronising farmers' markets or making use of delivery schemes, you can drastically cut your contribution to food miles and put fresher, better food on your table.

Locally produced food has other benefits as well:

- **Fresher, riper, better-tasting** Produce that is purchased in the supermarket or a big-box store has been in transit or cold-stored for days or weeks, whereas produce that you purchase at your local farmers' market has often been picked within 24 hours of your buying it. This freshness not only affects the taste of your food, but also the nutritional value, which inevitably declines during long storage times. In addition, because local produce doesn't have to stand up to the rigours of shipping, it can be allowed to ripen naturally on the tree or vine and sold ripe and ready to eat.

- **Seasonal** By eating with the seasons, we are eating foods when they are at their peak taste, are the most abundant and the least expensive.

- **Full of variety** Supermarkets are only interested in selling 'name-brand' fruit and vegetables such as romaine lettuce, Red Delicious apples and russet potatoes. Local producers have more freedom to try growing new varieties that might have a shorter shelf life or don't produce high yields, and so don't make it to a large supermarket.

- **More personal** Buying direct from the farm or at a farmers' market means that you get to know the people who grow and sell your food. Knowing some of the story of your food can be an important part of enjoying a meal, but equally important is the fact that knowing the person who grew your food provides you with a failsafe and actual person to speak to should you find the produce (or bread, or fish or meat) below standard. This kind of immediate person-to-person contact is good for you and good for the food producer.

- **The key to responsible land development** When you buy locally, you give those with local open spaces – farms and pastures – an economic reason to remain open and undeveloped.

Eating organic

The increased demand for organic food has been the result of many shifts in consumer consciousness. Food scares such as bovine spongiform encephalopathy (BSE or mad-cow disease) and foodborne diseases have affected consumer confidence in conventional farming. Greater awareness of environmental issues has made many people make the ethical choice of eating organic foods. Also, the increasing use of alternative therapies that rely on organically grown foods has helped to renew interest in the quality of the food we eat.

Interestingly, there have been few human studies into the benefits of organic foods. So, we can only guess at how beneficial they may be, and whether consumers of organic foods are truly healthier than those who consume conventionally produced foods. However, even if there were research to prove the superior health of organic consumers, the nutrient content of the food would be only one element in their total health picture. Consumers of organic foods may also, for instance, be more active. They may walk or cycle instead of taking the car. They may restrict their use of hazardous chemicals in the home. They may be better able to manage stress.

Nevertheless, one review of what research there is found that when all the data are taken together, there is a clear trend supporting the notion that organic foods are indeed more nutritious. For instance:

- Organic food contains, on average, higher levels of vitamin C and essential minerals such as calcium, magnesium, iron and chromium.

- In a review of 41 studies from around the world, organic crops were shown to have statistically significantly higher levels of vitamin C, magnesium, iron and phosphorus. Spinach, lettuce, cabbage and potatoes showed particularly high levels of minerals.

- *Nitrate* levels in organic foods are, on average, 15 per cent lower than in conventionally grown foods. Scientists at Glasgow University found a link between the levels of nitrates in vegetables and throat cancer, the numbers of which have trebled over the last 20 years and claim more than 3000 lives a year. They believe that an increase in the use of nitrate fertilisers since World War II may be one of the major reasons for the rise in this cancer.

Slow food

In his best-selling book *Fast Food Nation*, author Eric Schlosser writes of the growing costs of our 'love affair' with fast foods. 'Fast food,' he argues, 'has triggered the homogenization of our society … has hastened the malling of our landscape, a widening of the chasm between rich and poor, fuelled an epidemic of obesity, and propelled the juggernaut of American cultural imperialism abroad.' This must-read book documents how fast food has lured us into choosing diets that are deficient in nearly everything except calories, and into supporting practices that are deceptive in every aspect – from advertising to flavouring – as well as systems that degrade nearly everyone and everything involved.

As a result, for many of us, the shopping, preparation and eating of food have become just one more rushed chore in an already packed day. Yet, according to the Slow Food movement, it doesn't need to be that way.

The Slow Food movement began in Italy in 1986 as an act of resistance against fast food. Since then, it has expanded globally to 100 countries and now has 83,000 members in the US, Europe, Japan and elsewhere. Its view is that processed fast food is not only changing the physical landscape through intensive farming, but is

▶

also eroding the way of life that revolved around the producing and eating of great food in a relaxed, sociable way.

As an antidote to this loss of the pleasures of sharing good food, its members are keen to 'protect the pleasures of the table from the homogenisation of modern fast food and life'. They want to know where their food comes from and how it is produced. They want local foods produced by someone they know and trust, and they want to help motivate other ordinary people into taking control of how they live, work and eat.

By promoting 'gastronomic culture', Slow Food is committed to promoting the diversity of local and regional quality food that is produced and marketed in a way that protects traditional foods at risk of extinction, and guarantees farmers a fair price while protecting the environment and the natural landscape.

Even if you are not a committed food campaigner, you can embrace the principles of slow food in your everyday life by considering some of the suggestions at the end of this chapter.

- Organic vegetables have higher levels (between 10 and 50 per cent) of secondary nutrients. These include antioxidants that help to mop up harmful free radicals implicated in cancer.

- Deficiencies in certain vitamins and minerals can lead to a variety of symptoms, including muscle cramps and depression.

- Between 1940 and 1991, trace minerals in conventional UK fruit and vegetables fell by up to 76 per cent; US figures showed a similar trend.

- In a survey of organic vegetable soups, researchers found that they contained almost six times as much salicylic acid as non-organic vegetable soups. This acid helps combat arteriosclerosis (hardening of the arteries) and bowel cancer, and is responsible for the anti-inflammatory action of aspirin. It is naturally used by plants as a defence against disease.

Supporters of organic food also point out that organically grown foods contain more secondary metabolites than conventionally grown plants. Secondary metabolites are substances that form part of plants' immune systems and which also help to fight cancer in humans.

But the claim for the superiority of organic foods is not based on nutrient content alone. In some ways, the nutrient-content argument may even be misleading as it's not what is in organic foods, but what is not in them that is more important – pesticides and, according to the prevailing regulatory standards for organic processed foods, the full range of worrying additives. But this brings us to the thorny question of whether organic convenience food is in keeping with either the spirit or letter of organic principles.

Organic junk food

A significant proportion of the organic market is now made up of convenience foods. As the market booms, there is a genuine risk that the kind of commercial success demonstrated in recent years by organic foods will attract people with the wrong motives and wrong values to take up organic farming.

A quick look at the supermarket shelves will also confirm that the majority of organic items stocked in any supermarket are convenience foods. Pre-prepared sauces, beefburgers, chips, pizza, ice cream, peanut butter, jam, sausages, chicken paste and chocolate are all big sellers. It is highly unlikely that any of these foods are substantially better for you (or more nutritious) than their conventional counterparts.

Unfortunately, there's no basic difference in the processing of some organic foods and non-organic foods. Many organic foods are not really produced in the traditional way at all. They're still produced using conventional industrial methods. For instance, organic bread can still use highly refined flours. Manufacturers of organic products are also using preservatives such as sugar. In fact, some organic biscuits have more sugar and fat in them than a conventional biscuit.

Focusing on nutrient counts and a lack of pesticide residues is important, but it also narrows our vision. The boom in organic food has come about largely because of clever marketing on the part of the big supermarkets. They have sold us the idea that buying organic is something healthy which you don't have to change your lifestyle to do. In reality, buying better food, be it local or organic, will require a shift in your mindset and your scheduling. As these giant retailers fall over themselves to package and shift more and more organic convenience foods, another issue has emerged. Many countries already have a strict definition of organic, but what we really need is a better definition of 'food'.

What is good food?

What is it that makes food 'good'? Since food is central to so much of our social experiences as well as the foundation for continuing good health, this question is worth pondering.

For some, quality is defined by what you pay for food; for others, it is defined by how fresh it is or whether it's organic. In fact, good food is defined by a number of factors, some of which may seem like a Utopian ideal in the food desert we now occupy. And while every meal you eat may not meet these high criteria, it's still worth aiming high. For food to be 'good', it must be:

Authentic. In other words, it should not have been synthesised or adulterated during its production, processing or storage. It must be what it promises to be and what consumers expect it to be – for example, the brown colour of brown bread is real, not just a synthetic colour added to white bread.

Sensual. Food should feel good to eat. It should combine taste, smell, texture, look and feel. Think of the incomparable blend of sensations when you bite into a genuinely ripe peach or eat a freshly caught fish. If you can't recall these sensations, you've been away from genuinely good food for too long.

Functional. How appropriate is a specific food to its purpose? For example, different varieties of potatoes are more or less suitable for boiling, baking, roasting or frying. When we are denied variety in our diet, the functional quality of food in making a dish special disappears.

Nutritious. How does what you eat benefit your body? Good fresh food has enormous value for its protein, fat and carbohydrate contents as well as its levels of vitamins, minerals, trace elements, beneficial enzymes and live organisms (as found in live yoghurt).

Ethical. Everything you eat has social and political implications. Food should be produced in such a way as to protect and honour

▶

the planet and the people on it. Instead, the industrialisation of food has had negative impacts on human rights, animal rights and the environment. How much rainforest was destroyed for the hamburger you're eating? Did a farmer in Ghana go bankrupt producing your favourite chocolate bar? Pondering these questions makes it increasingly hard to justify eating according to the fast food habit.

▶ RETURN TO REAL FOOD

The more we learn about the toxic potential of modern foods, the greater the need for a new food culture that values wholesomeness, nutrition, freshness and flavour. Raising our expectations of food and embracing these values has the knock-on effect of protecting the natural environment, treating animals humanely, protecting our soil, and respecting the farmers and food-industry workers who are involved in the food-production process. It also leads to a stronger preference for foods that are produced locally.

Getting back to good food is much easier than you think. Consider these tips:

Eat the best quality you can afford. Avoid junk foods (such as biscuits, sweets and sodas), which are not only chock-full of artificial colours and other additives, but are also of little nutritional value – high in calories, sugar, fats and/or sodium. This is especially good advice for children, who are the main consumers of junk food and at increased risk of health problems involving additives. In addition, while frozen foods may be convenient, freezing destroys vital nutrients, and there is even some indication that refrigeration causes similar effects.

Eat freshly prepared. Consider removing the microwave from your kitchen. If you only use it to heat coffee, or cook potatoes or prepackaged meals, you probably don't need it. Getting rid of your microwave will also vastly improve the quality of the food you eat, as food that has been microwaved has fewer nutrients in it. In addition, proteins such as those found in meats are significantly altered during the microwave process. Eating food directly from the microwave may also mean ingesting food that is still giving off radiation; this is why users are advised to let food 'sit' for a few minutes afterwards – to let all this radiation disperse.

Eat natural. If it comes in a box or tub, or tray or jar – or if it's a colour you don't normally see in nature, think twice before putting it in your mouth.

Eat variety. This may limit your exposure to any one additive – safer in the event that it turns out to have long-term health risks.

Eat seasonally. It is less expensive, provides greater variety in the diet and will reduce your exposure to the antifungal and antibacterial chemicals commonly used to extend the shelf life of products grown out of season or shipped halfway across the globe.

Eat slowly. If it's a choice between a burger bar or the local café or restaurant, ditch the burger bar. If it's a choice between wolfing down a sandwich at your desk or sitting on a park bench, go to the park. Wherever possible, try to sit down and enjoy your meal, and teach your children to do the same.

Eat what you like. Be guided by your taste buds, and be aware that the more you change your eating habits, the more your taste will start to return to normal. Cravings for salty, sugary, highly processed foods will disappear and, with them, the tendency to overeat foods that are not good for your health.

chapter **6**

toiletries and cosmetics

WE USE THEM TO MAKE US FEEL GOOD, smell good and look good. We
spend vast amounts of money on them – globally more than $200
billion (£110 billion) a year – and with that investment comes a lot of blind
faith that the hair products and skin products, toothpastes and make-up
will somehow improve us. Whatever your head may know, your heart still
wants to believe that there is some instant magic in the toiletries and cosmetics you buy that will – at least for a little while – make you younger,
sexier, more beautiful and more vibrant than before.

The magic of all the toiletries and cosmetics we buy is strong, and the
promises on the front of the package so seductive that most of us never
bother to look on the back to find out what's actually in all these products
we buy. Even if you do check the label of your favourite cosmetics, the
chances are that all you will see is an incomprehensible alphabet-soup of
words.

It's easier, and certainly more comforting, to believe in magic than it
is to learn to makes sense of the often impenetrable labels on personal-
care products. But the effort might just be worth making since, whatever
the front of the package come-on is, the truth is that achieving a cosmetic quick-fix requires a cocktail of largely synthetic ingredients, which
are known to cause, among other things, cancer, central-nervous-system

disruption, birth defects and immune damage.

The chemicals in personal care products are a particularly insidious form of pollution because they enter the body through multiple routes. We can swallow them, inhale them and absorb them through the skin as well as through the mucous membranes in the eyes, mouth and nose. In addition, cosmetics commonly contain emollients (oils and fats), solvents (for instance, propylene glycol) and humectants (such as glycerine) which, while relatively harmless in their own right, increase the skin's permeability which, in turn, increases the amount of other, more toxic ingredients in the mix that is absorbed into the bloodstream.

While many people assume that the government oversees the safety and efficacy of cosmetics and toiletries, most regulatory agencies do not require manufacturers to demonstrate that their products are either safe or effective.

Such regulations as there are do little to protect consumers. While regulators have approved more than 3000 ingredients for cosmetic use in Europe, many more substances find their way into our cosmetics and toiletries through loopholes in the law – for instance, those that allow products to contain traces of contaminants and other banned substances that are difficult to remove during or after manufacture.

In an ideal world, we would all be able to judge the safety of a product by its labelling. Sadly, manufacturers are inconsistent in their labelling practices and many actively resist full disclosure of ingredients on their labels because of the fear of customer backlash. What this means is that, on any supermarket shelf, you will find some products where the labels are printed on the container, and others where they are listed on peel-away labels stuck on the underside of the product. Others print them on the packaging (which is often thrown away without as much as a glance), and some use vague wording or, worse, don't list all of their ingredients or only make the ingredients list available on request at the point of sale. What this means is that it's currently difficult for all but the most motivated among us to make good decisions about what products are safe.

Where the problem starts

When it comes to cosmetics and toiletries, certain types of ingredients, such as preservatives, perfumes and colours, are known to be a significant cause of skin reactions. In fact, skin reactions are the most frequently reported adverse effect of using cosmetics, with between 10 and 30 per cent of adults experiencing skin problems from exposure to preservatives and fragrances in cosmetic products.

There is evidence to suggest that the number of people experiencing skin reactions to cosmetics is increasing. At this time, more than 80 per cent of those who develop reactions to cosmetics are healthy individuals without any prior skin problems.

It can be fairly easy to pinpoint the cosmetic causes of skin reactions such as dermatitis. But tracking the causes of more significant or longer-term problems like depression and migraines, and even cancer, is a much more difficult task. And yet, as research into cosmetic ingredients advances, scientists are finding that many of the same substances that can cause short-term problems are also long-term poisons. Skin reactions, then, could be seen as the body's early-warning system kicking in and telling you to stop using particular products or to avoid certain ingredients.

Preservatives

Preservatives by their very nature are designed to kill things. Specifically, they work by killing cells and preventing their dissemination, and are intended to prevent the growth of bacteria and fungi – mainly, *Candida albicans*, *Pseudomonas aeruginosa*, *Escherichia coli*, *Aspergillus niger* and *Staphylococcus aureus* – which can potentially cause serious infections on the skin and in the body.

The problem is that human skin also comprises living cells, so preservatives, even if used in small quantities, present a risk to the integrity of the skin and, should they be absorbed into the bloodstream, to the rest of the body, too. For this reason, most cosmetic preservatives have restrictions on their use – usually limiting them to a small percentage of the total formula.

For cosmetic formulators, finding new preservatives is complicated because, to be considered effective, a preservative has to fulfil several criteria. It must be:

- Effective across a wide range of microbes.

- Long lasting, in that it continues to keep the product free from contaminants for the life of the product.

- Rapid acting, at the first sign of contamination.

- Non-sensitising (it won't cause an allergic response).

- Non-toxic and non-irritating.

- Compatible with the other ingredients in the mix.

- Stable (it won't break down during storage and stays active across a wide pH range).

- Inactive, except as an antimicrobial (it won't interact with other ingredients).

- Soluble, so that it mixes well with whatever base (water or oil) it's in.

- Acceptable in odour and colour.

- Cost-effective.

No single preservative, synthetic or natural, fulfils all of these criteria, which is one reason why manufacturers often use several different preservatives in a single product. Another reason is solubility: some preservatives are water-soluble and some are oil-soluble; in a water-oil emulsion such as a hand lotion, formulators need to use both types.

The most commonly used cosmetic preservatives belong to a family of chemicals known as alkyl hydroxy benzoates, or **parabens**. Look on any cosmetic ingredients label and it's likely you will find *methylparaben, ethylparaben, butylparaben* and *propylparaben* listed, either singly or, more often, in combination.

All the most commonly used preservatives can cause dermatitis and other skin reactions – some more so than others. Parabens are universally recognised as skin sensitisers. But, in late 1998, researchers at Brunel University in the UK published a study that identified parabens as oestrogen mimics as well, each with a different oestrogenic potency. Methylparaben was the least potent, followed by ethylparaben, propylparaben and, finally, butylparaben. In studies of breast tumours, traces of parabens were also found in every single sample, suggesting that this oestrogenic effect is not just an artifact of the lab.

After parabens, **Kathon CG** – the main constituents of which are *methylisochlorothiazolinone* and *methylchlorothiazolinone* – is the most common preservative ingredient used in cosmetics. Like parabens, it too is a common allergen.

But not so long ago, a study from the University of Texas Health Science Center found that Kathon CG was also mutagenic – in other words, capable of causing genes to mutate. This study was the first to test commercially available products containing this preservative. The researchers noted that, when a product is both a sensitiser and a mutagen, then it also has the potential to cause cancer and that 'more adequate testing for its cancer-causing potential is needed'. Since then, laboratory studies have found that methylisochlorothiazolinone is also a neurotoxin.

Fragrances

The addition of '*parfum*' (in the EU) or 'fragrance' (in the US) is a particularly thorny issue for consumers because most of us will never know which fragrance chemicals are in the products we use. Manufacturers are allowed to simply list them under simple, shorthand names that belie the often hundreds of different ingredients that are involved in producing a single scent. (Even the simplest fragrances can contain between 30 and 50 ingredients.)

The fragrance portion of a product is thought to account for as much as 15 per cent of all allergic reactions in eczema patients, and this trend is increasing. And while synthetic fragrances are the most commonly used and, thus, the most commonly implicated, emerging evidence suggests that natural fragrances may also cause allergic reactions.

But most fragrance chemicals are potentially more damaging as they are composed of neurotoxic solvents associated with central-nervous-system (CNS) disorders such as multiple sclerosis, Parkinson's disease, Alzheimer's disease and sudden infant death syndrome, many of which have been labelled as toxic waste by the US Food and Drug Administration. It's not just adult cosmetics that are a problem. Play make-up and perfumes aimed at children often contain unacceptably high levels of these substances.

According to the 1991 US Environmental Protection Agency (EPA) report *Health Hazard Information*, the 20 most common fragrance ingredients make up a toxic soup that no thinking person would volunteer to be exposed to. Among these chemicals, seven – 1,8-cineole, beta-citronellol, beta-myrcene, nerol, ocimene, beta-phenethyl alcohol and alpha-terpinolene – are completely lacking in safety data. Among the rest:

- **Acetone** is on the 'hazardous waste' lists of several government agencies. It is primarily a CNS depressant that can cause dryness of the mouth and throat, dizziness, nausea, lack of coordination, slurred speech, drowsiness and, in severe exposures, coma.

- **Benzaldehyde** acts as a local anaesthetic and CNS depressant. It can cause irritation to the mouth, throat, eyes, skin, lungs and gastrointestinal (GI) tract, causing nausea and abdominal pain. It can also cause kidney damage.

- **Benzyl acetate** is an environmental pollutant and potential carcinogen linked to pancreatic cancer. Its vapours are irritating to the eyes and respiratory passages, and it can also be absorbed through the skin, causing system-wide effects.

- **Benzyl alcohol** is irritating to the upper respiratory tract. It can cause headache, nausea, vomiting, dizziness, a fall in blood pressure, CNS depression and, in severe cases, death due to respiratory failure.

- **Camphor** is a local irritant and CNS stimulant that is readily absorbed through body tissues. Inhalation can irritate the eyes, nose and throat, and cause dizziness, confusion, nausea, muscle twitches and convulsions.

- **Ethanol** is on the EPA's 'hazardous waste' list. It causes CNS disorders and is irritating to the eyes and upper respiratory tract even in low concentrations. Inhalation of its vapours has the same effects as ingestion, including an initial stimulatory effect followed by drowsiness, impaired vision, loss of muscle coordination and stupor.

- **Ethyl acetate** is also on the EPA's 'hazardous waste' list. It's a narcotic, and is irritating to the eyes and respiratory tract, and can cause headache and stupor. It's defatting effects may cause drying and cracking of the skin. In extreme cases, it may cause anaemia with leucocytosis and liver or kidney damage.

- **Limonene** is a carcinogen as well as a skin and eye irritant and allergen.

- *Linalool* is a narcotic and cause of CNS disorders. It can produce sometimes fatal respiratory disturbances, poor muscular coordination, reduced spontaneous motor activity and depression. Animal tests indicate that it may also affect the heart.

- *Methylene chloride* was banned in the US by the FDA in 1988, but no enforcement is possible due to trade-secret laws that protect the chemical-fragrance industry. It is on the 'hazardous waste' lists of several government agencies. It is a carcinogen and CNS disrupter; it's absorbed and stored in body fat; it metabolises to carbon monoxide, thereby reducing the oxygen-carrying capacity of the blood. Other adverse effects include headache, giddiness, stupor, irritability, fatigue and tingling in the limbs.

- **alpha-Pinene** is a sensitiser, and can damage the immune system.

- **gamma-Terpinene (*g-Terpinene*)** causes asthma and CNS disorders.

- **alpha-Terpineol (*a-Terpineol*)** is highly irritating to mucous membranes; aspiration into the lungs can produce a pneumonitis or even fatal oedema; it can also cause nervous excitement, loss of muscle coordination, hypothermia, CNS and respiratory depression, and headache. Scientific data warn against repeated or prolonged skin contact.

In the EU, certain fragrance ingredients with a high potential to cause allergic reactions must now be listed separately on the product label. These are:

- Amyl cinnamal
- Amylcinnamyl alcohol
- Benzyl alcohol
- Benzyl salicylate
- Cinnamyl alcohol
- Cinnamal
- Citral
- Coumarin
- Eugenol
- Geraniol
- Hydroxycitronellal
- Hydroxymethylpentylcyclohexenecarboxaldehyde

- Isoeugenol
- Anisyl alcohol
- Benzyl benzoate
- Benzyl cinnamate
- Citronellol
- Farnesol
- Hexylcinnamaldehyde
- Lilial [2-(4-tert-butylbenzyl)propionaldehyde]
- D-Limonene
- Linalool
- Methyl heptine carbonate
- gamma-Methylionone [3-methyl-4-(2,6,6-trimethyl-2-cyclohexen-1-yl)-3-buten-2-one]

Penetration enhancers

Your skin absorbs up to 60 per cent of chemicals in products that come into contact with the skin, and sends them directly into the bloodstream. Scientists estimate that it takes as little as 26 seconds for some substances to go from the skin to every major organ of the body. This is why nicotine or birth-control patches are so effective.

But the job of estimating how little or how much of a particular product actually enters the body is complicated. It is made more so by the fact that certain ingredients, while considered inert or generally recognised as safe (GRAS), may enhance the skin penetration of other, more toxic chemicals.

These ingredients are known as penetration enhancers. Emollient or moisturising ingredients that are easily absorbed into the skin act as penetration enhancers. And so, too, do things like microscopic liposomes and nanosomes, which are forms of nanotechnology designed specifically to drive ingredients deeper into the skin. Others, such as solvents used in perfumes, and detergents used in shampoos and shower gels, can alter the structure of the skin in some way, usually by dissolving its protective oily barrier – in this way, allowing other chemicals in the mix to penetrate deeper into the skin. Because the skin is laced with tiny blood vessels, these chemicals will also eventually find their way into the bloodstream and internal organs.

The list of ingredients that can act as penetration enhancers is incredibly long, but often includes:

- **Ionic compounds** such as ionic surfactants, *sodium lauryl sulphate*, sodium carboxylate, sodium hyaluronate and sodium ascorbate.

- **Solvents** such as *acetone*, ethanol, *limonene*, *polyethylene glycol* (*PEG*), *propylene glycol* (*PPG*), *xylene*, *acetamide* and trichloroethanol.

- **Fatty-acid esters** such as butyl acetate, diethyl succinate, *ethyl acetate*, and some *isopropyl*, *methyl* and *sorbitan* compounds.

- **Fatty acids** such as capric acid, *lactic acid*, linoleic acid, linolenic acid, *oleic acid* and *palmitic acid*.

- **Complexing agents** such as liposomes, *naphthalene*, classical and non-ionic surfactants, and nonoxynol.

Carcinogens

Most of us are aware of the allergenic potential of cosmetics and toiletries, and manufacturers work hard to reduce the irritation factor of most of their products. But what may come as a shock is that there are longer-term risks associated with the continual use of cosmetics and toiletries. Many, for instance, contain known carcinogens.

Manufacturers argue that these ingredients are only present in small amounts and so could not possibly be harmful, and without the long-term research which manufacturers are unwilling to fund, the possibility that cosmetic use could lead to cancer is difficult to prove. Nevertheless, some types of cosmetics such as hair dyes are already being linked to higher rates of specific cancers among users (see page 145).

According to Dr Samuel Epstein, chairman of the Cancer Prevention Coalition, there are two classes of major cancer-causing ingredients in our cosmetics and toiletries.

The first class includes those ingredients that are carcinogenic in themselves – these are known as 'frank' carcinogens. The second group are called 'hidden' or co-carcinogens. These chemicals, while not carcinogenic in themselves, may under certain conditions – for instance, when mixed together – develop cancer-causing properties or increase the carcinogenic potential of other chemicals. Over 40 'frank' carcinogens and more than 30 'hidden' carcinogens are commonly used in everyday beauty products and toiletries – even those intended for children.

Frank carcinogens

This list comprises mostly the synthetic coal-tar dyes commonly used to colour cosmetics and hair dyes, as well as solvents and preservatives that appear on almost every cosmetic label. As an eye-opening exercise, check for yourself if any of your favourite products contain any of the following ingredients:

- Benzyl acetate
- Butyl benzylphthalate
- Butylated hydroxyanisole (BHA)
- Butylated hyroxytoluene (BHT)
- Crystalline silica
- D&C Green 5 (CI61570)
- D&C Orange 17 (CI12075)
- D&C Red 2, 3, 4, 10, 17*
- D&C Red 8, 9, 19, 33 (CI15585, CI45170, CI17200)
- Diaminophenol
- Diethanolamine (DEA)
- Dioctyl adipate
- Disperse Blue 1 (CI64500)
- Disperse Yellow 3 (CI11855)
- Ethyl alcohol
- FD & C Blue 1, 2 (CI42090, CI73015)
- FD&C Blue 4*
- FD & C Green 3 (CI42053)
- FD & C Red 4, 40 (CI14700, CI16035)
- FD&C Red 10*
- FD & C Yellow 5, 6 (CI19140, CI15985)
- Fluoride
- Formaldehyde
- Glutaral
- Hydroquinone
- Methylene chloride
- Nitrophenylenediamine
- Phenyl-p-phenylenediamine
- Polyvinylpyrrolidone
- p-phenylenediamine
- Pyrocatechol
- Saccharin
- Talc
- Titanium dioxide

* Now banned from cosmetics in the US and Europe

Hidden carcinogens

In general, these can be broken down into three main categories: formaldehyde releasers; nitrosamine precursors; and contaminants. Formaldehyde releasers and nitrosamine precursors are generally preservatives, solvents, carriers and detergents/surfactants. These are always listed on the label.

Formaldehyde is a skin irritant and known carcinogen, so products with these ingredients on their own carry a certain amount of risk. But when formaldehyde releasers and nitrosamine precursors are mixed in the same formula, they can produce potent cancer-causing agents called nitrosamines. Studies show that between 42 and 93 per cent of toiletries and cosmetics on the shelf contain these compounds, which are quickly and easily absorbed into the skin from both leave-on and wash-off products. Check the labels of your favourite cosmetics for these formaldehyde-releasing substances:

- 2-bromo-2-nitropropane-1,3-diol (Bronopol)
- Diazolidinyl urea
- DMDM hydantoin
- Imidazolidinyl urea
- Metheneamine
- Quaternium-15
- Sodium hydroxymethylglycinate

Nitrosamine precursors are among the most dangerous chemicals that we put in and on our bodies in the name of beauty each day. They belong to a family of hormone-disrupting chemicals, and are almost always found in products that foam, including bubble bath, body washes and shower gels, shampoos, liquid soaps and facial cleansers. Some of the most common of these ingredients are:

- Bromonitrodioxane
- Bronopol (2-bromo-2-nitropropane-1,3-diol)
- Cocamide DEA
- Cocamide MEA
- DEA oleth-3 phosphate
- DEA-cetyl phosphate
- Diethanolamine (DEA)
- Lauramide DEA
- Linoleamide MEA
- Metheneamine
- Monethanolamine (MEA)
- Morpholine
- Myristamide DEA
- Oleamide DEA
- Padimate-O (octyldimethyl para-amino benzoic acid)
- Pyroglutamic acid
- Stearalkonium chloride
- Stearamide MEA
- TEA lauryl sulphate
- TEA-sodium lauryl sulphate
- Triethanolamine (TEA)

Once added to the product, these chemicals readily react with any nitrites present to form the carcinogenic nitrosamine NDELA (*N*-nitrosodiethanolamine). Nitrosamines are also one of the major carcinogens in cigarettes, and are also found in cured meats. In the 1970s, nitrosamine contamination of bacon and other cured meats became a worldwide public-health issue. As a result, the nitrosamine content of cured meats has dropped drastically in recent years. However, the nitrosamine content of toiletries remains alarmingly high. In a single shampoo, you could absorb 50 to 100 mcg of nitrosamine through the skin. A typical portion of bacon would supply only 1 mcg of the chemical.

Nitrites get into personal-care products in several ways. They can be added as anti-corrosive agents or be present as contaminants in the raw materials. They can also result from the presence of formaldehyde-releasing chemicals in the mix.

The long shelf life of most toiletries increases the risk of this carcinogenic chemical reaction. Stored for extended periods at raised temperatures, nitrates will continue to form in a product, accelerated by the presence of certain other chemicals such as formaldehyde, paraformaldehyde, thiocyanate, nitrophenols and certain metal salts.

Inadequate and confusing labelling means that consumers may never know which products are most likely to be contaminated. However, according to a 1980 FDA report, approximately 42 per cent of all cosmetics were contaminated with NDELA, with shampoos having the highest concentrations. In two reports released in 1991, 27 out of 29 products tested were contaminated with NDELA.

While manufacturers plead that DEA and its relatives are safe in products that are designed for brief or discontinuous use, or are washed off, there is evidence from both human and animal studies that DEA is quickly absorbed through the skin. Also, this argument does not explain why these chemicals crop up regularly in body lotions and facial moisturisers, which are not washed off.

As far back as 1978, the International Agency for Research on Cancer (IARC) concluded that *N*-nitrosodiethanolamine should be regarded for practical purposes as if it were carcinogenic to humans. The IARC maintains this position on NDELA even today.

In 1994, the US National Toxicology Program similarly concluded in its *Seventh Annual Report on Carcinogens* that: 'There is sufficient evidence for the carcinogenicity of *N*-nitrodiethanolamine in experimental animals'. They noted that, of over 44 different animal species in which NDELA compounds have been tested, all were susceptible, and that humans were most unlikely to be an exception to this trend.

But the response of the cosmetic industry to the problem of nitrosamine formation in their products has been to put even more chemicals, such as preservatives and antioxidants, into the products we use in an attempt to slow or inhibit the formation of NDELA. Yet, none has been proved adequate against the possible nitrosating agents found in everyday cosmetics.

Contaminants

Carcinogens can get into your toiletries in other ways as well. Contaminants end up in cosmetics due to careless processing of the starting materials and, as such, are not listed on the label:

- Aflatoxin, in peanut oil and flour

- *Arsenic*, in *coal-tar* dyes, polyvinyl acetate, *PEG* (polyethylene glycol) compounds

- Chloroaniline, in chlorhexidine

- Crystalline silica, in amorphous (powdered) silicates used in toothpastes and make-up

- *DDT*, *Dieldrin*, Endrin and other organochlorine pesticides, in lanolin, hydrogenated cottonseed oil, quaternium-26

- DEA (*diethanolamine*), in DEA-cocamide/lauramide condensates, quaternium-26

- 1,4-*dioxane*, in ethoxylated alcohols, including *PEGs*, *polysorbate* 60 and 80, nonoxynol and chemicals with 'eth' in their names (such as choleth-24, ceteareth-3, laureths)

- Ethylhexylacrylate, in *acrylate* and methacrylate polymers

- *Ethylene oxide*, in PEGs, *oleths*, ceteareth-3, *laureths*, polysorbate 60 and 80, nonoxynol

- *Formaldehyde*, in polyoxymethylene urea

- Lead, in *coal-tar* dyes, polyvinyl acetate, *PEG* (polyethylene glycol) compounds.

In addition to these, many of today's toiletries are based on compounds called ethoxylated alcohols. Ethoxylates can be contaminated with the carcinogen 1,4-dioxane. Commonly used ethoxylates include polyethylene, polyethylene glycol (PEG), *polyoxyethylene*, and 'eth' compounds such as *sodium laureth sulphate* and those with 'oxynol' ingredients. Polysorbate 60 and 80 may also contain these contaminants.

In one 1991 study of a range of products including shampoos, liquid soaps, sun creams, bath foams, moisturising lotions, aftershave balms, cleansing milks, baby lotions, facial creams and hair lotions, more than half the products contained dioxanes at levels potentially harmful to human health.

■ BATH SOAPS AND BODY WASHES

These days, most of us don't use soap at all – for anything. Instead, we use body washes, bath foams, baby wash and shower gels, facial washes and scrubs, all of which rely on complex modern detergents – often the same ones used in heavy industry – to wash away simple dirt.

The difference between soap and detergent is rather like the difference between cotton and nylon. Soap and cotton are produced from natural products by a relatively small modification. However, detergents and nylon are produced entirely in a chemical factory. Detergents have a greater impact on the environment than soaps, both from the waste stream they generate during their manufacture and in their lesser biodegradability.

The detergents we use every day are part of a larger group of chemicals called surfactants (short for 'surface-active agents'). Surfactants work by changing the properties of water. For instance, they can lower the surface tension of water, making it 'wetter' and better able to interact with other cleaning agents in the mixture. Detergents have similar properties to surfactants and may also add foaming ability. Both detergents and surfactants can be synthesised from either plant or petrochemicals. There is no difference between the detergents that are in your household-cleaning products and those that you use in your bath. It is simply a matter of concentration.

Detergents, which replaced simple soap in our hygiene routine soon after World War II and which form a major part of most bath products, were originally developed for industrial use in hard-water areas where they were thought to clean more efficiently. Since then, research has shown that simple soap and detergent perform equally well in most types of waters, although hard water appears to increase the potential of both types of cleaners to irritate the skin.

Manufacturers also boast that, unlike soap, detergents do not produce precipitate – the scummy substance that floats on the water or sticks to the side of the bath or shower. This is not strictly true: all washing products produce some degree of precipitate and claims about precipitate simply serve to illustrate how much manufacturers rely on aesthetics rather than effectiveness to sell their products.

The problem can arise during the rinse. In hard-water areas, both types of cleaners can be difficult to wash off, and old-fashioned soaps even more so. However, genuine castile soap, made with a high percentage of coconut oil, appears to rinse equally well in both types of water.

Having said this, even among detergents, there is a wide variation in both effectiveness and ecological impact. Those based on plant materials are somewhat kinder to the body and environment than those based on petroleum. And while, for some industrial applications, detergent is an appropriate choice, it is totally unnecessary, and potentially toxic, when used to clean the body.

Soap is a simple, effective and largely natural cleanser. It is a simple substance that is made in a one-step process that creates little waste in its manufacture, and little waste in its use. To make soap, all you need is fat or oil and a strong alkali solution.

BATH BARS

That good old bar in the bath or shower is the mainstay of most people's personal-care regime. While they may all look the same, manufacturers claim significant differences in terms of effectiveness and mildness among their products. There is a genuine basis for such claims. For example, glycerine-based soaps are among the mildest on the market, while deodorant and antibacterial soaps are among the harshest and most irritating to skin.

Most bath bars are made from synthetic and semi-synthetic detergents, including **sodium tallowate** – made from animal fats – and **sodium palmate**, **sodium palm kernelate** and **sodium cocoate** which, although of vegetable origin, can be highly processed and retain none of their original vegetable characteristics. They can also contain **glycerin** (a humectant), water softeners such as pentasodium, **disodium EDTA** and **tetrasodium EDTA**, skin conditioners such as stearic acid and rinse aids such as **sodium chloride**, as well as **parfum** and synthetic colours.

BUBBLE BATHS AND BODY WASHES

Of all the available bath products, bubble baths, which are highly fragranced, have the greatest potential to cause skin irritation, allergic skin reactions and headaches.

Milder detergents

Soap is a simple, effective and largely natural cleanser. Detergents can only be produced synthetically, and the damage they can do to skin, hair, eyes and mucous membranes varies according to how harsh and denaturing they are. If you are determined to buy detergent-based body-care products, you can make safer choices by choosing those with ingredients that have a milder action on the skin and/or which don't contain potential carcinogens. Avoid shampoos, bodywashes and foam baths with ingredients that contain the acronyms DEA, TEA or MEA, and look instead for those that are based on the following milder detergents:

- Amphoteric-2
- Amphoteric-20
- Amphoteric-6
- Cocamidopropyl hydroxysultaine
- Cocoa betaine
- Cocoa glucoside
- Decyl glucose
- Decyl polyglucose
- Lauryl betaine
- Lauryl glucoside
- Polysorbate-20
- Polysorbate-40
- Sodium cocoyl isethionate
- Sodium lauraminopropionate
- Sorbitan laurate
- Sorbitan palmate
- Sorbitan stearate

However, a bigger problem with using bubble baths is that they can irritate more than just your skin. Regular bubble bath use is associated with a high rate of urogenital infections. The harsh detergents in these products can strip away protective oils from sensitive areas of skin as well as strip away the mucus that lines the genitourinary tract. Removing this natural protection allows bacteria to take hold and cause infection. Children are particularly vulnerable, and bubble baths are a major cause of urogenital infections in babies.

In the US, bubble baths are now obliged to carry a health warning, advising users to follow directions carefully, and that prolonged use can cause skin irritation and raise the risk of urinary tract infections.

Body washes come in liquids, gels and foams but, essentially, they are the same product containing the same basic ingredients as a bubble bath. Soaking in any bath product will prolong its contact with your skin, increasing the risk that chemicals will be absorbed. Hot water also increases your skin's permeability and helps to vapourise some of the chemicals in the product, making them more easily inhaled. So both bubble baths and shower gels have the potential to penetrate into the skin and lungs.

Your bubble bath or shower foam is likely to contain detergents like *sodium laureth sulphate* and *cocamidopropyl betaine*, preservatives such as tetrasodium EDTA, *methylchloroisothiazolinone* and *methylisothiazolinone*, and humectants such as *propylene glycol* or *butylene glycol*. If your bubble bath contains cocamide DEA (or similar compounds ending with DEA, TEA or MEA) along with formaldehyde-forming substances such as *2-bromo-2-nitropropane-1,3-diol* (bronopol or BNP), *DMDM hydantoin, diazolidinyl urea, imidazolidinyl urea* and *quaternium-15*, you shouldn't be using it because it is likely to contain cancer-causing nitrosamines (see page 110 for more information).

▶ TRY THIS INSTEAD ...

Most bath products are frankly unnecessary. Anything that produces a lot of foam has been made to appeal to your emotions and senses rather than to your desire to be clean, as foam adds no cleaning ability. However, manufacturers constantly add more detergent and additional foam-boosters to produce the foam that they believe consumers can't possibly live without. The increased concentration of detergent creates the need for conditioners and other additives, generating an even more complex cocktail of ingredients in the attempt to limit any skin reaction to the detergents.

The best alternative is to stick to bath bars, avoid bubble baths altogether, and limit your use of bath foams and shower gels. If you are looking for the mildest way to clean your skin, then:

Always opt for vegetable and glycerine-based soaps over harsher petrochemical-based varieties.

Buy real soap made from at least 70-per-cent vegetable oil. Many healthfood shops stock such soaps, or they can be ordered from specialist suppliers.

Choose a liquid castile soap instead of a body wash. Liquid castile soaps (such as those made by Dr Bronner) foam beautifully, and are made from enriching oils such as coconut, hemp and olive. They are usually fragranced with essential oils (but check the label), and even come unscented so you can add your own fragrance.

If you must have bubble baths, have them less often and make sure the room is well-ventilated to avoid inhaling too many chemicals.

For the more ambitious, making your own bath products means you can have exactly the right scent to suit your mood on any given day. It also ensures that you are not soaking in or inhaling a bathtub full of potentially harmful chemicals.

Use essential oils to fragrance your bath. To help them disperse in the water, mix 4–10 drops of essential oil in 15 ml of milk (semi-skimmed or whole). The fat in the milk will distribute the oils evenly around the bath. Alternatively, mix in a carrier oil such as almond or grapeseed. Choose oils that match your skin type: for **greasy skin**: lavender, orange, lemon, clary sage, neroli, cypress, ylang-ylang, bergamot; for **normal skin**: palma rosa, geranium, lavender, Roman chamomile, jasmine, neroli, ylang-ylang, frankincense, sandalwood, patchouli; for **sensitive skin**: geranium, lavender, German chamomile; for **dry or damaged skin**: geranium, lavender, German chamomile, Roman chamomile, clary sage, naiouli, thyme linalol, myrrh, or a blend of eucalyptus and lemon or peppermint.

A fragrant mineral bath. No need to buy expensive brands. Add a generous handful of Epsom salts and a few drops of your favourite essential oil (mixed in a carrier oil as above). Epsom salts can be purchased at any chemist in large 3-kg bags for a fraction of the cost of name brands that are essentially the same thing. For a bit of a fizz in the bath, add a handful of bicarbonate of soda as well. Epsom salts are a good way to encourage the skin to release accumulated toxins so, in addition to being pleasant and safe to soak in, they are therapeutic as well.

Make your own bath bomb. Commercially made bath bombs often have dubious chemicals and colours in them. Instead, if you want your bath to fizz nicely, mix 3 tbsp (45 mg) of bicarbonate of soda with 1¹/₂ tbsp (22 mg) of citric acid in a bowl together with 8–10 drops of your favourite essential oil. Drizzle a scant teaspoon of water over the dry ingredients and mix well. This is enough for one large bath bomb. You can press it into a mould (an old film cartridge or an ice-cube tray will do) and store in a plastic bag for later. Or you can use it right away by sprinkling the mixture in the bath just as you are getting in.

Have a herbal bath. Brew up a strong infusion of your favourite herbal tea and mix this into your bath water. Good choices include peppermint, chamomile, lavender and limeflower.

For dry irritated skin, try making your own herbal wash bag. Cut the foot off of an old pair of tights, about six inches from the end. Fill the pouch with a handful of oatmeal, some soothing herbs such as chamomile or lavender, and 2 tbsp (30 mg) of finely ground almonds. Tie a knot in the open end of the pouch. You can now use this in the bath or shower. One wash bag will last one day at most – keep it in the fridge in a plastic bag if you intend to use it morning and night, but don't try to store it for longer than this as it can accumulate bacteria. When wet, it will produce a lovely creamy liquid that will clean and nourish your skin without drying it. This is great for adults, but it's also good for babies and children who have dry skin.

■ DENTAL CARE

Brushing your teeth several times daily will keep them clean, clear the mouth of plaque-forming bacteria and freshen the breath. In pursuit of a dazzling smile and a fresh mouth, there is now a staggering variety of toothpaste products, including family toothpastes, whitening toothpastes, children's toothpastes, tartar-control toothpastes, toothpastes plus mouthwash, gels, creams and stripes, and mild mint, freshmint, baking soda and herbal toothpastes, each one claiming to do something specific and/or unique.

But while there is such a wide variety of dentifrices on the market, most are basically the same – there is no advantage of gel toothpaste, for example, over cream formulas. And while many toothpastes appear to make grand claims about what they can do for your teeth, look closely at the wording on the label next time you buy. It won't actually say it will prevent plaque or tartar buildup. Instead, it says it 'fights it' or 'can help prevent' it. This is a convenient way of sounding like you are making a medicinal claim (and thus encouraging the trust of the purchaser) when you really aren't.

While it may make your mouth feel fresh, toothpaste is not actually necessary for cleaning your teeth. Dry brushing can do the job just as effectively.

Tartar-control toothpastes cannot remove existing tartar. Likewise, those pastes that claim to prevent gum disease cannot treat existing gum disease. In both cases, a trip to the dentist is necessary. Smoker's toothpaste, which claims to remove stains, can be highly abrasive. Excessive abrasion on the teeth can damage tooth enamel and cause the gums to recede.

The problems of dental decay and gum disease are very real and impact on more than just the mouth. Periodontal disease is strongly linked to other conditions such as heart disease. Indeed, your risk of developing heart disease is much higher if you have poor oral health than if you smoke or have high cholesterol. One theory for why this is suggests that oral bacteria can enter the bloodstream, attach to fatty plaques in the coronary (heart) arteries and contribute to clot formation.

Another possibility is that the inflammation caused by periodontal disease increases plaque buildup, which may contribute to swelling of the arteries. Researchers have found that people with periodontal disease are almost twice as likely to suffer from coronary artery disease as those without periodontal disease. Poor oral health also raises your risk of stroke, peripheral vascular disease, osteoporosis, respiratory diseases, diabetes and preterm pregnancy.

But brushing, like so many daily tasks, can sometimes be boring, so major manufacturers have begun to advertise toothpaste in a way that suggests it is a beauty or luxury product rather than simply an aid to personal hygiene. One major brand even promises to provide noticeable improvement for all five signs of healthy teeth – fewer cavities, less tartar, healthy gums, naturally white teeth and fresh breath – in much the same way that antiwrinkle creams fight the 'seven signs of ageing'.

By turning basic daily necessities into more attractive, premium purchases, manufacturers are encouraging consumers to buy more – and buy them at a higher price. This has the knock-on effect of drawing attention away from the product ingredients.

Looking at the label on a typical toothpaste tube, you might wonder why you would want to put this product in your mouth at all. In a market crowded with alternatives, each brand has to make bigger claims about what it can do. And to back up these claims, more and more chemicals are added. Should you be worried? Probably.

Hard to swallow

Several of the 'active' ingredients in toothpaste are worrying. The industrial-strength detergent **sodium lauryl sulphate** (SLS) is a suspected gastrointestinal or liver toxicant. There is also concern that, by irritating and stripping away the protective mucous membrane of the mouth, SLS could increase the incidence of mouth ulcers and may also be involved in an increased risk of oral cancer.

Triclosan is one of the most common antibacterial agents used in toothpaste. It is often found in antibacterial/antiplaque formulas, and there is evidence that it can help reduce plaque buildup. However, although tartar-control formulas may prevent 40–50 per cent of new tartar buildup, they can do nothing for plaque that is already present.

Triclosan, like SLS, is an irritant, and there is some evidence that the two substances can combine synergistically to become an even more powerful irritant. Triclosan is also associated with a rise in 'superbugs', bacteria that are resistant to many kinds of antiseptics and antibiotics (see 'Antibacterial Cleaners', page 199).

Sensitive-tooth formulas contain nerve-deadening chemicals such as **strontium chloride** or **potassium nitrate**. But don't expect these toothpastes to work immediately, like they do on TV – most people won't notice any improvement for four to six weeks. If your teeth are very sensitive, you'll need a trip to the dentist to rule out an underlying problem such as a cracked tooth or gum disease.

Certain abrasives, such as **silica**, are also potentially harmful. Recent studies have shown that fine granules of this mineral can build up under the surface of the gums, causing granulomas – small nodules of inflamed tissue. Other fine-grained abrasives can have a similar effect, leading to symptoms that can mimic gingivitis, but which may also leave the gums more vulnerable to infection.

Many toothpastes also contain glue-like substances, such as PVM/MA copolymer, that keep the active ingredients in contact with the teeth even after rinsing.

Fluoride myths

Without doubt, the most controversial ingredient in toothpaste is *fluoride*. Many of us still buy fluoride-containing toothpastes believing that the chemical protects teeth. There is, however, little convincing scientific evidence to support this. In fact, fluoride is a systemic poison, and there is enough in the average-sized tube of family toothpaste to kill a small child if ingested. For this reason, both the American Food and Drug Administration (FDA) and the Swedish National Food Administration now require that toothpaste containing fluoride should be labelled with a special 'poison' warning.

Studies have shown a clear relationship between mouth cancer and fluoride intake in both animals and humans. For instance, benign squamous papilloma, which appears as a white patch on the inside of the mouth and is the precursor of squamous cell carcinoma, can also be triggered by fluoride exposure.

Fluoride can cause sensitivity/allergic-type reactions, and is now a suspect in a host of illnesses, including gastroesophageal reflux disease (GERD), bone problems, diabetes, thyroid malfunction and mental impairment. Fluoride exposure from toothpaste, supplements and water before the age of six is also an important risk factor for dental fluorosis, which leads to mottled and discoloured teeth.

Young children have a tendency to swallow toothpaste and, with it, the toxic fluoride. This may be because they are too young to control the swallowing reflex, or it may simply be that the sweet flavours and pretty colours make toothpaste as appealing as candy to swallow.

For both these reasons, it is now widely accepted that family toothpastes, which generally contain the highest amounts of fluoride (around 1500 ppm, or parts per million) are unsuitable for children under the age of eight.

More recently, fluoride has been found to activate and interfere with substances known as G-proteins – chemical messengers that play a vital role in the activities of hormones and neurotransmitters. By activating G-proteins, fluoride may actually be promoting gingivitis (gum disease) – thus contributing to the range of diseases associated with that problem.

WHITENING TOOTHPASTES

These toothpastes work in two ways – either by bleaching the teeth with chemicals such as *hydrogen peroxide* (which can be a slow process), or by using gritty particles to scrape away stains. Such toothpastes are popular among smokers and among those with low self-esteem. However, the abrasive action is harmful to your teeth. Although the jury is still out on chemical bleaching, problems have been observed.

At best, whitening toothpastes may produce a mild cleaning or bleaching action that only lasts as long as you keep using the product. At worst, they can make your teeth painfully sensitive to heat and cold, or they may irritate your gums and permanently destroy tooth enamel. Concern has also been expressed that the new chemical whiteners are still something of an unknown quantity. Peroxide, for instance, is highly reactive and may interact with other chemicals in the paste to form new, harmful chemicals.

The low-down on dental floss

Although we think of flossing as a recent development in dental care, evidence gleaned from the skulls of prehistoric humans suggests that we have been flossing in one way or another for a very long time. In the 1800s, floss was made of fine unwaxed silk thread. Now it is made of thin nylon string.

Some holistic dentists have expressed concerns that modern dental floss can be contaminated with mercury-containing antiseptics. Certainly, some flosses are impregnated with unnecessary flavourings derived from petrochemicals, and some are even coloured. Often, they are coated with waxes of petrochemical origin as well.

American naturopath Dr Hulda Clark has gone so far as to recommend that flossing is best done with a two- or four-pound monofilament fishing line (doubled and twisted for strength). She also suggests that the thin plastic used for most shopping bags is also serviceable. Tear off a thin strip and roll it slightly to make a quick, effective floss.

If you don't fancy that or don't have a fisherman in the family, you might just try to be a little more aware of the types of dental floss you use. Choose one without flavour or colour, and don't over-floss. It can wear a groove in your teeth and tear up your gums, making them more susceptible to infection.

MOUTHWASH AND BREATH FRESHENERS

The traditional purpose of a mouthwash is as an antiseptic gargle to help remove germs that can lead to bad breath. Today, mouthwashes come in many more complex forms that purport to fight plaque, strengthen teeth, fight tooth decay and freshen breath – in addition to killing germs. The result is a complex mixture of chemicals that, in the long run, may do more harm than good.

Although mostly water, there are several problems with the current crop of mouthwashes. First, most contain *alcohol*. Using an alcohol-containing mouthwash is associated with an increased risk of throat and mouth cancers. This is because alcohol is drying, changes the pH of the mouth, and strips away the protective mucous membrane in the mouth and throat. Although in a low concentration, most mouthwashes also contain *fluoride*. Drinking alcohol- and fluoride-containing mouthwash is a major source of poisoning among young children.

Breath fresheners – often sprays – are concentrated forms of mouthwash. Typically, they contain more alcohol than water, as well as *isobutane*, *glycerin*, sweeteners such as *saccharin* or *sorbitol*, flavourings and even colours. Because they are so high in alcohol and are not rinsed out of the mouth, regular users are at an increased risk of throat cancer. And incidentally, using a spray will not stop you having bad breath.

With good oral hygiene, mouthwashes and breath sprays are never necessary. A healthy mouth simply has no odour. If you are experiencing a problem with persistent bad breath, it could be because of gum disease or some other underlying infection. This problem is most effectively addressed by a trip to the dentist.

▶ TRY THIS INSTEAD …

Remember that it's not the paste, but the brush that cleans your teeth. Equally, it's not how hard you brush, but how long and how thoroughly. Brushing hard and fast won't clean your teeth better, and it may damage your gums. So, instead of just running the brush quickly over your teeth and hoping the toothpaste (or mouthwash) will catch what you don't, consider spending at least a minute (if not two) in gently but thoroughly brushing your teeth every morning and night.

The type of brush you use is also important so, for optimal dental health, invest in a good one with lots of filaments packed tightly together. A soft-to-medium brush is fine for most people (very few really need a firm brush), and the angle of the head is mostly immaterial. Many a weird-shaped brush has been developed in recent years – largely to try to make up for the lazy way in which most people brush their teeth. However, there is little evidence that they are substantially better than a standard straight-handled brush. Replace your toothbrush regularly at the first signs of wear.

If you still want to use commercial brands of toothpaste, consider these options:

Use less. In spite of what you see on TV, you only need a pea-sized amount of toothpaste (about a quarter of the advertised amount) to clean your teeth. And while children are advised to use a pea-sized amount, they can clean their teeth adequately with half this amount – in other words, just a 'smear'.

Dilute it. Turn toothpaste into a cream by diluting it with cooled boiled water. Store it in a small squeeze-top bottle. It will still foam and clean well.

Use a low-fluoride toothpaste. Among the brands aimed at adults, a low-fluoride content is around 500 ppm. Several children's brands contain even less, and there is nothing (apart from aesthetics) stopping the whole family from using a children's paste to clean their teeth.

Buy a fluoride-free brand and, if you can, one that is SLS-free. In most large supermarkets and chemists, it will be almost impossible to find a toothpaste that is fluoride-free *and* SLS-free. Healthfood stores will stock a wider range; but check the labels of 'natural' alternatives for detergents and other dubious chemicals.

Alternatives to conventional toothpastes are not hard to find; they are plentiful in healthfood shops, by mail order and on the Internet, and they are beginning to be sold in supermarkets, too. However, a quick scan of many ingredient labels will show that many of the so-called alternatives are not very 'alternative'. Many contain SLS and may also contain fluoride. Some also contain contentious preservatives such as **parabens**, a potential hormone disrupter.

While chalk or baking soda (**sodium bicarbonate**) can be substituted for silica, essential oils for Triclosan and **glycerin** for more harmful humectants such as propylene glycol, the basic mixture is the same. The trick with toothpaste alternatives is to read labels and find one with a basic mix that is as natural as possible while still providing the degree of effectiveness, the feel in the mouth and the taste that you are used to.

Very few toothpastes are free from worrying chemicals of one sort or another. If you feel strongly that you shouldn't put anything in your mouth that you aren't prepared to swallow, then brushing regularly with a tiny amount of baking soda or food-grade **hydrogen peroxide** will clean your teeth adequately. Hydrogen peroxide gives the bonus of gently whitening your teeth.

Baking soda is a useful mild abrasive and comes with antibacterial properties. Since undiluted, straight bicarbonate of soda can be hard on tooth enamel (particularly as you get older and enamel begins to soften), try dissolving a teaspoonful in a little water first, and then dipping your toothbrush into the liquid frequently during brushing (do the same when using hydrogen peroxide).

Since baking soda doesn't taste great, you can try making it more palatable by mixing the dry powder in a small, airtight container with a few drops of peppermint oil. Mix together well and then store for use as and when you need it.

It's also rather easy to make your own toothpaste and mouthwash.

Simple toothpaste can be made from bicarbonate of soda, vegetable glycerine and essential oil of peppermint, lemon or fennel.

As a general rule, use 1 part of liquid to two parts of bicarbonate of soda – for example, 50 ml (4 heaped tbsp) of glycerine to 100 ml (8 heaped tbsp) of bicarbonate of soda. You may have to play with the proportions until you get just the consistency you like. Add five drops of the essential oil of your choice to pep up the flavour. Shake well before use.

This mixture can be stored in a small squeezable or pump dispenser (such as those used for travel), which can be purchased at most large chemists. Use it sparingly. Don't be tempted to make more than about 50 ml at a time. Although the essential oils will act as preservatives, when making your own toiletries, it is always safest to make small amounts as needed rather than risk the product going off.

Another way of making this mixture up is to substitute a natural mouthwash – one without alcohol, fluoride, chemical preservatives, flavours or colours – for the glycerine. Mix this with bicarbonate of soda in approximately the same ratio as above.

Simple mouthwash The simplest mouthwash is a couple of drops of peppermint oil or sage tincture in a cup of water. To make around 100 ml of a more complex blend, you need:

15 ml (1 tbsp) lavender tincture
15 ml (1 tbsp) Calendula tincture
10 ml (2 tsp) aloe juice
30 ml (2 tbsp) cooled boiled water
30 ml (2 tbsp) vegetable glycerine
5 drops peppermint essential oil

Mix the ingredients together and pour them into a bottle. This mixture will keep for up to six months. If you have an infection in the mouth or gums, substitute Echinacea, myrrh or goldenseal tinctures for the lavender.

■ DEODORANTS AND ANTIPERSPIRANTS

Deodorants were the first products to be developed to help combat the problem of body odour. They are basically strong perfumes that mask the odour produced by bacteria in your armpits. Antiperspirants, which prevent sweat from leaking out of the armpits, were developed later. Nowadays, there is a huge range of antiperspirants, deodorants and antiperspirant/deodorants on the market in a variety of formulations, including creams, roll-ons, solids and sprays. A quick look at the labels will tell you that there isn't much of a difference among the ingredients in any of them.

Antiperspirants and deodorants typically contain a range of moisturisers, solvents, preservatives (such as **parabens**), synthetic perfumes and antibacterial agents such as **Triclosan** (which can be absorbed through the skin, and which has been shown to cause liver damage in animal experiments).

While nobody wants to go around smelling like a compost heap (and nobody enjoys being around someone who does), it's worth asking what price we are paying for trying to stay shower-fresh all day long.

Finding an answer to this question became more urgent in 2002, when UK researchers highlighted the potential risks associated with preservatives known as parabens (or para-hydroxybenzoic acids) in deodorants. The researchers at the University of Reading found traces of parabens in every single tumour sample taken from a small group of women with breast cancer.

Parabens are used in a wide variety of cosmetics, and the scientists suggested that the chemicals had seeped into body tissues after being applied to the skin, probably via deodorants. These findings are worrying because parabens are oestrogen mimics and this makes them potential triggers for the growth of human breast tumours.

Aluminium worries

But before bad news about parabens came out, it was the aluminium content of antiperspirants that was a major cause of concern.

Most antiperspirants contain some form of aluminium, most commonly, *aluminium chlorohydrate, aluminium zirconium tetrachlorohydrex GLY, aluminium chloride, aluminium sulphate* and *aluminium phenosulphate.*

No one knows exactly how aluminium compounds work to reduce underarm wetness. They may prevent sweat by clogging the sweat ducts which, in turn, increases the pressure inside of the ducts due to the sweat building up. It is thought that this pressure buildup then causes the sweat glands to stop secreting.

Alternatively, they may cause perforations in the glands so that the sweat seeps out into the surrounding tissues rather than coming out through the surface of the skin. Or they may block the transmission of the nervous impulses that activate sweat glands.

Whatever the mechanism, aluminium is absorbed through the skin, however superficially. The recently acknowledged link between Alzheimer's disease and aluminium has raised a furious debate as to whether or not it is safe to put aluminium compounds into deodorants. Unfortunately, this is not a question that has benefited from much scientific evaluation. Only one study reports an association between Alzheimer's and a lifetime's use of deodorant. No other studies have been conducted that refute or confirm these findings.

Nevertheless, other evidence from looking at the incidence of breast cancer among 400 American women suggests that it may be the combination of underarm shaving and deodorant use that allows chemicals to seep into breast tissue. In this study, women who shaved three times a week and applied deodorant at least twice a week were almost 15 years younger when diagnosed with cancer than women who did neither. The researchers suggested that aluminium compounds could act as a breast-cancer trigger.

Certainly, aluminium-based deodorants are a major cause of skin irritation and, for this reason alone, should be approached with caution by users. Aluminium zirconium products have been shown to cause granulomas (small nodules of chronically inflamed tissue) under the arms with prolonged use.

▶ TRY THIS INSTEAD ...

Body odour can be caused by bacteria in your armpits, but it can also be coming from what's inside your body – for instance, what you eat, and how 'polluted' your body is by toxins and allergens.

If you can, try to avoid aluminium-based antiperspirants. Aluminium is

Alum vs aluminium

Rock crystals are the newest alternative to aluminium-containing antiperspirants. Some of these are made from magnesium sulphate while others are made from alum. These products often claim to be 'aluminium-free' or 'free of aluminium chlorohydrate', yet alum by its other name is aluminium sulphate. Manufacturers suggest that aluminium sulphate has a much higher molecular weight than aluminium chlorohydrate – which is true – and so cannot be absorbed through the skin. However, this may be too simplistic. While aluminium chlorohydrate has a lower molecular weight, it is also less soluble in water (or sweat).

Sulphates, on the other hand, are highly soluble in water, and alum may break down into its component parts more readily in a sweaty armpit. Does this mean that the aluminium will be absorbed into the skin? Without the emollient ingredients found in most conventional formulations, it is unlikely, but it would be reassuring if there were more conclusive research evidence to enlighten us.

highly toxic, and there is too little evidence of safety with aluminium-containing products applied to the skin. The presence of ingredients such as magnesium oxide and zinc oxide will buffer the irritant properties of aluminium- and zirconium-based compounds, but they, too, can cause skin irritation.

In addition, when selecting conventional antiperspirants and deodorants:

Avoid aerosols, which surround you and those in your immediate area with a cloud of easily inhaled and toxic chemicals. Aerosols can contain planet-poisoning *hydrochlorofluorocarbons* (HCFCs), as well as the neurotoxic and reproductive toxins propane, butane and isopropane.

Switch to a solid or stick variety. Because it is less emollient, it is less likely to aid the absorption of ingredients into the skin. Sticks also tend to produce less irritation.

Never apply antiperspirants or deodorants to broken or newly shaved skin. The chemicals in them will be much more easily absorbed into your system if your skin is broken in any way.

Avoid coloured products. The colouring won't help you stay drier, and the coal-tar and petrochemical-derived colours used in these products are easily absorbed into the skin and can be carcinogenic.

Avoid products containing quaternium-18, which can cause rashes even beyond the area of application.

Your healthfood shop may sell deodorants based on plant extracts and essential oils (but remember to read the label to find out what is really in them). Some also sell crystal deodorants (made from mineral salts). These can be very effective, but always check what they're made of – some are aluminium-based (see box, page 130). Don't buy crystal deodorants with labels that are in any way unclear about the mineral used.

If you are feeling more ambitious, you can make your own anti-perspirants and deodorants from a few simple ingredients.

Dust under your arms with plain cornstarch. If you don't sweat heavily, this may be all you need.

Try a simple astringent such as witch hazel, which helps to temporarily contract the tissues around the sweat glands, may be all some people need (but do not apply to broken skin as it may sting).

A mixture of unflavoured vitamin C powder or citric acid and water works well for some people. Mix one-quarter of a teaspoon of powdered vitamin C or citric acid to a pint of water. Dab this sparingly under your arms after a bath, or spritz a little on from a spray bottle. If you can't wait around for it to dry, dust with cornstarch afterwards.

For a more ambitious spray, the owners of Neal's Yard, one of the UK's most respected natural toiletry manufacturers, recommend the following:

    6 tbsp (90 ml) witch hazel
    2 tsp (10 ml) vegetable glycerine
    2 drops each of clove, coriander and lavender essential oils
    5 drops each of grapefruit, lime and palma rosa essential oils
    10 drops of lemon essential oil

Mix the witch hazel and vegetable glycerine together, then add the essential oils. Shake well. Store in a dark glass or plastic bottle with a spray top. The mixture will last for up to six months.

To make an effective foot deodorant, all you need is 2 tbsp (30 ml) of witch hazel and 5 drops each of lavender and grapefruit essential oils. Blend the ingredients together, store in a spray bottle (preferably made of dark-coloured glass or plastic). Spray regularly onto clean feet. Shake before applying. This mixture will keep for up to two months.

For a simple foot powder, use cornstarch. If you want a powder that perfumes and deodorises, mix 5 drops each of lemon and coriander essential oils in with the cornstarch. Store the perfumed mixture in an old talcum-powder dispenser or similar type of container.

BODY SPRAYS

Body sprays serve no useful function. They are not deodorants, they are not quite strong enough to be perfumes and they can't stop you from sweating. Nevertheless, the market for body sprays, for men and women, has expanded exponentially in recent years.

Advertising for such products suggests that using them will make you more attractive to the opposite sex, or give you the courage to do wild and outrageous things. In reality, they are likely to give you a headache (which may stop you from doing wild and outrageous things), cause you to become forgetful, tired and listless, and may even make the people around you feel sick as well.

Body sprays are mostly solvents, propellants and fragrances. The perfumes can cause allergic reactions, headaches, dizziness, fatigue and a range of mental symptoms; the solvents and propellants are neurotoxic, and have been implicated in reproductive problems such as miscarriage and birth defects.

▶ TRY THIS INSTEAD ...

The best alternative of all is to bin these unnecessary and expensive items. If you must add yet another fragrance to your body, try to keep it as natural as possible.

Use food-grade flower waters. Rose and orange flower waters can be purchased in any supermarket or chemist. While not chemical-free, these have somewhat fewer nasties in them than conventional body sprays. Either splash them on or transfer them to a spray bottle and spritz on.

You can make a pleasant body spray from water and essential oils. Try mixing 5 drops each of lavender, sage, lemon, rosemary and grapefruit essential oils with 3 drops of peppermint oil into 10 ml of vodka. Shake to mix, then add 100 ml of white vinegar. Leave this mixture to sit for an hour or so to fix the scent.

Next, add the scented mixture to 500 ml of spring or filtered water and shake again.

You can also substitute natural vanilla essence for the essential oils. By learning more about essential oils, you can make an infinite number of light splashes and sprays to suit your every mood.

TALC

Talcum powder is a traditional mainstay of freshness. We use it liberally on babies' bottoms, and to absorb perspiration on hot summer days and nights. A few of us are old enough to remember our mothers having special dishes of talc in the bathroom which had big, inviting powder-puffs to help you dust your body – and most of the bathroom floor – with the stuff.

But time marches on, and the romantic illusion of talc has taken a huge knock.

Talc, or magnesium silicate, is made up of finely ground particles of stone. As it originates in the ground and is a mined product, it can be contaminated with other substances. Asbestos is a good example, and recent reports of the talc used in crayon manufacture being contaminated with this poisonous substance have caused alarm to every parent whose child has ever sucked on a crayon.

The harmful effects of talc on human tissue were first recorded in the 1930s. More recently, a report from the US National Toxicology Program concluded that talc is carcinogenic.

An ominous series of studies has linked talc to ovarian cancer; in these cases, talc was found in a number of ovarian and uterine tumours as well as in ovarian tissue. It has since been confirmed that talc, either placed on the perineum (or on the surface of underwear or sanitary towels), can reach the ovaries by ascending the fallopian tubes. It is now estimated that women who frequently use talc have three times the risk of developing ovarian cancer compared to non-users.

The talc used in the manufacture of condoms carries a similar risk. In the 1960s, the medical journal *The Lancet* reported the first case of a woman who had a significant amount of talc in her peritoneal (abdominal) cavity. Laboratory tests confirmed that the talc in her body matched that found on her husband's condoms. The authors concluded that talc had travelled up through the fallopian tubes and became implanted in her abdomen. Talc sprinkled on diaphragms may also be implicated in such problems.

Talc use is also associated with respiratory problems. Because it comprises finely ground stone, it can lodge in the lungs and never leave. Babies whose mothers smother them in talc have more breathing difficulties and/or urogenital problems than other infants. Women are also at risk since, even if they don't use talcum powder on their bodies, they are likely to be using cosmetics (face powders, eyeshadows, blushers) that are talc-based.

▶ TRY THIS INSTEAD ...

Don't use products containing talc. Giving up body powders is relatively easy. Giving up your eyeshadow may be less so (try applying it with a damp sponge to minimise fallout). Whatever you can do to cut your exposure to talc will benefit your health.

Make your own. You can quickly and easily make a very efficient and inexpensive body powder based on cornstarch. Combine one part of baking soda to eight parts of cornstarch. Mix these up in a blender and add 10–15 drops of your favourite essential oil (optional). Store in an airtight container (either a jar or an old talc container, or you could recycle one of those Parmesan cheese shakers).

Babies' bottoms do not need talc or any other powder to stay fresh. Instead, let your baby go without nappies as often as possible, or investigate cotton nappies, which allow the skin to breathe and have been shown to cause less nappy rash than disposables.

Use talc-free condoms, but be aware that many talc-free condoms contain other particles, such as vegetable starches, silica (another carcinogen), mica, diatomaceous earth and *Lycopodium* (club moss) spores. *Lycopodium* can be contaminated with talc, sulphur and/or gypsum, and is linked with inflammation of the soft tissues. It is not known how many chronic 'women's problems' may be the result of an overuse of talc or, indeed, allergy to the latex used in condoms, or other contraceptives such as the diaphragm and all the paraphernalia that go with them (spermicidal jellies, foams, creams and lubricants).

FEMININE DEODORANTS

Feminine deodorants and douches are totally unnecessary. The majority are bought and used simply out of a media-fuelled paranoia, which makes women worry that the people around them can detect any faint odours coming from their genitals.

If you really have a problem with strong and unpleasant vaginal odours, go to your doctor to sort out the underlying cause of the problem. You may have a low-grade vaginal infection that can easily be cleared up.

Ironically, the use of feminine deodorants – which are no different from most body sprays – can cause the very vaginal infections that may be the cause of unpleasant odours. More worryingly, in one study involving nearly 700 women over three years, researchers found that those who used vaginal douches more than once a week experienced a fourfold risk for cervical cancer. It did not matter which preparation was used, since all douches alter the chemical balance of the vagina, making the cervix more susceptible to bacterial infection and tissue changes.

Feminine deodorants are almost always aerosols, which means that you inhale harmful chemicals when you use them, and they are always highly perfumed. Douches contain harsh detergents, perfumes and colours, none of which should be coming into contact with this delicate part of your body.

▶ TRY THIS INSTEAD ...

Have a little confidence in yourself and toss these toxic products in the bin where they belong. In addition:

Bathe daily. When you wash your genitals, do not apply soap directly. It is too harsh and may dry out delicate skin. Use the foam or bubbles from your soap to gently clean yourself.

Wear cotton underwear, which allows air to circulate and discourages the bacteria that can cause unpleasant odours.

If you are experiencing vaginal itching or soreness, see your doctor and sort out the real problem. It is unlikely to be something which you can simply wash away with a douche.

If you must douche, use a simple mixture of distilled white vinegar in one pint of water, which will have less of an impact on the vaginal microflora. Even so, use this very infrequently.

■ HAIR CARE

How many different types of shampoo have you tried in your lifetime? And how often have they fallen short of what they promised to do? If you have had more than your fair share of shampoo failures, it could be because there are only a limited number of cleansing agents considered suitable for use in hair-cleaning products. If you are unsure of the truth of this statement, compare the expensive designer brands with their cheaper cousins. Often, the only genuine difference between them is the price.

The main function of a shampoo is to clean the hair. Its function is so simple that advertisers have to work doubly hard to make it sound more complicated and exciting than it actually is. Thus, using a particular brand brings with it the promise of harmony, a lust for life, nourishment and adoration by members of the opposite sex. Some shampoos are apparently so remarkable that they not only clean your hair, but give you an orgasm as well. But underneath all the puffery, a shampoo is just a bottle of highly coloured, highly perfumed, detergent.

The word 'shampoo' is derived from 'chapo', a Hindi word meaning to massage or knead. The first shampoos were simple solutions of soap invented by British hairdressers during the heyday of the Empire. Modern shampoos, however, are usually a mixture of several different detergents and surfactants, typically *sodium lauryl sulphate* (SLS), *ammonium lauryl sulphate*, *monoethanolamine* (MEA) lauryl sulphate, *diethanolamine* (DEA) lauryl sulphate and *triethanolamine* (TEA) lauryl sulphate.

Generally the strongest detergent is used in the greatest measure, then milder detergents/surfactants, which modify the harshness of the first detergent, are added. These other detergents/surfactants can also add foaming ability and conditioning properties.

For the formulator, the choice of detergent for any particular shampoo is as much a matter of aesthetics as it is about cleaning. For instance, SLS is not very soluble in cold water, and so it cannot be used to make shampoos that look 'clear'. For these shampoos, other compounds such as ammonium lauryl sulphate or TEA lauryl sulphate are used. Some shampoos have extra ingredients in them to make them produce more foam, even though foam doesn't clean your hair.

Carcinogens in the mix

As detailed on page 110, a number of common ingredients in shampoos, such as **2-bromo-2-nitropropane-1,3-diol** (bronopol or BNP), **DMDM hydantoin, diazolidinyl urea**, imidazolindinyl **urea** and **quaternium-15** break down into **formaldehyde** during storage. When formaldehyde-forming agents mix with amines such as **diethanolamine** (DEA), **tri-ethanolamine** (TEA) and **monoethanolamine** (MEA), they form carcinogenic N-nitrosodiethanolamine, or NDELA.

Nitrosamine formation is particularly problematical in shampoos, as we use them so frequently and in such great quantities. It is estimated that, when you wash your hair with a shampoo contaminated with NDELA, your body absorbs more carcinogenic nitrites than if you had eaten a pound of bacon.

A further problem is that products containing the milder laureth detergents (as in **sodium laureth sulphate** and **ammonium laureth sulphate**) can be contaminated with the carcinogen 1,4-dioxane. Laureth compounds are part of a larger family of chemicals called ethoxylated alcohols. Many of these, including **polyethylene glycol** (PEG), polyethylene, **polyoxyethylene**, oxynol and other *eth* chemicals (as in laur*eth*) can be contaminated with 1,4-dioxane. Products containing **polysorbates** 60 and 80 can also be contaminated with this chemical.

The contamination of the raw materials used to create sodium laureth sulphate was noted as far back as 1978, and has been confirmed in a recent review. Yet, little has been done to address the issue.

As manufacturers fall over themselves to make a more 'scientific' and 'improved' shampoo, the list of chemical ingredients grows. The latest published research reveals that the preservatives **methylchloroisothiazolinone** and **methylisothiazolinone** (which together are called Kathon CG) have the potential to cause nerve damage and skin cancer.

Using hot water to shampoo your hair actually increases the rate of absorption of these chemicals into your body, so if you don't like cold showers, choose your shampoos carefully.

▶ TRY THIS INSTEAD ...

Hair care begins with what you eat, not what you wash with. Hair is 95-per-cent protein, so if your hair is limp, consider whether your protein intake is adequate.

Hair also needs to be thoroughly wet before shampooing. This helps to spread the shampoo evenly throughout the hair. For really clean hair, you need to rinse thoroughly but, in the 'wash-and-go' culture, this is a step which most of us rush through. In addition:

Read the label. Find a shampoo with the fewest possible ingredients to limit your exposure to toxic chemicals. Don't buy products that contain formaldehyde-forming agents and amines.

Use less. Sounds obvious, but most of us use far too much shampoo to get the job done. Shampooing once, using half what you normally use, will clean your hair perfectly well. Always tip your head well back when rinsing to avoid any getting onto your eyelids or into your eyes.

It is not easy to make a shampoo based entirely on natural ingredients. At some point, detergent must be added. But you can make mixes that are less concentrated and which expose you to fewer harmful chemicals in each wash. So:

Dilute it. Mix your shampoo with an equal amount of water, and put this mixture in an old *and well-rinsed* shampoo bottle. Adding a little bit of table salt (about 1 tsp/100 ml of liquid) will help to thicken the mixture.

For a variation on the diluting theme, try this: half-fill an old shampoo bottle with your regular shampoo. Top up with an equal amount of water or a strong herbal infusion (such as chamomile) mixed with 1 tsp of coconut oil (this comes as a solid, but will melt in the hot infusion). Olive and jojoba oils are also good choices. Add 1–2 tsp of table salt to thicken the mix or, alternatively, add 1–2 tsp of sodium bicarbonate to soften the water and aid rinsing (dissolve this in water or tea *before* mixing). This mixture will still foam well, and clean and condition your hair, too. Always give it a shake before using, as the ingredients in some shampoo mixtures will separate when the mix is altered.

Use a castile soap. These come in both bar and liquid forms. Because of their high oil content, castile soaps will wash and condition your hair. Alternatively, use a pure vegetable-oil soap (these can usually only be found at specialist suppliers). These types of soaps can also be used on the body, saving you money as well as being safer.

DANDRUFF SHAMPOOS

Dandruff shampoos are made with detergents to which antiflaking agents such as *coal tar*, zinc pyrithizone, *salicylic acid* and *selenium sulphide* are added. While they can relieve itching and decrease flaking, no dandruff shampoo can control dandruff completely.

Sulphur and salicylic acid work by breaking the flakes into smaller, less noticeable pieces. It is thought that coal tar, selenium sulphide and zinc pyrithizone can slow the production of flakes. Beyond this, little is known of how, exactly, antidandruff shampoos work.

Of all the antiflaking agents, zinc pyrithizone and coal tar are considered to be the most effective for controlling dandruff.

All antiflaking agents have some side-effects. They can be irritating to both the skin and eyes. In particular, salicylic acid, an ingredient of aspirin, can be severely irritating and is poisonous if swallowed. Coal tar is a known carcinogen, and can be an irritant when inhaled or when it comes into contact with skin.

▶ TRY THIS INSTEAD ...

Dandruff is caused by a fungus, and is most effectively treated from within. Effective dietary measures include cutting out sugar and yeasty foods, supplementing with B-complex vitamins and probiotics (*acidophilus* and *bifidobacteria*), and making sure that you drink plenty of water each day.

Externally, a more natural alternative is to make an effective antidandruff lotion with 1 tsp each of rosemary and thyme essential oils, mixed into 100 ml (3.5 fl oz) of apple juice and 2 tbsp (30 ml) of cider vinegar. Apply this at bedtime or on days when you can let your hair dry naturally to help keep dandruff at bay.

CONDITIONERS

Have you ever noticed how shampoo bottles always recommend that you use a conditioner afterwards? This is because the detergents used in shampoos are often so harsh that you need to use a conditioner to repair some of the damage done by their use. Healthy hair rarely needs conditioning. Hair damaged by detergent use (and other assaults) almost always does.

All shampoos, no matter how 'mild', will strip away the protective layer of sebum (natural oils produced by the scalp) that coats your hair. Stripping the sebum away exposes the outside layer of the hair, known as the cuticle. The cuticle is made up of translucent overlapping cells that are arranged like the shingles on a roof. When these cells are disturbed, they can rub against each other and become damaged, resulting in the social horror of flyaway hair. Stripping away the sebum also leaves the cuticle (the inner part of the hair shaft) vulnerable to damage from other chemicals used on the hair.

Many shampoos contain conditioning agents that smooth down the cuticle and cover it with a synthetic version of sebum.

Conditioners, whether used separately or incorporated into your regular shampoo, do not repair hair. They cannot penetrate the hair shaft and make it stronger. Instead, they coat the hair with chemicals that temporarily glue the damaged hair shaft down – giving the illusion of healthier hair.

A typical hair conditioner will contain *triethanolamine* (TEA), film-formers like *polyvinylpyrrolidone* (PVP), various silicones such as *dimethicone*, humectants like *propylene glycol* and *glycerin*, *quaternium compounds*, preservatives like *DMDM hydantoin*, *disodium EDTA*, *methylchloroisothiazolinone* and *methylisothiazolinone*, and *parfum*.

▶ TRY THIS INSTEAD ...

The most sensible alternative is not to use a conditioner at all. You can see from the examples above that many shampoos (even the ones that are not specifically 'conditioning' shampoos) contain some conditioning ingredients. If you follow the advice for using or making milder shampoos, you shouldn't need a conditioner.

If you do continue to use conventional conditioners, once again, the best advice is to use less. You can do this in two ways: first, only use a conditioner once or twice a week; or second, put less on your hair at each washing. This can be hard to do straight from the bottle, so try diluting it instead. To do this, half fill a well-rinsed conditioner bottle with regular conditioner, then top it up with water. Shake before use.

Alternatively, consider these more basic options:

Regular trimming, and keeping the use of hair-destroying things like rollers, curling irons, hairdryers and lots of drying styling gels to a minimum will also help keep hair looking good.

Condition before you wash. Contrary to what we have been encouraged to do, this is the best way to keep hair soft and manageable. Rubbing good-quality oil through your hair a half-hour or so before you shampoo or, better still, at night before bed will provide the same conditioning action as the hazardous ingredients in your usual conditioner.

Good choices for conditioning oils include olive oil for deep conditioning and coconut, jojoba or almond oil for light-to-medium conditioning. Add 2 tbsp of honey to 100 ml (3.5 fl oz) oil to help 'repair' split ends. Leave on for half an hour before shampooing.

After shampooing, rinse with diluted cider vinegar (which is pH neutral) to remove detergent deposits and lightly condition the hair.

Styling products

Most hairstyling products are used to make up for poor-quality haircuts and the damage caused by year after year of abusive practices such as harsh shampoos, hairdryers, heated rollers and styling wands.

Like shampoos, many of us tend to collect half-used pots, tubes and bottles of the stuff – a good indication that they never quite do what they are supposed to. Apart from poor performance, most styling products contain dubious chemicals, which your hair, skin and lungs would be better off without.

HAIRSPRAY

Hairspray is essentially plastic dissolved in a solvent and put into a pressurised can or pump spray. It works by gluing strands of hair together so that they form a stronger structure that can then hold a style. Recently, it has been reported that hairspray also contains **phthalates** – hormone-disrupting chemicals which are used to keep plastics soft and pliable.

Many women find it hard to believe that hairspray is just liquid plastic. If you are one of them, try this test. Spray your usual hairspray onto your bathroom mirror and leave it to dry. If you spray a thick-enough layer, you should be able to peel it off in a single sheet. But even if you don't, you will be able to scrap off little shavings of plastic – the same stuff that you deposit on your hair and into your lungs each time you use hairspray.

Hairspray also contains ingredients such as **alcohol (denatured)**, **dimethyl ether**, **VA/vinyl butyl benzoate/crotonates copolymer**, **aminomethyl propanol**, **cyclopentasiloxane**, **dimethicone copolyol**, **PPG-3 methyl ether** and **parfum**.

Perhaps unsurprisingly, there is a medical condition known as hairdresser's lung – a respiratory disease that is caused by chronic exposure to hairspray. Even though the average consumer is unlikely to develop this disease, using hairspray regularly can do other nasty things to your health. Your nose is lined with tiny hairs that filter out dirt and pollution from the air you breathe. When hairspray gets into your nose and onto these little hairs, they become sticky and begin to attract and trap dust and pollution until they become saturated with dirt – at which point, they can no longer filter pollutants effectively.

Other distressing side-effects of hairspray use include nail abnormalities. When you spray and then style your hair using your fingers, the spray is deposited on your nails, where it can cause the new nail to grow poorly or predispose it to infection. Breathing difficulties and contact dermatitis after hairspray use are also common complaints.

HAIR GEL

Like hairspray, hair gel is a type of resin or plastic. Hair gels are generally more concentrated than hairsprays, which is why you can use them to make your hair stay in so many different gravity-defying shapes. Common ingredients include *polyvinylpyrrolidone* (PVP), PVP/dimethyl-aminoethylmethacrylate copolymer, *laureth*-23, *triiso-propanolamine*, *carbomer*, methicone copolymer, polyquaternium-4, *propylene glycol*, preservatives such as *parabens*, *DMDM hydantoin*, *disodium EDTA*, *diazolidinyl urea*, *phenoxyethanol*, *parfum* and even synthetic colours.

▶ TRY THIS INSTEAD ...

Apart from not using it, there are very few alternatives to things like hairspray and gel. The best alternative is to stop buying hairstyling products and use the money you save on getting a really good haircut. With well-cut hair, you shouldn't need to apply lots of glue to keep your hair in place. Do this, and you may find that you and your hair live happily ever after.

Try reserving the use of hairsprays and gels for when you really need them, like on special occasions, when you need your hair to stay in place. In addition, when purchasing hairsprays, gels and other styling agents:

Read the label. Try to buy products with the fewest and least toxic ingredients.

Use pump sprays in favour of aerosols. You are still at risk of inhaling the noxious chemicals in the mixture, but you will be avoiding inhaling toxic propellants as well – a small step in the right direction.

HAIR DYES

In a culture obsessed with youth and beauty, grey hairs are the enemy, and today's hair dyes are marketed as being as good for your self-esteem as they

Hair today, gone tomorrow

Depilatories, which come in gels, creams, lotions, aerosols and roll-ons, are chemical razor blades. Usually, they contain a highly alkaline chemical such as *calcium thioglycolate* that dissolves the protein structure of the hair, causing it to separate from the skin surface. The problem is that skin and hair are similar in their composition. What damages one can also damage the other. For this reason, if you use depilatory creams, it is especially important to follow the directions, not leave them on for too long and not reapply them too regularly.

are for your hair. But, underneath the advertising hype is a disturbing amount of data linking regular hair dye use with a range of different cancers.

To achieve luscious shades of chestnut brown, coppery red, mahogany or black, permanent hair dyes must first chemically damage your hair. Under a microscope, the cuticle of human hair looks like overlapping fish scales. The pigment molecules that give hair its colour are stored in the central cortex of the hair, beneath the scaly layer. Before the colour can penetrate the hair shaft, the cuticle must be 'opened' so that the chemicals can get into the natural pigment molecules.

Permanent hair dyes consist of two components: colour and developer. The colour component usually contains a range of synthetic dyes and intermediates such as **ammonia, diaminobenzenes, phenylenediamines, resorcinol** and **phenols.**

Mixed with the developer – usually **hydrogen peroxide** – the colour component begins to oxidise to produce a particular colour. The ammonia in the mix causes the hair shaft to swell, forcing the cuticles apart and allowing the mix to deposit the new colour underneath. The process of oxidation takes time, which is why the formula usually looks one colour when you first apply it and another when you rinse it off.

Toxic ingredients like **diaminotoluene** and diaminoanisole were removed from hair dye products some 20 years ago, but it is likely that a heavy past use of dyes containing these chemicals is the cause of some cases of breast cancer today. But a quick scan of the label on most hair dyes reveals that they still contain chemicals, most commonly **phenylenedi-amines**, that are just as harmful. The type of phenylenediamine used depends on the end colour, thus:

- para-phenylenediamine (black)
- para-toluenediamine (brown)
- ortho-phenylenediamine (brown)
- para-aminophenol (reddish-brown)
- ortho-aminophenol (light brown).

Other hair dye ingredients that have proven carcinogenic in at least one animal species include: **4-chloro-m-phenylenediamine, 2,4-toluenediamine, 2-nitro-p-phenylenediamine** and **4-amino-2-nitrophenol. Coal-tar** dyes have also been found to cause cancer in laboratory animals, yet no warning is required for these either.

These ingredients and their variations (usually HCl or hydrochloride, or sulphates such as para-phenylenediamine sulphate) are powerful irritants, and have been implicated in severe allergic reactions (phenylenediamines are also mutagenic, causing DNA mutations and foetal abnormalities in animals). Other irritant ingredients include **hydrogen peroxide, resorcinol** and 1-naphthol. Hair dye sold in the EU containing any of these ingredients should carry a warning: *Can cause an allergic reaction. Do not use to colour eyelashes or eyebrows.*

In the US, products containing 4-methoxy-m-phenylenediamine (4-MMPD, 2,4-diaminoanisole) must also carry a warning: *Contains an ingredient that can penetrate your skin and has been determined to cause cancer in laboratory animals.* However, no such warning is required for this ingredient in the EU.

Other hair dye ingredients such as chlorides are highly irritating to the mucous membranes. Chloride fumes can irritate the lungs and eyes, and cause burns or rashes on the skin. Hair colours also contain several penetration enhancers known to aid the absorption of other toxic chemicals into the bloodstream. These can include **propylene glycol, polyethylene glycol**, fatty acids such as **oleic, palmitic** and **lauric acid**, and isopropyl alcohol to name but a few.

More cancer

Both human and animal studies show that the body rapidly absorbs the carcinogens and other chemicals found in permanent and semi-permanent dyes through the skin during the more than 30 minutes that dyes remain on the scalp. So, if you use permanent, semi-permanent, shampoo-in or temporary hair colours, you are increasing your risk of developing cancer.

Problems with hair dyes were first noted in the late 1970s, when several studies found links between the use of hair dyes and breast cancer. In 1976, one study reported that 87 out of 100 breast-cancer patients had been long-term hair dye users.

In 1979, another study found a significant relationship between the frequency and duration of hair dye use and breast cancer. Women who started dying their hair at age 20 had twice the risk of 40-year-olds. Those at greatest risk were the 50 to 79-year-olds who had been dying their hair for years, suggesting that the cancer takes years to develop.

A year later, another study found that women who dye their hair to change its colour, rather than masking greyness, were at a threefold risk of developing breast cancer.

Research continued and, in the early 1990s, Japanese and Finnish studies also linked hair dye use with breast cancer. More recently, a jointly funded American Cancer Society and FDA study found a fourfold increase in relatively uncommon cancers, including non-Hodgkin's lymphoma (NHL) and multiple myeloma, among hair dye users.

A more recent Harvard study suggested that, compared with women who never dyed their hair, women who dyed their hair one to four times a year had a 70-per-cent greater risk of ovarian cancer. Women who used hair dye five times or more per year had twice the risk of developing ovarian cancer compared with women who never did so.

As if this wasn't enough, a study in the February 2001 edition of the *International Journal of Cancer* found a link between long-term hair dye use and an increased incidence of bladder cancer.

But it is the link with otherwise uncommon cancers that causes the greatest concern, and may well be the best evidence of hair dye toxicity.

Evidence suggests, for example, that if you use hair dye, you may be increasing your risk of NHL and multiple myeloma by anywhere from two to four times over that of a non-user. Some researchers even believe that hair dyes may account for as many as 20 per cent of all cases of NHL in women.

Other data from the US National Cancer Institute (NCI) shows that women who used permanent hair dyes had a 50-per-cent higher risk of developing NHL and an 80-per-cent higher risk of multiple myeloma than non-users.

In this NCI study, other cancer risk-factors, such as a family history of cancer, cigarette-smoking, and herbicide or pesticide exposure, did not change the risks calculated for hair dye use. However, the risk increased with the number of years of use, and for women using black, brown or red colouring products.

As a general rule, the darker the shade of the dye, the higher the risk of breast cancer; thus, women who use black, dark-brown or red dyes are at the greatest risk.

In all fairness, there are problems with studies into hair dye and cancer risk. Some involved small numbers of women who worked in the cosmetics industry. Historically, this group of women are exposed to the known carcinogens in hair dyes – *diaminotoluene*, diaminoanisole and *phenylenediamines*, *coal-tar* dyes, the *dioxane* found in detergents, solvents, nitrosamines and *formaldehyde*-releasing preservatives – in much greater concentrations than the rest of us. However, taken together, they do point towards an increased overall risk that may be unacceptable.

Men are at risk, too

While women were once the main users of hair dyes, use among men has increased dramatically in the last few decades and, with it, the incidence of rare cancers. According to the NCI, hair dye use is responsible for a 90-per-cent increased risk of multiple myeloma among men.

This result echoed that of an earlier NCI study, which showed that men who had used hair dyes had a twofold risk for NHL and almost double the risk of leukaemia.

No problem?

Hair dye manufacturers continue to defend the safety of their products, suggesting that any risk is 'minimal'. It is true that some studies dispute the cancer risk. One, which involved 1500 male and female hair dye users in San Francisco, found no increased incidence of NHL. The weight of the evidence, however, suggests a need for caution.

One difficulty is that there are large variations in the chemical content of hair dyes. This means that, when an association is found, it is difficult to know which ingredient or mix of ingredients is the culprit. In addition, cancer is a slow-developing disease in humans. By the time it surfaces, it is difficult to prove beyond a shadow of a doubt that one particular exposure was the cause. This is, of course, good news for manufacturers, who can continue to produce potentially toxic products with impunity and without risk of litigation – but bad news for the rest of us.

▶ TRY THIS INSTEAD ...

If you intend to keep dyeing your hair, consider these safer options:

Read the label. If you dye your hair, use the safer alternatives that are currently on the market. These should not contain phenylenediamines (though many so-called natural hair colours do). Never buy products that are in any way unclear about their ingredients.

Read the label again. This time look for dyes. Avoid products which use colours like Acid Orange 87, Solvent Brown 44, Acid Blue 168 and Acid Violet 73, as these are also carcinogenic.

Don't dye your hair too often. Leave the maximum amount of time between applications.

Leave hair dyes on the head for the minimum required time.

Hair colourants made entirely from plant-based ingredients are the safest choice; however, these are few and far between. Pure herbal hair dyes will need to be left in the hair significantly longer then synthetic dyes, but have the advantage of conditioning the hair while they colour.

> **Go natural.** In a world of look-alike bleached blondes and unnaturally red redheads, you'll probably be the standout.

■ MAKE-UP

Many women would argue that make-up is just a bit of fun – a harmless pleasure that makes them feel good about themselves. But the make-up which women put on their faces each day – and wear for long hours at a time – is anything but a benign enhancement to beauty.

There is nothing unique about the ingredients in your favourite make-up. On the whole, these will be exactly the same as the ingredients in your face cream, and bath and hair products.

By the time a woman has made-up her face, she has covered her skin in *mineral oil*, a carcinogen, and preservatives such as *parabens* (a sensitiser and oestrogen disrupter), *Kathon CG* (a sensitiser, mutagen and suspected carcinogen) and *diazolidinyl urea* (another sensitiser). She will also have exposed herself to synthetic colours, many of which are known carcinogens and allergens; fragrance, the ingredients of which are sensitisers, central-nervous-system disrupters and carcinogens; plasticisers such as *polyvinylpyrrolidone* (PVP), also a carcinogen; surfactants such as *tri-ethanolamine*; film-formers such as *dimethicone* and *polytetrafluoroeth-ylene* (PTFE, or Teflon); *talc*, which is carcinogenic when inhaled and commonly contaminated with heavy metals such as lead, and poisons such as *arsenic*; synthetic waxes derived for petroleum (also potentially carcino-genic); and sunscreens, which are sensitisers as well as oestrogen mimics.

Preservatives

In addition to parabens and Kathon CG (the risk of which are detailed elsewhere in this chapter), most types of make-up also contain the preser-vative *butylated hydroxyanisole* (BHA) – a chemical that is easily absorbed into the skin and which has been designated a human carcinogen by the US National Toxicology Program.

Eye make-up, especially mascara, can sometimes contain mercury-based preservatives such as *phenylmercuric acetate* and *thimerosal* (the same controversial preservative used in childhood vaccines). These are toxic and damaging to the eye. Mercury-based preservatives can also be found in a wide range of toiletries, including soap-free cleansers, antiseptic sprays, make-up remover and eye moisturisers.

Thimerosal is not always listed on the label by that name, but may instead be called by any of its many synonyms, including mercurochrome, merthiolate, sodium ethylmercurithiosalicylate, thimerosalate, thiomeros-alan, merzonin, mertorgan, ethyl (2-mercaptobenzoato-S), mercury sodium salt, merfamin or [(o-carboxyphenyl)thi] ethylmercury sodium salt. A glance at this complicated list, and it's easy to see how the use of mercury in a product used on the eyes has escaped the attention of the vast majority of us.

Carcinogens

Liquid formulas like foundations are prey to the same problems as shampoos and other toiletries. That is, they often contain the same carcinogenic nitrosamines found in shampoos and foam baths. The longer the product has been on the shelf, the higher the risk of nitrosamine formation. Mascara – especially those that promise to extend lashes – can contain any number of carcinogenic plasticisers, including polyurethane.

Another common ingredient, *silica*, is usually touted as a natural skin-enhancing mineral – in spite of the fact that cosmetic silica is synthesised in the lab. In 2000, crystalline silica (sometimes called crystalline quartz, the same ingredient found in cat litter and scouring powders) was added to the National Toxicology Program's list of carcinogens.

While silica can be used in any cosmetic formulation, it is the easily inhaled powdered products such as face powder and eyeshadow that are the most risky. The concern here is that the amorphous hydrated form of silica commonly used in cosmetics can be contaminated with carcinogenic crystalline quartz. However, it is impossible to tell which silica-containing products are contaminated in this way, so using any silica-containing product is a game of chance.

Most make-up, even powder formulas, contains some form of mineral oil. Mineral oil is what binds powders together, and also provides the basis for liquid formulations and lipsticks. Mineral oils were first recognised as carcinogens in 1987. Listed as *paraffinum liquidim* (the stuff that baby oil is made from) or *petrolatum* (petroleum jelly), these highly refined oils have a chequered history. Mineral oils are also thought to increase the photosensitivity of the skin, making it more prone to sun-induced damage and skin cancer.

Because the mineral oils used in cosmetics are highly refined, scientists cannot say conclusively how dangerous they are to humans. The thinner the oil, as in *paraffinum liquidim*, the more risky they are thought to be because of the high levels of volatile hydrocarbons that thin oils contain. The National Toxicology Program's Ninth Report on Carcinogens notes that analyses of mineral oils used for medicinal and cosmetic purposes reveal the presence of several carcinogenic hydrocarbons known as polycyclic aromatic hydrocarbons. These include benzo[b]fluoranthene, benzo[k]fluoranthene and benzo[a]pyrene.

Toxic metals

Amazingly, cosmetics can also contain toxic metals, most commonly as contaminants in pigments and talc. One Finnish study that looked at 88 brands of eyeshadow found that 75 per cent of the products tested contained detectable levels of at least one of the following elements: lead, cobalt, nickel, chromium and arsenic.

In this investigation, the elements found in the cosmetics were impurities in the ingredients rather than listed ingredients – a problem seen in many cosmetics. While the researchers felt that, in most cases, these levels were not enough to cause allergic reactions, another study in the UK found that chronic exposures to very low levels of arsenic – lower than those in the Finnish study – were capable of causing hormonal disruption.

Colours

Most of us would avoid foods that contain artificial colours. Yet, each day, women paint their faces with a range of artificial colours known to cause health problems in both the short and long term.

Artificial colours may be carcinogens (indeed, all coal-tar dyes are considered carcinogenic); others may contain hidden carcinogenic impurities in some batches, but not in others, depending on the source of the raw materials. What's more, contact dermatitis and irritation can also be caused by cosmetic pigments such as artificial colours.

Checking for harmful dyes in cosmetics is a complex business, made more difficult by the fact that, in Europe, these colours are usually listed by their INCI (International Nomenclature for Cosmetic Ingredients) numbers – usually 'CI' followed by five numbers. (This, in turn, is different again from the name given to the same ingredient when used as a food colouring, when it's usually an 'E' followed by a number; see table, below.)

New colours are being developed all the time, but not with an eye on safety. For example, one of the newest – FD&C Red 40 (also known as Allura Red, CI16035 and, in foods, as E129) – is a popular addition to eye-shadows. It was approved and has been in use since 1994 despite the fact that the safety testing was all funded and performed by the manufacturer. Nevertheless, the National Cancer Institute reports that p-credine, a chemical used in the manufacturing of FD&C Red 40 is a carcinogen.

Certain carcinogenic colours are now banned from use in both US and European cosmetics; these include D&C Red 2, 3, 4, 10 and 17, FD&C Red 10

Common name	US	Europe	E number
Alizarin Cyanine Green F	D&C Green 5	CI61570	-
Pigment Orange 5	D&C Orange 17	CI12075	-
Rhodamine B	D&C Red 19	CI45170	-
Acid Red 33	D&C Red 33	CI17200	-
Pigment Red 53 sodium salt	D&C Red 8	CI15585	-
Pigment Red 53 barium salt	D&C Red 9	CI15585	-
Acetate Blue G	Disperse Blue 1	CI64500	-
Acetate Fast Yellow G	Disperse Yellow 3	CI11855	-
Brilliant Blue FCF	FD&C Blue 1	CI42090	E133
Indigo Carmine	FD&C Blue 2	CI73015	E132
Fast Green FCF	FD&C Green 3	CI42053	E143
Ponceau SX	FD&C Red 4	CI14700	E124
Allura Red	FD&C Red 40	CI16035	E129
Tartrazine	FD&C Yellow 5	CI19140	E102
Sunset Yellow	FD&C Yellow 6	CI15985	E110
Titanium dioxide	Pigment White 6	CI77891	E171

and FD&C Blue 4. Nevertheless, these still regularly appear in cosmetics that have been illegally imported from other countries.

While a single use of a single make-up product may be 'safe', your total daily exposure of all coloured products – soaps, shampoos, conditioners, shaving cream, toothpaste and deodorants (and don't forget juices, cereals, pastries, coffee creamer and even vitamins) – may add up to an unacceptable risk.

▶ TRY THIS INSTEAD ...

When it comes to make-up, it may be a case of choosing your poison carefully. If the rest of your lifestyle is relatively toxin-free, the appropriate use of well-chosen make-up may not add significantly to your total toxic load. When you buy or use cosmetics, follow these simple guidelines to help you choose the safest ones.

Start on the inside. Beauty really does come from within. It starts with a nutritious diet, adequate rest and periodic breaks from stress. Without these basics, no make-up in the world will make you look beautiful.

Read the label. It is essential to get into the habit of looking at the ingredients in your cosmetics. Do not rely on claims of 'all natural', 'organic' or 'cruelty-free'. These claims are meaningless. The only thing that tells the true story of the cosmetic is the ingredients list. Once you have identified an ingredient or ingredients that you wish to avoid, keep its name on a card or list that you can take with you when you shop. Remember also that price is no guarantee of safety or quality. Sometimes the cheaper brands contain fewer toxic ingredients. Only the label will tell you for sure.

But also, don't put too much faith in the label. Don't just buy a product because it was safe last time you looked. By the time you are ready to replace your eyeshadow or lipstick, it may be made from completely different ingredients. Manufacturers are continually reformulating their products, often according to what ingredients are available and least expensive at the time. In addition, many ingredients labels – for instance, those used on eyeshadows and lipsticks – list the colours for the entire range rather than the specific product you are buying. For these reasons, some products say 'may include ...' or the symbol '+/-' before a list of ingredients, making it impossible to make sensible choices about safety.

Avoid cosmetics that are pearly, glittery, opalescent or frosted. These are among the most dangerous since, to achieve this effect, manufacturers add ingredients such as pure aluminium, mica and even fish scales. Used near the eye, these particles can flake off and cause corneal damage. Ingested aluminium, in particular, is linked to Alzheimer's disease. Stick to matte colours, blot well and shine up your lips with a over- or undercoat of shea butter or natural oils.

Choose lip gloss (which has a lower volume of colouring ingredients) rather than lipstick for everyday wear, *but be aware*. Conventional lip glosses contain less colour, but are high in phenol, a poisonous substance that is easily absorbed into the delicate tissue of the lips (aided by the addition of petrolatum, a petroleum-derived moisturiser, as well as other wetting agents). Phenol ingestion can cause nausea, vomiting, convulsions, paralysis, respiratory collapse and even death; minute amounts are linked to skin rashes, swelling, pimples and hives.

Seek 'safe' colours If you are looking for products with less harmful colours, one easy way to work your way through the maze is to remember that, in cosmetics, a number that begins with 'CI75' is considered a 'natural' colorant, even though some of these are highly synthesised. Anything else may be considered suspect. Those beginning with 'CI77' indicate an inorganic substance used as colouring (such as iron oxides and natural carbon, but more toxic aluminium and barium sulphate also fall into this category).

Avoid all perfumed cosmetics and especially avoid lip products with a sweet taste. Often, these include saccharin (a suspected carcinogen) and phthalic anhydride (made from another suspected carcinogen, naphthalene), an irritant that can cause headaches, nausea, vomiting, diarrhoea and confusion, and has been linked to kidney and brain damage in infants. All the more remarkable is that it is commonly used in 'play' and 'fun' make-up aimed at young girls.

Choose products without sunscreens. Chances are, you are wearing your make-up indoors anyway. Don't be fooled by claims of natural sunscreens. There is no such thing. The only effective sunscreens are synthetic chemicals that add to your toxic burden.

If you don't need to wear make-up, don't. Many women wear make-up for the most trivial occasions, a trip to the supermarket or bank, picking the kids up from school, weekends at home or walks in the park. Get out of the habit. Get used to the way you look without make-up, and give your skin and your system a break. If you can't stand to go out without something on your face, stick to the basics – a swipe of carefully chosen mascara and a bit of lipstick or gloss is fine for everyday wear.

■ SKIN CARE

Moisturisers are an integral part of many women's beauty routine. While most moisturisers promise miraculous effects, they really have just one basic function – to maintain the water balance in the most superficial layers of the skin. This area of the skin, known as the stratum corneum, is made up of cells that are being constantly shed and replaced by new cells emerging from the deeper layers of the skin.

The stratum corneum is approximately 30 per cent water. Two-thirds of this is bound to biological tissues and usually does not change unless there is a serious skin condition such as eczema or psoriasis. But the remaining water content rises and falls according to what's going on in the environment – for instance, dry weather conditions, overwashing, or exposure to central heating, air-conditioning and certain chemicals.

The word is misleading since 'moisturiser' would seem to indicate that it will put water into the skin. But no moisturiser, no matter how expensive or how many ingredients it contains, can do this. Even if your moisturiser could push water back into your skin, it would be quickly disseminated throughout the rest of your body rather than be held there for an indefinite period.

Moisturising ingredients work in two ways to help slow this water loss.

Humectants such as *propylene glycol*, *glycerin* and *urea* act like water magnets, drawing moisture from the atmosphere and keeping it near the skin.

Emollients are generally fats, oils and waxes that form a barrier on the surface of the skin. For years, moisturising creams and lotions relied on emollients like *lanolin* and mineral oil to produce this protective barrier. Today, synthetic derivatives of vegetable oils such as *isopropyl palmitate* and *hexyl laureate* are more common, as are a range of synthetic film-formers such as *dimethicone* and *Teflon* (PTFE or polytetrafluoroethylene).

Do they work?

Moisturisers are mixtures of oil and water and, to keep these two opposing substances bound together and to make sure the product has a long shelf life, a cream or lotion will contain a raft of emulsifiers, stabilisers and preservatives. To make it nice to use, it will also contain perfumes and colours. If the cream also claims other properties such as improving wrinkles, further ingredients are added.

So, what starts out as a simple emulsion quickly becomes a cocktail of harmful ingredients such as *paraffinum liquidum*, *triethanolamine*, *propylene glycol*, quaternium-15, *carbomer*, *dimethicone*, *trisodium EDTA*, BHA (*butylated hydroxyanisole*), *parabens* and *parfum*. The emollients in the mix also act like penetration enhancers – ingredients that aid the absorption of other more toxic substances into the skin and eventually the bloodstream.

Hardly surprising, then, that moisturising creams can and do cause problems like allergic reactions, skin irritation and contact dermatitis, characterised by redness, itching, burning and stinging sensations. Used over the long term, they can also create the very problem they are intended to solve by actually increasing water loss from the skin.

Toxic ingredients

Some moisturising ingredients can actually damage the skin. Humectants such as *alpha-hydroxy acids* (AHAs such as *lactic acid* or *glycolic acid*) act like chemical peels, thinning the stratum corneum and, ultimately, accelerating water loss. If your moisturiser includes fruit acids, or AHAs, it may cause premature ageing of your skin as well as increased susceptibility to damage from the sun's ultraviolet rays.

Many emollients trap dirt and sweat under the skin and some, like petrolatum, degrade the skin's natural protective barrier, making it more vulnerable to bacteria and viruses.

Film-forming ingredients like **Teflon** (*PTFE*) and **dimethicone** are now routinely added to body-care products without any comprehensive evaluation of their safety. Teflon contains the potential carcinogen PFOA (perfluorooctanoic acid), and some silicones are known tumour promoters, and accumulate in the liver and lymph nodes. Both are non-biodegradable.

Several of the ingredients commonly used in body lotions can make the skin more permeable, allowing more toxic ingredients to be absorbed into the body. There is also some evidence that moisturisers can make the skin more susceptible to damage caused by the synthetic detergents used in many facial and body-care products.

Particularly worrying are the newer moisturisers that make use of nanoparticles, which slip into the spaces between skin cells before releasing their active ingredients. No research has been conducted to show how much more of these substances is absorbed into the bloodstream with these particles so, if you want to avoid them, look for words like 'liposome' or 'nanosome' on the label.

While the cosmetics industry loudly trumpets the benefits of moisturisers, most of their effects are unsubstantiated and/or temporary. Healthy skin begins on the inside, and nothing you put on your skin will be as effective as sorting out your diet, your sleep, your stress levels and your environment. Unless you have an underlying skin condition that requires medical attention, you probably don't need a regular moisturiser.

BODY LOTIONS, OILS AND GELS

The ingredients of a typical body lotion are not much different from those of a hair conditioner. And basically, the two products perform the same function – replacing natural oils with synthetic ones, and then coating the skin with a thin waterproof layer.

While body oil may seem like a simpler alternative, many are based on mineral oil. Some, like baby oil, are 100 per cent **mineral oil** (parafinum liquidim), with added perfume.

Mineral oil, a byproduct of the distillation of gasoline from crude oil, impedes the skin's ability to breathe, attract moisture and detoxify. It can also slow down cell renewal and promote premature skin-ageing. While it is used for its lubricant qualities that, in the short term, appear to make the skin softer, when used over the longer term, mineral oil can make the skin dry out. This is because mineral oil dissolves the skin's natural oils, thereby increasing water loss (dehydration) from the skin.

Any mineral-oil derivative can be contaminated with cancer-causing *polycyclic aromatic hydrocarbons* (PAHs). Mineral oils may also increase the skin's sensitivity to sunlight, and have been linked to an increased risk of skin cancer. *Petrolatum*, paraffin or paraffin oil and *propylene glycol* are all forms of mineral oil.

Among women who regularly switch toiletry brands or try new products, mineral oils have been shown to be the major cause of new skin irritation, including rashes and spots. There is no good reason for this kind of suffering to take place.

Because of the risks of mineral oils, manufacturers have switched to silicone-based oils and gels.

Silicones such as *dimethicone* (or dimethiconol), *cyclomethicone*, *cyclopentasiloxane* and *cyclohexasiloxane* are synthesised from silicon metal to produce water-repellent 'dry' oils and waxes. They add many of the 'feel-good' qualities associated with modern body-care products such as texture, silkiness, lustre and smooth application.

Silicones come in many forms. Film-forming silicones add spreadability and smoothness as well as water-repellence to products such as facial cosmetics, lotions, creams, antiperspirants and deodorants. In cosmetics like lipsticks, eyeshadows and blushers, silicone resins and gums provide longevity to help the product stay on the skin, and maintain its colour; in hairstyling products, they improve control.

Used as surfactants and conditioners in hair products, silicones add foam stabilisation to add shine, body and softness to the hair. Volatile silicones (that is, those that evaporate quickly) make aesthetically pleasing and effective antiperspirants and deodorants that don't leave a residue. Highly reflective silicones enhance the shine of surfaces such as skin and hair.

Silicones are also widely used in household cleaning products (including laundry detergents, fabric softeners, polishes and waxes).

On the whole, silicones allow the skin to breathe better than mineral oils, but question marks still hang over their long-term safety. While they increase the feel-good factor of a product, they are poorly absorbed by the skin, which raises some doubt as to how well the ingredients suspended in them will be absorbed. Some, like *dimethicone*, are also cancer-causing suspects.

▶ TRY THIS INSTEAD ...

If you're going to continue to use commercial moisturising products, choose those with the fewest ingredients and watch out especially for those that may be contaminated with carcinogens. It's the oil and wax contents of moisturisers that hold moisture next to the skin, so why not consider simple vegetable oils to maintain the skin's suppleness. They will do the same job at a fraction of the price, and you'll have the advantage of knowing exactly what you are putting on your face.

If your skin is occasionally dry, consider using natural oils after bathing or washing to temporarily seal in moisture. Natural oils contain all the nutrients natural to the plant or animal from which they come. Many, such as jojoba and emu, are amazingly similar to the oils in human skin and, as such, are non-irritating, don't clog pores and are deeply nourishing.

Effective moisturisers can be prepared on an 'as needed' basis by almost anyone from a simple mixture of vegetable or biological oils (coconut, jojoba, almond or emu) and plant 'butters' (shea or mango), water and glycerine. With practice, these can be made to suit different areas of the body in response to the skin's seasonal needs (heavier oils in winter, lighter ones in summer).

- Almond oil
- Aloe vera
- Apricot kernel oil
- Avocado oil
- Beeswax
- Castor oil
- Cocoa butter
- Coconut oil

- Grapeseed oil
- Hempseed oil
- Honey
- Jojoba oil
- Macadamia nut oil
- Mango butter
- Olive oil
- Rosa mosqueta oil

- Emu oil
- Evening primrose oil
- Glycerine

- Shea butter
- Squalene
- Wheatgerm oil

As a general rule, use lighter oils such as apricot kernel, coconut or jojoba oil for normal skins, and heavier oils such as avocado and evening primrose oil for older or drier skins. Rosehip oil is also considered a rich and nourishing oil for the face.

FACE CREAMS

Skin has a life of its own that most of us never hear about. Getting in touch with its natural rhythms, rather than bullying it into submission with lots of creams and potions, is the most straightforward path to a better complexion.

Flip through any magazine or browse in any shop and you will be confronted with a bewildering array of products that promise great skin all day, every day. But perfect unchanging skin is only the preserve of celebrities and models, who inhabit a world of perpetually good lighting, professional make-up artists and PhotoShop.

In reality, skin is a mirror, reflecting and reacting to what you eat and drink, and your exposure to environmental pollutants, allergens, cosmetic irritants and the elements. How well you sleep and the stresses you are under are also relevant to the way your skin looks from day to day.

In real people, it is in the nature of healthy, normal skin to change on almost an hourly basis. Studies show, for instance, that:

- Production of new skin cells is highest at midnight and lowest at noon.

- Oil production in the skin is twice as high at noon than it is at 2 a.m.

- Your skin is more likely to absorb what you put onto it – for example, topical medications – at 4 p.m. than at 8 a.m.

- You're more likely to have an allergic skin reaction in the morning than later in the day.

Normal skin changes are not problems that need to be fixed, and there's no getting round the fact that if you want great skin, there are no shortcuts and no miracle products. Acknowledging this means that you can stop obsess-

Hand and nail creams

Like body oils and lotions, hand and nail creams are essentially mineral oil-based. There is little difference between the ingredients of most body lotions and those that are supposed to be specifically for the hands, although hand creams tend to have even more emollients in them. Hands become dry and cracked because they are more exposed to the elements and more in use than almost any other part of the body. You also wash your hands more often, and expose them to detergents and other cleaning products more frequently every day as well.

While not as thin as facial skin, the skin on your hands is still thin enough to allow the penetration of noxious chemicals. To keep them soft and to avoid absorbing chemicals into your body, always use gloves when doing cleaning jobs, and substitute vegetable oils and vegetable oil-based creams for petroleum-based ones.

ing over the most minute and transient shifts in skin tone and colour, and adopt a more sensible approach to skincare that works from the inside out.

Adjusting your lifestyle to include sleeping longer, eating better, drinking more water and exercising more at different times of the month can help mitigate some of the natural changes that take place at skin level. But ultimately, accepting and working with these may make the difference between being at war, or making peace, with the way you look.

In spite of the fact that good skin begins on the inside, the skincare market is overflowing with choices that promise to keep you young and wrinkle-free as well as removing dirt, oil and make-up.

WRINKLE CREAMS

How skin ages is a complicated process that involves internal and external factors, some of which are within our control, but many of which are not.

Ageing causes decreases in collagen and elastin, the 'scaffolding' of the skin, causing the skin to wrinkle and sag. Gravity can also make loose skin around the eyes and jowls sag even more. Aged skin also appears more translucent because of the reduction in the number of pigment-containing cells (melanocytes). It is also thinner and more fragile, and at an increased risk of injury while being less able to repair itself. Your genetic inheritance is also influential, as are hormonal changes at menopause, although human studies have failed to conclusively link oestrogen decline and wrinkly skin.

An unhealthy lifestyle will also be reflected in your skin's condition. Prematurely ageing skin often mirrors the body's inefficiency in eliminating toxins and waste products. Addressing the source of the problem – for instance, through diet (see box, page 166) – rather than simply relying on topical creams and lotions is always advisable.

It has long been believed that sun exposure is the single biggest external cause of wrinkles. But is this true? Excess sun exposure can generate skin-damaging free radicals, leading to 'photoageing'. Ultraviolet-A (UVA) exposure is believed to be particularly harmful as it leads to the breakdown of the skin's collagen fibres.

But it can be difficult to differentiate between genetically normal wrinkles and those caused by the sun. In addition, a recent study challenged the received wisdom by suggesting that people with very wrinkled faces were 90 per cent less likely to get basal-cell carcinoma (BCC), the most common form of skin cancer, even though they had the same amount of sun exposure as cancer victims.

The key is the way that older, smooth skin repairs itself – by stimulating the production of transforming growth factor (TGF)-beta which, in turn, suppresses the immune system and promotes blood-vessel growth, both of which are risk factors for cancer. If confirmed, this would quash the broadly accepted idea that wrinkling is an indicator of sunlight-induced damage and, therefore, of skin-cancer risk.

Smoking also increases the breakdown of collagen as well as dries out the skin and reduces circulation, thus depleting the skin of oxygen and essential nutrients. Smoking may also lower levels of skin-protective vitamin A. Research shows that smoking 20 cigarettes a day for just a few years is equivalent to almost 10 years of chronological ageing – a much greater rate of damage then lifelong sun exposure.

Do wrinkle creams cause wrinkles?

Many women who scan food labels for harmful additives unthinkingly use toiletries that contain undesirable chemicals, believing that what we put on our bodies is not as influential to health as what we put in them.

Yet, facial skin is thinner than skin elsewhere, and may absorb toxic chemicals (such as petroleum byproducts, carcinogens such as nitrosamines and *formaldehyde*, solvents and oestrogenic preservatives such as *parabens*) at a much greater rate.

Our sun phobia means that it can be very difficult to find a commercial moisturiser that doesn't come with a sunscreen. Even some night creams now contain sunscreening agents! But increasingly, sun creams are being blamed for making us vulnerable to skin cancer. What's more, if you work outdoors, you will probably need more protection than a moisturising cream can give whereas, if you work in an office all day, an added sunscreen is just another unnecessary chemical.

In the attempt to look younger, many women remove the superficial layers of their skin with harsh exfoliants and chemical peels such as *alpha-hydroxy acids*, *glycolic*, *hydroxycaprylic* or *lactic acid*, passion-flower or citrus extract. Widely believed to improve the appearance of sun damage, offer UV protection and heal sunburnt skin, recent evidence suggests, however, that these chemicals and the products that contain them can actually cause premature ageing as well as increased UV susceptibility.

Better alternatives

Even among the many so-called natural alternatives, there are very few skincare products with documented scientific evidence of benefits. Most claims made in marketing these products are based on animal studies and the 'science' of guesswork.

The most important factor in a skin cream is its ability to moisturise. Mineral oils (*paraffinum liquidum*, *petrolatum*) have been largely abandoned in favour of semi-synthetic lipids (fats and oils) and their constituents, including ceramide, *hyaluronic acid*, cholesterol, triglycerides, *phospholipids* and *glycerin*. Synthetic humectants (ingredients which draw water to the skin) include *propylene glycol* and *glycerin* (which can be animal or vegetable in origin). Many also include silicones (*dimethicone* and various siloxanes).

Natural vegetable oils are more compatible with the skin, much less drying than mineral oils and better absorbed than either mineral oil or silicones. Good examples include almond, coconut, jojoba, soya, carrot, wheatgerm, macadamia, olive and avocado oils. Some animal-derived oils such as squalene and emu also make good alternatives. These oils are more than just vehicles for other ingredients; they often have skin-boosting qualities of their own – for instance, they are high in essential fatty acids, and vitamins A, D and E. These fatty acids temporarily strengthen cell membranes, slowing down the formation of fine lines and wrinkles, and helping the skin to resist attack from free radicals. Beeswax and soya wax are good alternatives to silicones, while vegetable glycerine and honey are effective, natural humectants.

Added antioxidants may also help. A handful of studies suggest that coenzyme-Q10 (ubiquinone) smoothes wrinkles, although published research in this area is scant.

Vitamin E, either as alpha-tocopherol or as a tocotrienol, is an antioxidant that, added to a cream, can help prolong the product's shelf life. Some studies suggest it can also help to smooth superficial wrinkles if it is used continuously.

Vitamins C and E in combination probably work best against UVB damage. Vitamin E also can work synergistically with carotenoids. Other UV-protective nutrients (in the lab and in animals) include selenium, Ginkgo biloba extract and aloe vera.

Alpha-lipoic acid (ALA) scavenges both water and fat-soluble free radicals, sparing levels of vitamin C and E in the skin. ALA is rapidly available to skin cells and may also have some UV-protecting properties.

Many plant extracts, including those from cocoa and green tea as well as rosehip oil and horsetail, are also antioxidant.

MORE STUFF FOR YOUR FACE

The amount of stuff we put on our faces is simply staggering, and since facial skin is thinner than skin elsewhere, the potential for absorbing toxic chemicals is much greater. While most skincare products promise to help us look younger, prolonged use can dry and age the skin considerably. It may not show when you start using it at age 24, but by the time you are 54, the damage will be noticeable and mostly irreversible.

Acne treatments Teenagers often use products that boast antibacterial properties believing that they contain some sort of magic that will wash away spots. They won't.

Skin food

Diet can significantly affect the skin and its tendency to wrinkle. Researchers from Monash University in Australia studied the diets of 453 people (aged 70 years and over from Australia, Greece and Sweden) to find out if particular foods either predicted or were associated with skin-wrinkling. The findings strongly suggest that a high intake of fruit, vegetables and fish as well as certain healthy fats can reduce skin wrinkling.

FOODS THAT PROTECT AGAINST WRINKLES

- Higher total fat
- Monounsaturated fat
- Olive oil and olives
- Fish (especially fatty fish)
- Reduced fat milk and milk products
- Eggs
- Nuts and legumes (especially lima and broad beans)
- Vegetables (especially leafy greens, spinach, asparagus, aubergine, celery, onions, leeks and garlic)
- Wholegrain cereals
- Fruit and fruit products (especially prunes, cherries, apples and jams)
- Tea
- Water
- Zinc-containing foods (seafood, lean meat, milk and nuts).

FOODS THAT PROMOTE WRINKLES

- Saturated fat
- Meat (especially fatty processed meats)
- Full-fat dairy products (especially unfermented products and ice cream)
- Soft drinks and cordials
- Cakes, pastries and desserts
- Potatoes
- Butter
- Margarine

Typically, such products contain:

- **Harsh detergent/surfactants** such as *sodium laureth sulphate* (SLES), which can be contaminated with the carcinogen 1,4-dioxane, and/or the potential hormone disrupters *cocamide DEA* and *triethanolamine* (TEA).

- **PEG**, or polyethylene glycol, compounds are preservatives that can be contaminated with the carcinogen 1,4-dioxane. PEGs can also form carcinogens when mixed with DEA and TEA. *Pareth* is a surfactant that also belongs to the same family as PEG.

- *Phenoxyisopropanol* is an antibacterial agent, manufactured by combining carcinogenic phenol (*coal tar*) with the solvent *isopropanol*. It is an irritant, and allergic reactions are possible.

- *Carbomer* is a gelling agent that can be irritating to skin and eyes.

- *Parfum* does not clean the face, and can be a source of skin and airways irritation.

- **Colour** does not clean the skin, and is added only to appeal to the eye.

Cleansing lotions are often touted as a better way to clean make-up and grime from your face. Lotions and creams, we are told, can clean without stripping away the skin's natural oils (although products containing solvents will dissolve natural oils, usually replacing them with synthetic ones). The ingredients of most cleansing lotions are nearly indistinguishable from those of facial moisturisers. Moreover, even the simplest cleansing lotion can contain a range of suspect chemicals.

Liquid face washes are similar in their content to liquid body washes (see page 116), but contain slightly more water. Because liquids are more complex to make than solids, they generally contain more potentially harmful chemicals than detergent bars.

Exfoliating scrubs typically contain harsh detergents, emulsifiers and abrasives. An abrasive can be anything from ground fruit pits to talc to more worrying particles such as aluminium oxide. Others contain skin-drying agents such as alcohol. A simple face cloth will do the job just as well, so it's silly to invest in anything else. Exfoliants are a waste of money, may unnecessarily damage your skin through overenthusiastic use and will certainly add to your body's toxic burden.

Toners are now accepted as the necessary intermediate step between cleaning and moisturising. In fact, this step is an invention of the marketing world. Clean skin is as toned as it needs to be.

Many toners use *alcohol* to dry the skin and make it feel tighter. Others promise to close your pores, thus making your skin look younger and firmer. Unfortunately, your pore size is genetically determined, and pores neither open nor close. If they did, your face would wobble like a jelly throughout the day. What toner does is put astringent chemicals on your face to lower the skin temperature. This affects the underlying tissue that will temporarily contract, giving that characteristic 'tight' feeling which comes after using a toner.

▶ TRY THIS INSTEAD ...

Don't use special cleansers for your face – these are not much more than a mixture of dilute dish detergent and oil. Instead:

If you have spots, it's probably the result of hormones and a poor lifestyle. Getting plenty of sleep, drinking water rather than sodas, cutting down on the sugar and fat in your diet, investigating any food or other allergies (if the problem is really severe) and a little patience is the best way to tackle them.

Try to avoid liquid cleansers, which are more expensive and have more harsh chemicals in them.

Opt for glycerine-based soaps if you want to use a conventional bar – they are among the mildest.

Switch from detergent bars and cleansers to castile or pure vegetable oil soaps. These will clean your face and neck without stripping them completely of the skin's natural, beneficial and protective oils (and you won't need to invest in separate bars for your body and face either).

Whatever you use, remember to rinse well. Film left behind by neglectful rinsing can irritate the skin.

Forget about antibacterial cleaners. Simple soap and warm water are among the best antibacterials and the most effective ways to keep your face clean. They are also less expensive and unlikely to have as many suspect chemicals in them.

To remove make-up and city grime, use almond or jojoba oil on a cottonball, then rinse with warm water. Follow with a cool rinse or mild astringent such as witch hazel.

You can tone your face simply and easily by splashing cold water on it. If you absolutely need to buy something to 'tone' your skin, buy simple products like distilled witch hazel or try using a weak solution of cider vinegar in distilled water.

SHAVING CREAM

Wet-shaving with a blade is one of the oldest ways of removing unwanted hair (from any part of the body). There is now a wide variety of shaving creams or foams on the market for both men and women. They look nice, feel nice and some even smell nice. But they can contain some not-so-nice ingredients, for example: *triethanolamine* (TEA) and *lauramide DEA*, PEG-150 distearate, BHT and *imidazolidinyl urea*, *parabens*, quaternium-15, *paraffinum liquidum*, and propellants such as *isobutane* and *propane*.

▶ TRY THIS INSTEAD ...

A wet shave should be a *wet* shave. Getting the hair thoroughly wet before shaving means you can use less cream or foam to get the job done. Modern shaving creams are loaded with lubricants because most men and women skip the essential wetting part of the shave. In addition:

Use a shaving soap. It won't really be a soap (unless you buy it at a specialist natural healthcare shop), but a detergent bar. However, you will be able to avoid the problems associated with solvents and propellants found in shaving foams. Use a brush to get lots of foam unless you have very dry skin. The shaving brush may irritate dry skin, so soap up on your hands first before applying the foam to your skin.

Use shaving oil. More and more companies are making these nice oils that usually contain added essential oils to smooth and soothe the surface of the face while shaving. Opt for vegetable-oil bases rather than mineral oils.

Buy an electric shaver. The shave won't usually be so close, but it avoids a lot of unnecessary exposure to harsh chemicals.

SUN CREAMS

Sun exposure and the use of sunscreens is one of the most complex and contradictory areas of skin health. On the one hand, exposure to the fresh air and sun is vital for a healthy body. Sunlight, for example, is an important source of vitamin D, necessary for the development and maintenance of bones and teeth. But, at the same time, too much sun exposure can raise your risk of skin cancer.

Relying on sunscreens as your sole means of protection is fraught with problems since the protection they offer is never guaranteed. In addition, most commercial sun creams contain a mixture of harsh and harmful chemicals that come with their own risks. For example, some of the chemicals in sunscreens are thought to cause disruption or permanent damage to the nervous, immune and respiratory systems. Young children may be especially susceptible to sunscreen chemicals and their toxic side-effects. Among the most harmful are **benzophenones**, which can cause allergic reactions, and **PABAs**, which have been shown to form carcinogenic nitrosamines when mixed with other chemicals.

The effectiveness of any sun cream depends on its UV absorption, its concentration, formulation and ability to withstand swimming or sweating. As a general rule, the higher the sun protection factor (SPF), the greater the number of chemicals in a sun lotion or cream. It is not uncommon for sun creams to contain three or more sunscreen agents as well as perfumes, insect repellents and a host of other chemicals besides. Though many of the ingredients used in sunscreens have been tested individually, studies of the long-term effects of combinations of sunscreen agents, applied liberally over an extended period of time, are rare.

There are two main types of ultraviolet rays: UVA and UVB. The SPF factor in your sun cream is for UVB protection only. Most UVB rays are filtered out by the ozone layer. Those that do get through stimulate the skin's pigment to produce melanin, our natural defence against sunlight. UVA rays are not filtered out by the ozone layer and penetrate the skin at a deeper level, so they have the potential to cause more skin damage. Gauging UVA protection is a little more difficult, though most creams now put UVA information on their labels as well.

Some experts believe that, when exposed to UV rays, sunscreens like oxybenzone can break down into chemicals that destroy or inhibit the skin's own natural defences against sunlight. This leaves it vulnerable to damage by the free radicals produced by exposure to sunlight. Free radicals are the toxic byproducts of metabolism. Free-radical damage to the skin is implicated in skin cancer, premature ageing and other signs of damage to the skin.

Similarly, sunscreens such as *padimate-O* are thought to absorb harmful UV rays. But, as scientists point out, once absorbed, this energy has to be released somewhere – usually directly onto the skin, where it is metabolised into free radicals that can actually increase the risk of skin cancer.

What's in your sun cream?

There are two basic types of creams available on the market today: chemical sunscreens, which act by absorbing UV light; and chemical sunblocks, which reflect or scatter light in both the visible and UV spectrum. Both types are associated with skin irritation.

These are the most common chemical sunscreens:

- *Benzophenones* are common skin sensitisers that can provoke allergic reactions in some individuals. Common benzophenones include *oxybenzone*, *dioxybenzone* and *sulisbenzone*.

- *PABAs* are formaldehyde-forming chemicals that can form carcinogenic nitrosamines when combined with amines such as DEA, TEA and MEA in the mixture. PABAs can cause skin irritation. Common PABAs are p-aminobenzoic acid, *ethyl dihydroxypropyl PABA*, *padimate-O* (ocyl dimethyl PABA), *padimate-A* and *glyceryl PABA*.

- **Cinnamates** are common skin irritants. This group of chemicals includes *cinoxate*, *ethylhexyl-p-methoxycinnamate*, *octocrylene* and *ocytl methoxycinnamate*.

- *Salicylates* are also skin irritants associated with a high rate of dermatitis among users. Those commonly used in sun creams include *ethylhexyl salicylate*, *homosalate*, *octyl salicylate* and neo-homosalate.

- Other common sunscreen agents include *methyl anthranilate, digalloyl trioleate* and *avobenzone* (butyl methoxy-dibenzoylmethane).

- The most commonly used chemical **sunblocks** are *zinc oxide, titanium dioxide* and *red petrolatum*.

Bear in mind that, in addition to sunscreens, sun creams also inevitably include all the same ingredients as in body lotions such as mineral and other synthetic oils, PEGs, TEA and other surfactants, preservatives and fragrances (see page 158).

Faking it

There are two ways to get a tan without exposure to the sun: using a sunbed or applying fake tan.

Sunbeds produce UV radiation, just like the sun. In fact, a sunbed can be even more dangerous than the sun. It's estimated that 20 minutes in a solarium can be equivalent to approximately four hours in the sun.

Sunlight contains a mix of UVA and UVB radiation, and some of this is filtered out by the ozone layer. Sunbeds produce mainly UVA radiation, which penetrates deeper into your skin. They produce less UVB radiation than the sun.

People using sunbeds are less likely to use a sun cream to protect themselves against UV radiation. Goggles are essential – as with sunshine, the combination of UVA and UVB can result in eye damage by burning the cornea. Long-term exposure can result in irreversible damage and cataracts. Sunbeds can also speed up thinning of the skin, the development of wrinkles, and other changes usually associated with ageing.

In the 1950s, the first self-tanning product came onto the market. There

Natural sunscreens?

Read labels for natural and 'organic' sunscreens carefully. Usually, they are simply the same old ingredients with added plant extracts and oils. Can the addition of these natural ingredients really prevent sunburn? No, of course not. For example:

- Aqua – water does not prevent sunburn.
- Glycerin – a lubricant used in moisturisers to make them feel good and go on more smoothly. It has no sun-blocking ability, but can dry the skin, making it more vulnerable to sun damage.
- Octyl palmitate – a relative of vitamin C. There is no evidence that it offers protection from the sun.
- Retinyl palmitate – also known as pro-vitamin A or pro-retinol, this has no evidence of sun protection.
- Tocopherol acetate – a relative of vitamin E, again this has no evidence of any effect as a sunscreen.

Other ingredients including aloe vera, carrot oil, chamomile, borage oil and avocado oil used as fillers, stabilisers or preservatives. They are seldom present in high enough quantities to protect or nourish your skin, and none has any proven sun-blocking capacity.

are now hundreds of cosmetic products marketed as safe and effective alternatives to direct sun exposure. But while products like these are widely promoted as a safe alternative to sun exposure, there are inevitably problems associated with them.

First of all, self-tanning lotions offer little protection from UV radiation. So, if you're taking a trip outside in the sunshine to show off your new fake tan, you'll still need to use a sun cream. Next, it's worth considering how self-tanning products work to colour your skin.

The most effective products contain a chemical called dihydroxyacetone (DHA). This sugar derivative has been the staple active ingredient in self-tanners for many years. It can smell bad, and it can sometimes turn you a strange shade of orange but, more important, it has never been fully evaluated for safety.

DHA is not a dye. It imparts temporary colour to the skin through a 'free-radical'-generating chemical reaction with the amino acids in superficial layers of the skin. The way it works is not dissimilar to the way exposure to the air can turn a cut-up apple brown.

Some products use another chemical, erythrulose, in addition to the DHA. Erythrulose works identically to DHA, but develops more slowly. The two chemicals used together may produce a longer-lasting effect.

Both dihydroxyacetone and erythrulose can cause contact dermatitis, but there is a greater irony here that won't be lost on those who have ever skimmed a women's magazine. Most anti-ageing creams, for instance, include ingredients that help fight the damaging skin-ageing effects of free radicals, known to promote premature skin-cell death.

Using a fake tan means volunteering for this kind of damage to your skin. A 2004 laboratory study in the journal *Mutation Research* underscored this fact with the finding that DHA interferes with the normal cell cycle in human skin, induces DNA damage and accelerates cell death within 24 hours of application. This alarming study was one of only very few attempts to explore how safe fake-tan promoters are; erythrulose, for example, has never been fully evaluated for long-term safety.

Fake-tan products also suffer from the same plethora of toxic ingredients as body lotions. Often, they include numerous film-formers – not just silicones, but the plasticiser tri-C14-15 alkyl citrate (which is often found in food packaging). These make application easier, but also act like plastic wrap on the skin, preventing it from eliminating toxins.

▶ TRY THIS INSTEAD ...

Recent research published in the *British Medical Journal* suggests that individuals who use sunscreens may actually be at an increased risk of developing skin cancer. This is because high SPF creams give sun-worshippers a false sense of security, encouraging them to venture out during peak periods and to stay out in the sun much longer than would normally be considered safe.

It is also because of the mix of ingredients in sun cream, and the damaging effects they have on the skin. The only safe recommendation is not to rely on sunscreens as your sole method of protection. There is no doubt that sunscreens can be useful, but they should not be applied over large parts of the body for extended periods of time.

Around 80 per cent of our total lifetime's exposure to the sun comes during childhood. So, it is especially important to make sure children are protected against strong sunlight. If you want to teach your children good sun-exposure habits, lead by example. Research into children's voluntary use of sun creams, for example, suggests that they copy what their parents do. Consider these simple strategies for enjoying the sun:

Get out in the sun. If you want a glow that is truly healthy, then regular, moderate sun exposure is the only way to go. This doesn't mean foolishly baking in the sun for hours, but rather enjoying the sun as a natural part of your daily routine. Studies show that we all need approximately 15 to 20 minutes of sun exposure on our face, arms and legs each day to produce and maintain vital supplies of vitamin D. Staying out of the sun means that many of us don't get enough vitamin D, and this has led to the re-emergence of diseases like rickets, and contributed to spiralling rates of depression as well as cancers of the breast, prostate and colon.

Keep babies under six months old out of strong sunlight. Baby sun creams with a high SPF probably have the greatest number of toxic chemicals, and are definitely not suitable for the delicate and permeable skin of babies.

Limit time in the sun. It is probably best to avoid being out when the sun is at its strongest – between the hours of 11 a.m. and 2 p.m.

Cover up. When you and your children are going to be out in the sun for extended periods of time, make practical use of tee-shirts, sunglasses and beach umbrellas.

household products

I N THE LAST CENTURY OR SO, a greater understanding of the importance of home hygiene has been one of the most influential factors in improving health and longevity.

A clean home is a healthy home. By keeping your home clean, you are keeping levels of germs and allergens low, and this can help maintain your home as a haven where you can rest and your body can repair itself.

To maintain a clean home, most of us use an artillery of conventional detergents and antibacterial cleaners. Cruising the aisles of your local supermarket, it may seem that there is a huge selection of different household cleaners, each with its own special 'formulation'. But most household cleaners contain the same basic range of ingredients. You certainly don't need six specialist cleaners when one concentrated all-purpose cleaner will do most jobs around the home. Nevertheless, as a society, we are obsessed with the idea of specialist cleaning products.

As a result, we spend something in the region of £4.6 billion ($8.3 billion) globally each year on household cleaners. Laundry-care products account for half of our total spend on these products, with surface cleaners, dishwashing products and air fresheners following close behind.

While they may remove surface dirt and sometimes germs and, on occasion, make your home smell nice, these products can, ironically, end up making our homes less clean than they were before. This is because the ingredients found in everyday cleaning products contaminate the air and surfaces in our homes with a horrifying mix of carcinogens, hormone disrupters, neurotoxic solvents, mood-altering chemicals and reproductive toxins.

Any substance that comes into contact with your skin, or that you inhale, or wash down the drain and into the soil, will ultimately end up inside your body. Indeed, years of scientific research have shown that our homes are the most significant sources of exposure to toxic chemicals.

For instance, 25 years ago, a survey conducted by the US Environmental Protection Agency (EPA) found that the highest concentrations of 20 toxic or cancer-causing chemicals – such as toluene and benzene, both human carcinogens – were up to 50 times higher indoors than outdoors.

Many of the chemicals detailed in the EPA report can be found in your favourite bottle of all-purpose cleaner, as well as in your toilet cleaner, air freshener and dish detergent. The problem has become so great that scientists throughout the world consider household cleaning products one of the most important sources of indoor air pollution, and one of the most insidious threats to human health. They cite the fact that, as our use of these cleaners in our homes, schools and workplaces has grown over the last 60 years, the incidence of diseases like cancer and asthma has grown dramatically as well.

Your household cleaner is unlikely to be the only cause of this phenomenon but, as you begin to become familiar with the chemicals used in everyday cleaners, you may find yourself shocked at how often your favourite bottle or spray contains two or more known cancer-causing agents.

Of course, many people who are exposed to these environmental toxins do not reach the kind of high exposures that can lead to cancer or death. Instead, they may experience an array of subtle symptoms, including headaches, rashes or breathing difficulties which, while less dramatic, can be extremely debilitating. But it is still worthwhile asking whether, as there is no safe dose of a carcinogen, these products should be on the shelf at all.

Although it can be hard to change your thinking about household cleaners as anything other than benign, it's worth considering some of the problems – both real and potential – that they bring with them.

- **Nobody knows how safe or unsafe they are.** If a cleaning product has made its way onto the shelves of your local supermarket, most of us assume that it must be safe. Consumer surveys show that the vast majority – some 88 per cent of those asked – believe that household products have been tested for safety before they are sold, and 87 per cent think manufacturers are required to list their products' ingredients on labels. Neither of these assumptions is true.

  Household cleaning products are made using a variety of industrial chemicals, often referred to as high production volume, or HPV, chemicals. According to a 1998 EPA report, 43 per cent of the most widely produced chemicals have no basic toxicity data available at all, and just 50 per cent have even preliminary screening data. In fact, only a measly 7 per cent of HPV chemicals have a complete set of screening-level toxicity data.

  In the UK, the environmental group Friends of the Earth, in their 2000 report *Crisis in Chemicals*, noted that only 14 per cent of HPV chemicals in Europe have a full set of basic safety data, 65 per cent have incomplete safety data and 12 per cent have no safety data at all. What these figures mean is that no one can say for sure how safe or unsafe the chemicals in our household cleaners really are.

  And of course, once again, the problem of the cocktail effect rears its ugly head. When the chemicals in your favourite cleaner are tested for safety, they are done so individually, not in combinations. Yet, in household products, combinations of multiple chemicals are the norm and, yet again, manufacturers are not required to produce independent scientific confirmation that their cleaning products are safe for people or the environment before putting them on the shelf. Like the fox that guards the hen house, any testing that is performed is usually done by the manufacturer and, very often, the results are not made public.

- **They contain harsh and sometimes toxic chemicals.** The health and safety issues associated with cleaning chemicals are relevant to everyone. Most people these days spend as much as 90 per cent of their time indoors in homes, offices, schools and hospitals, and are in constant contact with the fumes of cleaning chemicals in the air and chemical residues on the surfaces they touch.

According to the US Consumer Protection Agency, over 150 chemicals found in the home are associated with allergies, birth defects, cancer and psychological disorders. Cleaning chemicals may be a significant contributor to indoor air pollution, causing eye, nose and throat irritation, headaches, dizziness and fatigue. A 17-year study by the EPA concluded that women who work in the home have a 54-percent higher death rate from cancer than women who work outside the home.

Knowing this, it would make sense to look on the labels of your favourite cleaners to check whether they contain any of these known toxins. Unfortunately, manufacturers of household cleaners are not required to list all the ingredients used in their products on the label – and they don't volunteer this information as it's considered a 'trade secret'. This means that you may never be able to identify whether your glass cleaner, dish detergent or spot remover contains chemicals that could harm you or your family and, if so, at what concentrations.

Nevertheless, independent studies have shown that the majority of household cleaners do contain harmful ingredients (see the table on page 181).

Many of these 'bioaccumulate' – in other words, they are stored in the body – to a level where they can cause ill health. Many are also highly volatile – they easily evaporate and can be inhaled. Others that are sprayed from aerosol cans or hand pumps release a shower of microscopic, easily inhaled particles. As the other chapters in this book show, many of these chemicals can be found in other types of products as well. Using potentially toxic cleaners is simply adding to the overall burden of these toxins in your home.

- **They are ecologically unsound** It may be only recently that we've begun to look at the impact that industrial chemicals have on human health. But there is a large and long-standing body of evidence of how these chemicals affect the environment. Over the years, volumes of data have been amassed regarding the environmental impact of the detergents, solvents and phosphates commonly found in household products. We know what happens to animals like frogs, birds and plants when we release these toxins into the air and waterways. We know the damaging effects of propellants and other toxic chemicals on the ozone layer.

Household horrors

While it is not so easy to avoid chemicals present in our water supply or the pollution spewing from factories and cars, it is possible to do something about the chemicals you use in your own home. The following is a list of 'red-flag' chemicals commonly found in cleaning products. Their worrying health effects provide plenty of good reasons to make the switch to the more natural alternatives given throughout this book.

Substance	Effect
Alcohol (including ethanol, methanol, isopropanol)	Nausea and vomiting if swallowed
Ammonia	Fatal when swallowed
Ammonium hydroxide	Corrosive; irritant
Bleach	Potentially fatal if ingested
Butyl cellosolve	Damages liver, kidney and nervous system
Chlorine	Number-one cause of poisonings in children
Formaldehyde	Highly toxic; a known carcinogen
Hydrochloric acid	Corrosive, eye and skin irritant
Hydrochloric bleach	Eye, skin and respiratory tract irritant
Lye	Severe damage to stomach and oesophagus if ingested
Naphtha	Depresses the central nervous system
Nitrobenzene	Causes skin discoloration, shallow breathing, vomiting and death
Paradichlorobenzenes	Irritates eyes, nose, central nervous system
Perchlorethylene	Damages liver, kidney and nervous system
Petroleum distillates	Highly inflammable; suspected carcinogen
Phenol	Extremely dangerous; suspected carcinogen; fatal if taken internally
Propellants	Central nervous system poisons; irregular heartbeat
Propylene glycol	Provokes immune response; main ingredient in antifreeze
Sodium hypochlorite	Potentially fatal
Sodium lauryl sulphate	Carcinogen; toxin; causes gene mutation
Sodium tripolyphosphate	Irritant
Trichloroethane	Damages liver and kidneys; narcotic

As our petroleum reserves diminish, another environmental concern has arisen. Many of the chemicals that are used in cleaning products are petroleum-based, contributing to the depletion of this non-renewable resource. For instance, it is estimated that, if every household in the US replaced just one 800-ml (28-oz) bottle of petroleum-based cleaner with an equivalent plant-based product, it would save 118,700 barrels of oil in one year – enough to heat 6800 average American homes.

In and among the tonnes of cleaning products we pour down the drain each year are toxic substances that are not processed adequately by sewage-treatment plants or septic systems. In a May 2002 study of contaminants in stream water sampled across the US, the United States Geological Survey (USGS) found persistent detergent metabolites (breakdown products) in 69 per cent of the streams tested; 66 per cent contained disinfectants.

The detergent metabolites detected were members of a class of

Wipe and waste

The single biggest revolution in cleaning has been the invention of the wipe. The convenience of wipes is such that, in the last decade, there has been an unprecedented boom in the use of disposable cloths of all kinds. Today, in any supermarket, along with hand wipes and baby wipes, you can buy self-tan and deodorant wipes, and make-up- and nail polish-removing, blackhead-clearing, car-washing, multisurface, disinfecting, furniture, floor, fridge and hob wipes.

Made from plastic, cellulose and polyester fibres pressed together and soaked in a cleaning fluid, the global retail value of wipes in 2004 was around £2.2 billion ($4 billion) and is expected to reach £3 billion ($5.3 billion) in 2006. Personal and cosmetic wipes account for around 65 per cent of this market, and even people who don't have babies are often seen buying packets of baby wipes to use as instant clean-ups anywhere. For US troops in Iraq, they were standard issue.

▶

Figures from North America suggest that if someone were to load all the disposable wipes purchased there last year onto 18-wheel trucks, the caravan would number 9000 trucks, stretch for 68 miles and would be carrying 83,000 tonnes of used convenience cloths.

Apart from catering to the damaged psyche of a throwaway society, wipes have other disadvantages: they are expensive, can't be flushed down the toilet and clog sewer systems when they are (even so, many manufacturers still omit relevant information on 'flushability' on their packets). They are also very slow to biodegrade. As is the case with disposable nappies, it is likely that all the wipes we've ever used are still festering somewhere underground. The environmental impact of this has yet to be studied.

chemicals called **alkylphenol** *ethoxylates* (APEs), including nonylphenol ethoxylates and octylphenol ethoxylates, surfactants that are added to some laundry detergents, disinfectants, laundry stain-removers and citrus cleaner/degreasers to make them more effective. When discharged in municipal waste water, nonylphenol and octylphenol ethoxylates break down into the oestrogen mimics nonylphenol and octylphenol, which are more toxic, and do not readily biodegrade in soil and water. The presence of synthetic oestrogens in water may be harming the reproduction and survival of salmon and other fish as well as humans.

As they circulate through the water supply, these chemicals threaten people, animals and the environment. For instance, male fish that are exposed to APEs in rivers have been found to produce female egg-yolk proteins, and laboratory studies have shown that, in humans, the APE p-nonylphenol triggers the growth of oestrogen-sensitive breast cancer cells.

The plastic bottles used to package cleaning products pose another environmental problem not only because they are derived from petroleum, but also because they contribute to the mounds of solid waste that must be land-filled, and to air pollution when they are incinerated.

The perils of being too clean

Cleaning the house can be harmful in other, more unexpected ways, too. For instance, by overcleaning an otherwise adequately clean home, we may be condemning our children to a future of chronic ill health.

Manufacturers of cleaning products prey heavily on parents' fears for the health of their children and loved ones. Yet, there's evidence of a link between early childhood infections and a lower risk of developing atopic diseases such as allergies, asthma and eczema. This idea is part of what is known as the 'hygiene hypothesis' – a theory that developed out of scientists' inability to explain why rates of atopic diseases among children in developed countries were escalating out of control.

The name 'hygiene hypothesis' is, of course, misleading since hygiene *per se* is not a bad thing and, indeed, better hygiene is responsible for many of the gains in human health. But obsessive measures towards cleanliness, killing germs and suppressing illnesses, however, are clearly creating more problems than they are solving (see 'Antibacterial Cleaners', page 198).

The theory goes that, by 'protecting' children from exposure to dirt and germs, and by preventing diseases from taking their course in childhood, we are inadvertently destroying the body's ability to respond appropriately to allergens, infection and other stimuli that actually help the immune system to mature and function properly.

During most of our evolution, and from the moment of birth, our bodies have been exposed daily to dirt and germs. It is thought that this exposure helped to forge and maintain the immune system's sophisticated network of chemical pathways and specialised cells. According to the hygiene hypothesis, without the early input of everyday dirt and germs, the immune system cannot respond appropriately when challenged.

The idea came into being in 1989, when David Strachan, an epidemiologist at the London School of Hygiene and Tropical Medicine, noticed that children from big families – where infections were likely to circulate freely – were less likely to develop atopic disorders (such as eczema, asthma and psoriasis).

Since then, the evidence in favour of this theory has continued to accumulate. A study by the Institute of Social and Preventive Medicine in Basel, Switzerland, published in the prestigious *New England Journal of Medicine* in 2002, looked at over 800 children aged 6 to 13. Researchers found that kids who lived in the dustiest environments, especially those who lived on farms, were less likely to suffer from asthma and hayfever.

As the hypothesis has evolved, scientists have found that it is not just exposure to dirt and germs that is protective. Being exposed to endotoxins – the waste products sloughed off by bacteria – also helps to 'train' the immune system.

What's more, the protective effect of small exposures to these challenges has expanded to encompass not just atopic diseases, but also immune disorders such as multiple sclerosis (MS), and type 1 (insulin-dependent) diabetes, and inflammatory bowel diseases such as ulcerative colitis and irritable bowel syndrome (IBS).

Safer cleaning: getting back to basics

Cleaning is a necessity. It is also a science, an art and an act of discipline. People who actually like to clean will also tell you that, on occasion, it has a spirituality all its own, that doing the dishes or scrubbing the floor can be both comforting and uplifting.

Of course, none of the information or suggestions in this book will make the regular routine of vacuuming the stairs or cleaning the bath any more appealing in itself. But making use of these simpler, greener alternatives will, in some cases, have an immediate impact on your health and environment. When you're not inhaling or absorbing risky chemicals into your body, you may find that your energy levels rise, and that nagging skin and respiratory symptoms disappear or at the very least improve. Since many of these chemicals can have a direct effect on the emotional centres of the brain, you may also find that your mood improves as well.

Sadly, it's become all too easy to rely on hazardous cleaning chemicals that end up giving us a clean, but not so healthy, home. Many of these products work very quickly and effectively, and this ease of use may leave you thinking that you are just too busy to make substantial changes in the way you take care of your home. You may be asking yourself if it will really make a difference to choose a 'greener' way to clean your home.

Most of us sympathise with the need to keep environmental pollution to an absolute minimum, but our resolve often disappears at the super-market, where brightly packaged products promise to transform our homes into spotlessly clean aromatherapy spas. What could green cleaning possibly have to offer that could compete with today's modern cleaning product formulations?

In fact, green cleaning brings with it a range of benefits:

- **It costs less.** By using readily available ingredients like baking soda and vinegar to clean your home, you will find you spend less on everyday cleaners.

- **Less backache.** When you make it yourself, there are no heavy bottles to carry home. Suddenly, bringing in the groceries becomes less onerous.

- **No heavy perfumes.** The fragrances used in cleaning products are significant triggers of asthma as well as headaches. Going fragrance-free may have the knock-on effect of improving your health.

- **Self-sufficiency.** Not having to rely on commercial cleaners is emotionally freeing. Suddenly, all those commercials that try to sell you toilet cleaner as a cure for a dead-end love life seem remarkably silly.

- **A cleaner home.** Instead of washing away dirt with toxic waste or masking unpleasant smells with other smells, you will be getting your home genuinely clean.

- **Nothing dangerous under the sink.** It's a much safer way to live, especially if you have children.

- **A cleaner planet.** You'll be doing your bit – relatively effortlessly – to keep the planet in good shape for future generations.

As many of the alternatives described here are both inexpensive and freely available, you might find a little extra change in your pocket each month. This means you can give yourself a treat while congratulating yourself on keeping both your immediate and the wider environment chemical-free.

Product manufacturers are aware of the increasing interest of consumers in natural cleaning products, and there are many good alternatives if you want to buy, rather than make your own, cleaning products. Natural ingredients are usually derived from citrus, and the oils are combined with minerals, salts, sodas and plant enzymes. Plant-based cleaners are often able to match the cleaning power of synthetically derived ingredients. Be aware, however, that many manufacturers simply add a citrus ingredient to an otherwise synthetic formulation so that a label claim can be made.

Unfortunately, there are no regulations governing this area, and many companies are free to make 'natural' claims that don't stand up to any real scrutiny.

▶ TRY THIS INSTEAD ...

It's always good to know how to make basic cleaning products with safe everyday materials.

If you are unsure as to where to start, then begin with the basics. The best way to keep your home clean is to not let grease and grime build up in the first place. A quick regular wipedown is still the best way to prevent surfaces from getting sticky, greasy and grimy. It will also make doing big jobs like ovens and hobs easier in the long run. However, not many of us can consistently reach this level of perfection.

Throughout this book, you will find simple, inexpensive and green alternatives to 'industrial strength' chemicals. To limit your exposure to chemicals in household cleaners, try the following options.

Dilute (and dilute again) Most liquid detergents and soaps can be made into useful all-purpose cleaners simply by diluting them. To make sure you're keeping exposure to a minimum of chemicals, try using an ecologically sound vegetable-based dish detergent or, even better, a liquid castile soap, well diluted in water.

Hot water Many people forget that hot water and steam are among the best, and most effective, household cleaners. In addition, it is usually the elbow grease, not the chemicals, that really gets the job done.

Steam A steam cleaner can be useful for really stubborn grease, and for quick cleanups on carpets. It is also a very effective disinfectant for sinks and toilets.

But effective cleaning has other rules as well. Whatever your approach, cleaning has its own set of rules. Follow these and cleaning will become, if not a source of enlightenment, at least a less onerous chore.

Make it yourself Most of us are used to buying our cleaning products off the supermarket shelves. When we think of alternatives, often the first place we look is back in the supermarket – where green alternatives are often pretty thin on the ground. Why not consider making your own? The simplest (and cheapest) ingredients are often all that is needed for the majority of household-cleaning jobs.

Baking soda Chemists call this white powder sodium bicarbonate ($NaHCO_3$). Your grandmother would probably have mixed it with water, called it 'a bicarb' and drunk it to cure heartburn. That should tell you something about how safe it is.

For cleaning, baking soda does a lot of different things:

- As a powder, it's a mild abrasive that can scratch off hardened dirt without scoring whatever it is you're trying to clean.

- It dissolves in water without leaving a gritty film like other scouring powders do.

And because it dissolves in water, baking soda gives you other benefits:

- It's a mild disinfectant with the ability to kill some bacteria and fungi.

- It helps to cut through grease.

- It softens water, thus helping your other cleaners to work and rinse off more effectively.

Vinegar Chemists might call vinegar a dilute solution of acetic acid (CH_3COOH). When table wine turns 'bad', it chemically changes into vinegar. You probably wouldn't drink it as a beverage, but you might mix it with a little olive oil and put it on your salad.

Vinegar is a mild acid that cuts through grease, and disinfects by killing many types of bacteria, yeast and moulds. It is also an efficient air freshener.

Soap Most people confuse soap and detergent. Chemists originally developed synthetic detergents as an alternative to soap where hard water (containing magnesium or calcium) or acid is present. The detergent that we buy from a store is really a synthetic that has been manufactured from a variety of mineral products like coal tar and petroleum.

On the other hand, soap – for example, traditional castile soap – is a mild detergent that is simple, and made from natural products like vegetable oils and animal fats. Used sparingly and under the right conditions, soap is gentle and a wonderful cleaning agent in that it has a minimal impact on the environment.

Borax This can be bought from most chemists and, while it is an effective cleaner, it should be used with caution because it can also be toxic at high levels.

- Borax is an effective water softener and can be used in home-made products to help soap work harder and rinse away better.

- It is an effective mould/mildew remover and disinfectant.

- It can whiten clothes and help prevent odours.

Microfibre cleaning cloths These new cloths are so useful that, once you begin to use them, you will wonder why you ever bothered to waste your money on anything else.

Water is the most powerful solvent in the world. The purpose of detergents is to bring more water in contact with whatever surface you are cleaning. Microfibres effectively do the same thing. Microfibres are finer than human hair and have a superior absorbency when compared to other cloths. The combination of these properties means that microfibre cloths have a greatly increased surface area, bringing more water into contact with the cleaning surface. Used as directed, they will leave most surfaces both clean and dry.

Many manufacturers have jumped on the microfibre gravy train recently, so you can afford to be choosey about the cloths you buy. The best ones are denser and generally more costly. However, they can be reused indefinitely, and the denser the cloth, the greater its surface area – and the more fibres there are to trap dirt.

And finally …

Elbow grease There's no getting around this one. Many of the recipes in this book work just as well as the more hazardous chemicals you've been using all this time. But occasionally, using non-toxic alternatives to conventional household cleaners means that, at least some of the time, you will have to scrub harder or longer.

Clues on the label

How do you know if the products you are using are toxic?

With any other type of product, you could check out the ingredients list on the label. But cleaning products don't generally have ingredients lists. Manufacturers have successfully pleaded their case for secrecy with the regulatory authorities. To list the ingredients would, they say, be revealing a trade secret, and this would be bad for business. This means that the concerned consumer who wants to know what's in their toilet or oven cleaner will need to learn to read between the lines.

Most countries have rules about specific safety labelling that must appear on products containing known toxins such as methyl alcohol, turpentine, petroleum distillate products and a variety of other common cleaning ingredients. Poisonous products, for instance, are usually marked with a picture of a skull and crossbones. In addition, the majority of commercially available cleaning products contain 'signal' words on their labels such as:

- Hazardous
- Corrosive
- Inflammable
- Warning
- Caution
- Danger
- Irritant

▶

These little clues on the bottle tell you that the product is dangerous. The best way to ensure that you don't use toxic, corrosive, inflammable products is to make your own from safe ingredients. But if you want to buy a product at the supermarket, it's important to check for these signal words on the label of any product you buy. In addition, remember to avoid buying any product that: a) does not clearly indicate what the active substance is; b) does not list hazards associated with the product (like 'highly irritating fumes' or 'toxic when ingested'); c) does not describe precautions you can take to avoid being harmed; and d) does not list necessary or appropriate instructions for first-aid treatment.

Cautions are there for a reason. If the instructions tell you to use a product in a well-ventilated area, it's not because the manufacturers are concerned that you aren't getting enough fresh air. It's because the product is harmful if inhaled. Likewise, if the label recommends that you wear gloves, it's not because the manufacturers are concerned you might break a nail, but because the product is a skin irritant or is easily absorbed through the skin.

Household cleaners

To fulfil the increasingly ambitious claims for their products, manufacturers rely on combinations of chemical compounds that can be harsh and highly toxic. Ask yourself, if a cleanser can instantly strip a kitchen tile of years of accumulated grease, what might it do to your skin or your body's cells or the natural environment.

Although it is impossible to avoid all the chemical culprits known to damage health, it does pay to learn which key ingredients are most problematical. As you read through the information that follows, you will notice how certain chemicals turn up again and again in a range of household cleaners. Armed with this information, you can then begin to take steps to limit what you buy or, better yet, make use of the suggestions for buying or making non-toxic alternatives. Your home will still be clean, and your health will improve immeasurably by doing so.

■ AIR FRESHENERS

In spite of their name, air fresheners do not freshen the air. Instead, they are one of the most concentrated sources of poisons and pollution in the home. While the accepted hype is that air fresheners remove unwanted odours and replace them with clean fresh smells, most do no such thing.

Air fresheners work in several ways. They can contain nerve-deadening agents designed to interfere with your ability to detect smells, or they can coat the nasal passages with a thin, undetectable oily film that also prevents odour detection. Alternatively, they can cover up one smell with another, more powerful, one. Rarely do they actually remove or break down unpleasant odours.

Air fresheners are often marketed as luxury items. And indeed, you wear a perfume and your husband has an aftershave but, typically, they contain synthetic fragrances as well as solvents and fixatives that are as common in most garages as they are in 'luxury' fragrances.

About 30–40 per cent of air freshener purchases are driven by what marketing departments call 'home-cleaning replacement'. Time-strapped, cash-rich people may clean less often or less thoroughly, and so use air fresheners to give the impression of a just-cleaned home. The rest is driven by the promise of luxury and a quick-fix mood-boosting experience.

Years ago, air fresheners were something that you sprayed into a room once in a while for effect. These days, you can plug them into an electric socket and have a continual release of strong perfume throughout your home. But the trend towards using continuous room perfumes means that your body never gets a break from exposure to these chemicals, and we simply don't know enough about the long-term effects of such exposure to deem this safe.

Air fresheners also provide a good example of how manufacturers leap onto current trends and use them for profit. For instance, many air fresheners now promise 'aromatherapy' for your home. It's all nonsense, and even if your air freshener doesn't make you feel sick in the short term, it may add to longer-term problems.

Animal experiments, for example, suggest that the chemicals in air fresheners may weaken the body's defences by making the skin more permeable. Allergic reactions to these products can range from sneezing and watery eyes to full-scale asthma attacks. Aerosol air fresheners contain neurotoxic propellants and can be harmful to the lungs if inhaled in high concentrations or over prolonged periods of time. Solids and plug-ins produce the same symptoms, and may be poisonous to children and pets if ingested.

In 1999, a British survey of 14,000 pregnant women concluded that the frequent use of household aerosol sprays and air fresheners was making women and babies ill.

The study, reported in *New Scientist*, found that women who used aerosols and air fresheners most days suffered 25 per cent more headaches and 19 per cent more post-natal depression than those who used them less than once a week. Babies under six months had 30 per cent more ear infections and more frequent diarrhoea if regularly exposed to aerosols and air fresheners. Early in 2005, the same team of scientists updated their findings in the *Archives of Environmental Medicine*, with much the same results. The researchers noted that the chemicals present in many aerosols, such as **xylene**, ketones and aldehydes, had already been associated with so-called 'sick-building syndrome', and that we now may be looking at a similar syndrome in homes.

Also in 2005, the European consumer group Bureau Européen des Unions de Consommateurs (BEUC) published a comparative study into home-fragrance safety. They looked at 74 different kinds of air-freshening products, including incense, natural products, scented candles, aerosols, liquid diffusers, electric diffusers and gels, and measured the concentrations of volatile organic compounds (VOCs) and aldehydes in the air after their use.

VOCs and aldehydes are potent neurotoxins that attack both the central nervous system (the brain and spinal cord) and peripheral nervous system (responsible for relaying sensory information to the brain, but also involved in controlling organs and muscles such as the heart, stomach and intestines). The study found that air fresheners released toxins such as acetaldehyde, styrene, **toluene, chlorobenzene, glycol ethers, phthalates** and artificial musk into the air. Traces of **formaldehyde** and **benzene** were also found.

In many cases, the total VOC emissions were much higher than the 'safe' dose of 200 mcg/m^3 (micrograms per cubic meter). In some cases, they were as high as 4000–5000 mcg/m^3.

Manufacturers defend their products by saying that, under normal use, the chemicals in air fresheners are safe. But in recent years, what constitutes 'normal use' has changed drastically. Instead of just an occasional spray, many of us now use continuous-release devices that release fragrance chemicals into the air all day long. What's more, air fresheners are not just found in homes, but in offices and shops, and in vacuum-cleaner filters, taxis and family cars.

As always, it is the cumulative or 'cocktail' effect – not just from air fresheners, but because of all the perfumed products we now use – that is crucial to the development of health problems.

YOUR AIR FRESHENER IS LIKELY TO CONTAIN ...

Para-dichlorobenzene (PDCB), *naphthalene*, *formaldehyde*, *sodium bisulphate*, *glycol ethers*, ethanol and other solvents, various propellants such as *hydrochlorofluorcarbons* (HCFCs), *butane*, *propane* and *isobutane*, disinfectants such as *cresol*, preservatives (such as *quaternary ammonium* salts) and petrochemical-based fragrances.

▶ TRY THIS INSTEAD...

You don't need air fresheners, and the best alternative is not to buy them at all. Simply keeping your home clean and well ventilated solves most odour problems. If your house is really smelly, then you need to get to the root of the problem – often animals, blocked drains, damp conditions, gas from your cooker or heater, off-gassing from new carpets, furniture or wallpaper, over-full bins and cigarette smoke – rather than just masking it.

To remove unwanted smells, consider some of these measures:

Buy pump sprays instead of aerosols. But don't kid yourself that these are much healthier. You will still be breathing in alcohols and perfumes as well as other chemicals. Pump sprays just mean that you avoid breathing in propellants – a baby step in the right direction.

Open a window. Fresh air is the best air freshener there is. To save money and environmental resources, we have all become accustomed to living and working in sealed premises. Unfortunately, sealing in the heat also seals in every smell, every chemical and gas that may be present in the environment. Unless you live in a dreadfully polluted space, opening a couple of windows to allow cross-ventilation is always the best way to get rid of a bad smell. Even in winter, this is unlikely to raise your heating bill significantly.

Buy houseplants such as English ivy, spider plants, peace lilies and philodendrons, which can help remove unpleasant odours and gases from your environment (see page 46 for a full list of air-freshening plants).

Make your own spray. A simple air freshener can be made by combining equal amounts of water and white vinegar in a spray bottle. Add 20–30 drops of your favourite essential oil (peppermint, lemon, pine and geranium are all good choices) and shake before using. As both vinegar and essential oils can be eye irritants, don't put your face in the area you have just sprayed, and never spray directly into your face.

Make your own room freshener with a 200-g (7-oz) box of baking soda and 10–15 drops of your favourite essential oils. Mix these well and place in a cardboard box (you can paint or decorate this) or a small dish. Alternatively, try placing a few cotton wool balls sprinkled with vanilla extract in an open dish or bowl, and leave these to freshen the room. This is only a short-term solution and, after a day or so, the smell of vanilla will dissipate and stop working. Nevertheless, this is useful after parties to cut through smoky smells, and also to freshen up small spaces such as closets and cars.

Use potpourri with caution. Most commercially prepared potpourris use petrochemical-derived fragrances. Look at the label and, if it says something like 'a blend of natural aromas' or 'natural' anything, it is probably not really natural at all, but 'nature identical'. If you want to avoid these, make your own potpourri, or buy an unscented variety and scent it with your own essential oils rather than the synthetic potpourri oil blends. These won't last as long, but they will be less harmful to your health.

Be careful when buying aromatherapy candles, also marketed as 'natural' alternatives to conventional air fresheners. Most use petrochemical fragrances instead of natural oils. Also, the candle itself is usually made from wax derived from petrochemicals. As this burns, it can release soot containing volatile chemicals and toxic metals into the atmosphere.

ALL-PURPOSE CLEANERS

All general-purpose cleaners work in essentially the same way to loosen grease and grime, and facilitate a clean rinse. For these products to live up to the promise of effortless cleaning, they usually have to be much stronger and more concentrated than necessary for everyday household use. In spite of this, few of them are significantly more efficient than simple soap and hot water for loosening everyday dirt and grime from household surfaces.

The ingredients in all-purpose cleaners are a combination of synthetic detergents, grease-cutting agents such as solvents, and bleaches and disinfectants. Depending on the mix of ingredients, these cleaners have been shown to be irritating to varying degrees to the skin, eyes, nose and throat, and can be corrosive if swallowed. Those that contain small amounts of phosphates are an environmental hazard.

Spray cleaners are basically the same mix of chemicals as liquid cleaners, though often in a less concentrated form. Although pump sprays don't contain aerosols, when you use them, you are producing a fine mist of chemicals that is easily inhaled and quick to enter the bloodstream. So, even though the product is less concentrated, you may take in more chemicals. Amazingly, for a product that is mostly water, spray cleaners are also more expensive to buy than standard liquid formulas.

Scouring powders and abrasive creams are a traditional standby for shifting greasy deposits in the kitchen and soapy scum in the bath. These products are generally made with strong bleaches or ammonia to make them work faster. When the dried bleach mixes with water, it produces chlorine fumes that are irritating to the eyes, nose, throat and lungs.

Dry powders also contain *crystalline silica*, which is an eye, skin and lung irritant, and carcinogenic when inhaled. It is all too easy to inhale silica particles when you sprinkle scouring powder in the sink or bath (and some of these types of cleaners are unsuitable for certain surfaces, like plastic, because they can scratch). Once inhaled, mineral powders – whether *talc*, *silica*, feldspar or quartz – lodge more or less permanently in the lungs.

YOUR ALL-PURPOSE CLEANER IS LIKELY TO CONTAIN ...

Detergents/surfactants, solvents such as ethanol, *isopropanol*, *butyl cellosolve* or glycols, disinfectants such as *ammonia*, *bleach* (sodium hypochlorite), *phenol* and *pine oil*, fragrances and colours. Abrasive or cream formulas contain fine particles of plastic, silica, calcite, feldspar or quartz. Most also contain undisclosed preservatives such as *quaternary ammonium compounds* and *EDTA*.

▶ TRY THIS INSTEAD ...

To limit your exposure to the chemicals in household cleaners, try the following options:

Limit your use of sprays (even pump sprays of mixtures you have made yourself) for hard-to-get-at places to reduce the number of chemicals you inhale.

For tough grease, make a strong solution containing:

> ½ tsp washing soda (also known as sodium carbonate, soda ash or sal soda)
> 2 tbsp distilled white vinegar
> ½ tsp liquid soap or dish detergent (or, alternatively, 1 tsp soap flakes)
> 2 cups hot water

Add a few drops of essential oil if you wish. This can be used neat or put into a spray bottle to help you get at hard-to-reach places. Always wear protective gloves when working with washing soda.

Try making a simple scouring powder from 200 g (7 oz) of bicarbonate of soda. That's all you need. Keep it in an airtight jar and use when you need to. It's that simple. If you like, add 10 drops of an essential oil and mix well to make a pleasant scent. Lemon, grapefruit, mandarin, tea tree, rose, peppermint or lavender are all suitable.

To make a stain-removing scouring powder use:

> 230 g (8 oz) bicarbonate of soda
> 90 g (3oz) borax
> 3 tbsp soap flakes (lightly crushed)

This will get rid of all but the most stubborn stains. To increase the bleaching power of this mixture, try adding 3 tbsp of sodium perborate (available at healthfood shops), a kind of bleach. Be sure to wear gloves when using this formula to avoid skin irritation.

An even stronger cleaner can be made with a mixture of liquid soap and trisodium phosphate (TSP). Add the following ingredients to 850 ml (1½ pints) of warm-to-hot water:

> 1 tsp liquid soap
> 1 tsp trisodium phosphate (TSP)
> 1 tsp borax
> 1 tsp distilled white vinegar

TSP is a strong skin irritant so you should wear protective gloves when using it. The benefit of using TSP in this particular mixture, apart from its effectiveness against grease and mildew, is that you know what chemicals you are actually using.

■ ANTIBACTERIAL CLEANERS

Over the last decade, our enthusiasm for fighting germs at home has become unstoppable. At the supermarket, we effectively take out insurance against germs by stocking up on a bewildering array of products that boast 'antibacterial action'. Nowadays, we can buy antibacterial hand soaps, laundry detergents, dish detergents, surface cleaners, toothpastes, mouthwashes and hand wipes. Antibacterial agents can be impregnated into clothing, furniture, blankets, insoles, the plastic lining of refrigerators, food-storage containers, shower curtains, rubbish bags, bins, chopping boards, and even high chairs and toys.

It is estimated that the worldwide market for antibacterial products is around £14 billion, and hospital use accounts for only 30 per cent of this. In the US – where the fight against germs has been vigorously embraced – consumers purchased around $540 million (£290 million) worth of antibacterial soaps, hand-cleaners and detergents last year. Indeed, some 75 per cent of liquid soaps and 29 per cent of bar soaps sold in the US now contain antibacterial agents.

Hygiene *per se* is not a bad thing and, indeed, better hygiene in homes is responsible for keeping us out of hospital, and better hygiene in hospitals has meant that, when we are sick or in need of surgery, it is safer and the recovery time shorter. If you have an ill or immune-compromised person in your home, taking extra care with hygiene is a necessity. But there is little that can be achieved with an antibacterial cleaner that can't be done much more simply and inexpensively with hot water and simple detergent. Also, there are now several good reasons to believe that using an antibacterial cleaner may do more harm than good.

No protection

In 2000, the American Medical Association (AMA) issued the startling statement warning that antibacterial soaps were no more effective against germs than common soap. The AMA based its opinion on several studies that showed that, while antibacterial hand soaps may initially kill more bacteria and viruses on the skin than regular soaps, within an hour or so afterwards, there is generally no difference in the number of germs on the skin. Hardly surprising, given that the average adult touches around 300 different surfaces every 30 minutes. Similarly, while antibacterial surface cleaners may initially remove more organisms than soap and water, within 90 minutes or so, there is generally no difference in the numbers of bacteria and viruses that have repopulated the area.

Knowing this provides a context for the results of a widely publicised study, originating from Columbia University in New York in 2004, which showed that people who used antibacterial soaps and cleaners developed cough, runny nose, sore throat, fever, vomiting, diarrhoea and other symptoms just as often as those who don't use antibacterial products. The researchers also pointed out that many of these illnesses are typically caused by viruses, against which antibacterial soaps and cleaners can provide no protection.

WHAT CAN YOU EXPECT FROM YOUR ANTIBACTERIAL PRODUCTS?

Products	Advantages	Disadvantages
Antibacterial handwashes and sanitisers	Kills almost 100 per cent of harmful germs within 15 seconds	You are recontaminated as soon as you touch something else
Antibacterial soaps and dishwashing liquids	Prevents growth of most bacteria, fungi and yeast	Does not kill them immediately; benefits only apply to hands, not dishes
Antibacterial sponges and scrubbers	Kills germs on sponges and scrubbers to eliminate odours	They do not destroy germs on any surfaces they come into contact with
Disinfectant spray	Kills bacteria, fungi and viruses; reduces surface-to-human transmissions of germs	As with all antibacterial products, continued use will produce resistant organisms
Surface cleaners	Kills household germs such as *Salmonella*, *E. coli* and *Streptococcus*	In some cases, it must be left on at least 10 minutes to have any antibacterial effect; surfaces become 'germy' again within half an hour
Triclosan/Microban embedded products (such as chopping boards, refrigerators)	Inhibits the growth of bacteria in the products	There is no evidence to show that it protects the person using the item

Resistance on the home front

Obsessive measures aimed at killing germs are problematical because 'germs' – that is, bacteria, viruses and fungi – are ancient and adaptable organisms. They are programmed to survive and, more often than not, instead of being killed by powerful chemical assaults, they simply evolve and become immune to them. Constant exposure to drugs such as antibiotics will eventually produce an organism that no drug will kill.

This ability to adapt is what has given rise to 'superbugs' such as methicillin-resistant *Staphylococcus aureus* (MRSA) and other resistant strains of bacteria that have become so prevalent in hospitals that many of us now fear having to stay in these institutions in case we become infected.

Indiscriminate use of antibiotics has received heavy and deserved criticism for provoking the rise of the 'superbug' in our hospitals. Less well publicised is the role that the exponential rise in the popularity of antibacterial household cleaners and toiletries in the last decade has had in producing antibacterial resistance at home. For years, scientists denied the impact of household antibacterials, but now, the latest evidence shows that you don't need to set foot outside your home to encounter a superbug.

In 2005, researchers in Oxford looked at MRSA cases in two Oxfordshire hospitals and discovered that around 25 per cent of serious cases were brought into hospital from the patient's home. How was that possible?

The answer is that, once upon a time, we approached hygiene with simple soap and water. Today, we use a variety of synthetic antibacterial chemicals – in particular, **quaternary ammonium compounds** and **chlorophenols** such as **Triclosan** – to keep the bugs at bay. Unlike soap and water, which works efficiently by physically loosening dirt and germs from surfaces and bodies, and washing them down the drain, antibacterial chemicals are designed to kill. In this, they are very like antibiotics and, perhaps not surprisingly, there is now a considerable body of scientific opinion that what is being touted on supermarket shelves as an antibacterial in household products is really an antibiotic, and that antibacterial chemicals used in the home are contributing to the growing threat posed by drug-resistant strains of bacteria.

In support of this idea, community-acquired MRSA (caMRSA) – a form of MRSA that arises in people who have had no contact with a hospital – is now being widely reported in the US, Britain, Australia and Canada.

Research is now showing that a whole range of antibacterial chemicals used as disinfectants in household cleaners, and as preservatives and active ingredients in personal-care products, are producing resistant strains of bacteria.

Studies from America and Japan have shown that household germs like Escherichia coli, Listeria monocytogenes, Pseudomonas aeruginosa, Enterococcus faecalis, Streptococcus pneumoniae and Staphylococcus aureus are already showing signs of resistance to common antibacterial cleaners. But worse than this, because our household cleaners work in the same way as antibiotics do, they can make bacteria resistant to true antibiotics. For instance, overuse of the common antibacterial agents **benzalkonium chloride, chlorohexidine** and especially **Triclosan** (a chlorophenol type of agent) not only produces resistance to these agents, but it also creates strong cross-resistance to penicillin-derived antibiotics as well.

The overuse of antibacterials like these in the home will eventually have the same devastating effect as overprescribing antibiotics in hospitals and clinics, producing increasingly resistant strains of bacteria that can't be killed and have the potential to make already sick people even sicker.

Bad for the environment, too

Most antibacterial chemicals are washed down the drain and one antibacterial in particular, Triclosan, is now among the most frequently detected compounds in our waterways. It is highly toxic to aquatic life, especially algae, and through our water supply, this chlorophenol works its way back into our bodies. A recent Swedish study found Triclosan in the breastmilk of 60 per cent of the women surveyed. This is a worrying finding, given that there are no human data to show that it is safe on ingestion.

And what happens when this antibacterial combines with chemicals in the wider environment provides further good cause for concern.

For years, manufacturers have reassured consumers that Triclosan breaks down quickly in the environment. But depending on where it is and what other chemicals it comes into contact with in the environment, Triclosan can break down into highly toxic compounds.

Evidence published in 2003 demonstrated that sunlight converts Triclosan into 2,8-dichlorodibenzo-p-dioxin, described as a 'mild' form of dioxin that nevertheless contributes to the already widespread dioxin contamination of our waterways and our bodies.

Dioxins are hormone-disrupting chemicals that mimic the action of natural oestrogen. In the body, oestrogen levels are generally low and finely balanced. However, in excess, oestrogen is a recognised carcinogen. Oestrogen mimics are particularly worrying because they can accumulate in the environment and in the body to produce the kinds of excesses that lead to cancer, reproductive and developmental problems, and immune-system damage.

The most well-known dioxin is the highly toxic 2,3,7,8-tetrachlorodibenzodioxin (TCDD), best known as a highly toxic impurity in Agent Orange, a neurotoxic herbicide used during the Vietnam War. Most dioxins share the toxic profile of TCDD, so the concept of a 'mild' dioxin is more of a public-relations exercise than a scientific certainty.

Moreover, Triclosan in the waterways can be altered further by repeated exposure to chlorine, for instance, in water-treatment facilities. If this chlorine-exposed Triclosan is then exposed to sunlight, it turns into a much more potent form of dioxin.

In 2005, research carried out at Virginia Tech University in the US found that the chlorine in tapwater and the Triclosan in some soaps and other products can react together to create harmful chloroform gas, which can be absorbed through the skin or inhaled. If inhaled in large quantities, chloroform gas can cause depression, liver problems and, in some cases, cancer.

YOUR ANTIBACTERIAL CLEANER IS LIKELY TO CONTAIN ...

Triclosan, phenol, benzalkonium chloride or *chlorohexidine*.

▶ TRY THIS INSTEAD ...

Overuse of antibacterial products of all kinds has become a substitute for good-hygiene practices such as washing hands thoroughly. You can't kill all the germs on your body, nor should you want to as some 'friendly' bacteria, for instance, help to keep the numbers of more harmful bacteria in check. What you can do is ensure that you are clean enough to be healthy. Consider the following alternatives to antibacterial soaps and cleaners.

Stop using antibacterial soaps and cleaners. Regular light cleaning with eco-friendly soap or cleaner and water is better than the occasional intense cleaning with strong biocides.

Use plain soap and warm water in preference to antibacterial soap.

Rinse and wring sponges and cleaning cloths well after use, and store where they can dry out thoroughly. Wash dish- and hand-towels regularly.

Don't buy antibacterial plastics such as cutting boards and storage containers impregnated with antibacterials such as Microban/Triclosan; these agents can leach into the stored foods.

Wipe up spills immediately. It's just common sense.

Hands are the most common vehicles for spreading germs. Wash your hands thoroughly after using the toilet, and before and after preparing food, and teach your children to do the same. Thorough handwashing is defined as 10–15 seconds of vigorous rubbing of the hands to produce a lather, followed by thorough drying. This is in stark contrast to most adults, who spend 3–5 seconds running their hands under water, and don't dry their hands thoroughly before leaving the bathroom or kitchen.

Hang hand and bath towels so that they dry thoroughly between each use. Wash all towels and facecloths regularly and dry thoroughly to remove any accumulated microbes.

■ BATHROOM CLEANERS

When cleaning your body, it's nice to know that you are doing it in a relatively clean space. What's more, in many busy households, the bathroom is sometimes the only private place and temporary refuge. For these reasons, many of us pay special attention to cleaning the bathroom even when the rest of the house is a mess.

But equally, because of the extra attention we pay to bathrooms, the smallest room in the house probably has a greater concentration of toxic chemicals in the air and on its surfaces than any other room in the house.

While it would be easy to think of the toilet bowl as the dirtiest place in the bathroom, this is usually not the case. Your toilet bowl has a constant flush of water running through it to keep it clean. Instead, the majority of really dirty jobs in the bathroom – such as the base of the toilet, the underside of the seat and under the rim, and the soapy scum that builds up in the tub or on the shower door – are usually the result of neglect. Some problems, like mildew on the tiles, are caused by poor ventilation, while others, like the mineral deposits that clog showerheads and make taps look unsightly, are due to living in a hard-water area.

There is a variety of specialist cleaners intended for use in the bathroom. But if you buy these, you may be wasting your time and money, as well as be fooling yourself as regards how much cleaner they really make your bathroom. You may also be exposing yourself to very harsh chemicals unnecessarily. Why risk it when nearly all bathroom-cleaning jobs can be done with everyday cleaners and a few special mixtures of non-toxic ingredients.

TOILET CLEANERS

We have become pretty obsessed with clean toilets in recent years. Spend a night in front of the TV, and you're likely to see commercials featuring animated toilet bowls singing about how happy they are now that they're using brand X, or cartoons showing flowers sprouting out of the bowl.

To keep the bowl fresh, there is a variety of liquids and powders as well as in-cistern and in-bowl devices that colour and fragrance the water as well as clean it and keep limescale at bay. They are all made from roughly the same harsh ingredients, The in-cistern and in-bowl types are perhaps the most risky as, every time you flush, you send a microscopic spray of easily inhaled chemicals into the air in your bathroom.

Toilet-bowl cleaners usually contain industrial strength cationic detergents such as **quaternary ammonium compounds** that, in addition to cleaning power, also act as mild disinfectants. Cationic detergents can be toxic and poisonous to ingest, and may cause nausea and, in extreme cases, coma. Cationics are also more easily absorbed by the skin, which is another reason why manufacturers recommend the use of protective gloves, and advise thorough rinsing should the product come into contact with skin.

YOUR TOILET CLEANER IS LIKELY TO CONTAIN ...

Petroleum-based detergents/surfactants, strong acids such as **muriatic** (**hydrochloric**) **acid** or **sulphuric acid** (**sodium bisulphate**), **oxalic** *acid*, *sodium hypochlorite*, calcium hypochlorite, *sodium carbonate*, sodium metasilicate, *phenols*, *ammonia*, *bleach*, *naphthalene*, *paradichlorobenzene* (PDCB), *5-dimethyldantoin*, *quaternary ammonium salts*, colours and fragrance.

Bleach safety

Liquid household bleaches are approximately a 5-per-cent sodium hypochlorite solution. Used properly, it can be a simple and effective disinfectant. However, chlorine bleach fumes can also be highly irritating to the skin, eyes, nose and throat. Contact with the skin can result in dermatitis. Ingestion can cause oesophageal injury, stomach irritation, and prolonged nausea and vomiting.

Bleach should never be mixed with any other cleaning solution. When mixed with acids such as ammonia, toilet-bowel cleaners, drain cleaners or even vinegar, it can release chloramine gas which can lead to coughing, loss of voice, a feeling of burning and suffocation, and even death.

▶ TRY THIS INSTEAD ...

Not even the darkest recesses of your toilet need attacking with this many detergents and disinfectants. Once again, it's not the cleaning products, but the tools you use with them that are important. So, the first thing to do is invest in a really good-quality toilet-bowl brush – one with stiff bristles – which can be stored in a unit that allows it to air-dry between uses. You can literally clean your toilet with any detergent and get the job done. A plain, diluted, vegetable-based dishwashing liquid or castile soap is ideal. Or try making a more sophisticated mixture.

Make a simple toilet cleaner with:

115 g (4 oz) vegetable-based dishwashing liquid or castile soap
2 cups baking soda

4 tbsp water

2 tbsp white vinegar

You can even add ½ tsp essential oil of peppermint, lemon, pine, tea tree or eucalyptus to give it a fresh, clean scent. Mix all the ingredients together (adding the vinegar last) and put them into a thoroughly rinsed squeezable bottle. This mixture can be used both inside and outside the toilet bowl.

To remove mineral deposits add a cup (250 ml) of white vinegar to the toilet bowl, then toss in a handful of baking soda. Let this bubble away for 10 to 15 minutes before giving the bowl a good scrub and flush.

An overnight soak A simple way to clean is to pour half a cup of borax straight into the bowl; use your brush to give the bowl a quick once-over, and leave it overnight.

Another overnight soak At night, place two effervescent 1000-mg vitamin C tablets (unflavoured), or a mixture of 2 tbsp each of citric acid and bicarbonate of soda, in the toilet bowl. In the morning, brush around the bowl and flush. This can help remove scum below the waterline.

If you still feel you must use conventional cleaners, make sure you put the lid down before you flush the toilet. That way, you won't be sending a spray of chemicals into the air every time you flush.

BATH AND SHOWER CLEANERS

These are usually nothing more than all-purpose cleaners (see above) plus a few extra ingredients, usually strong acids. Typically, they come as liquids, powders and creams. Their main job is to cut though the soapy scum that gets left behind on tubs, tiles and glass shower doors, although some of the newer products act like sealants, leaving a water- and dirt-repellent film on bathroom surfaces to help keep them clean. These products contain moisture-repellent nanoparticles that are 1/10,000th the diameter of a human hair. They are sold in pump bottles and aerosol cans.

Nanoparticles have never been tested for safety, yet they are increasingly being put into household products – in an uncontrolled medical experiment using humans as guinea pigs. Recently, the results of the experiment have begun to come in and, in 2006, the German government was the first to issue a health warning regarding the use of these novel household sprays.

Sealing sprays for glass and ceramics containing moisture-repellent nanoparticles and a propellant have provoked severe health disorders when dispensed from aerosol cans. Sprayed onto surfaces, they also dissipate into the air where they are easily inhaled. Doctors report that once in the lungs, the combination of nanoparticles and propellants disrupt the function of alveolar and bronchial tissues and, by extension, oxygen and moisture exchange. This has led to several cases of respiratory distress and, in severe cases, to accumulation of water in the lungs (pulmonary oedema), which has serious consequence.

To make using conventional bath and shower cleaners safe, never use aerosols, always wear gloves and make sure the room is well ventilated. Never use these products around food, children or animals. Once again, unless your bathroom is sorely neglected, you really don't need special cleaners to get the job done.

▶ TRY THIS INSTEAD ...

Use natural disinfectants. Both white vinegar and lemon juice act as mild disinfectants. Because they are acidic, they can be used to remove hard-water spots, dissolve mineral buildup and break down filmy soap residue without leaving a film of their own. They also act as deodorisers. Use 2 parts of water to 1 part of vinegar or lemon juice, or use undiluted for heavily soiled areas. Since both vinegar and lemon juice are acids, remember to wear rubber gloves if you are going to be using either for more than a few minutes. For scrubbing down the bathroom, a nylon scrubbing pad is a must.

Try a simple abrasive. Baking soda can be used neat to provide a mild abrasive action that is safe for tiles, countertops, sinks and tubs. Apply it with a damp cloth on surfaces or with an old toothbrush to reach hard-to-get-at places.

Consider buying shower curtains that are washable and wash them regularly to prevent soap and mildew buildup. If they get really scummy, spraying with undiluted distilled vinegar before washing will help remove soap residues. If you have a glass shower door, wipe it down after each use with a super-absorbent sponge cloth or, better yet, squeegee, which will be even more efficient. Wiping down tiles and glass doors regularly takes about 30 seconds and will prevent soap scum from building up.

LIMESCALE REMOVERS

Bathroom descalers are usually based on either *citric acid* or *phosphoric acid*. Citric acid is relatively mild and harmless, while phosphoric acid can cause skin and eye injuries.

▶ TRY THIS INSTEAD ...

Metal showerheads can be cleaned by boiling them for 15 minutes (or until the limescale deposits begin to soften) in ½ cup (125 ml) of white vinegar and 1 litre of water. This will remove all but the most stubborn mineral deposits. Scrub clean with an old toothbrush.

To clean a plastic showerhead, soak it in equal parts of white vinegar and warm water for one hour, then scrub clean with an old toothbrush.

To remove mineral deposits from around taps, lay a cloth soaked in hot vinegar on the fixture that needs cleaning. Let it stand for an hour or so, then wipe or gently scrub it off.

MOULD AND MILDEW CLEANERS

Mould and mildew can make your bathroom look and smell bad, and they are also a significant cause of respiratory problems. They are mostly a problem in bathrooms that are poorly ventilated but, instead of tackling them with fresh air, we attack them with strong fungicides. Mildew removers come in many forms, including in liquids which you rub on and then rinse off and, more recently, in sprays that you don't rinse off. They all contain the same basic ingredients. Among these are: *phenol* – a central-nervous-system depressor, skin irritant, circulatory-system disrupter and suspected carcinogen (see above); *kerosene* – which can dry the skin and cause lung inflammation; and *pentachlorophenol* – which is toxic when inhaled, absorbed or ingested and a known reproductive toxin associated with birth defects.

Most mildew cleaners only work in the short term. So, if you're going to use a short-term solution, why not make it a less toxic one?

▶ TRY THIS INSTEAD ...

Borax diluted in a little hot water and applied with an old toothbrush will remove mildew just as effectively. If the problem is really severe, leave the solution on for an hour or so before rinsing it off.

Think airflow Mildew is most likely to build up in damp places, so if you've got this problem, then poor ventilation may be the cause.

■ CARPET AND UPHOLSTERY CLEANERS

Most of us don't realise what effective dust and pesticide traps our carpets are. And yet, every time you tread on your carpet, you send a microscopic cloud of dust, dirt and chemicals into the air.

Along with everyday dirt, studies show that household carpets are reservoirs for volatile organic chemicals (VOCs) such as 4-phenylcyclohexene, tetrachloroethylene, *benzene*, *xylene*, *toluene*, styrene and methylbenzene, as well as tobacco smoke and heavy metals. Carpets also harbour pesticides such as heptachlor, *chlorpyrifos*, *aldrin*, *dieldrin*, *chlordane*, *atrazine*, *DDT*, orthophenylphenol, *propoxur*, *diazinon* and *carbaryl*. Infants and toddlers ingest two and a half times more of these noxious agents than adults do because they spend so much time sitting and playing on the floor. For this reason, keeping your carpet clean is probably more important than you know.

Whether carpet shampoos are the best way to keep carpets clean, however, is debatable. Carpet and rug shampoos are concentrated detergents that come in ready-to-use liquids, trigger sprays, powders and aerosols. They are formulated to wet the pile of the carpet, and take up superficial oil and grease. Applied to the carpet, they attract and trap soils, and then dry to a brittle powdery residue that can be vacuumed up.

All commercial carpet-cleaning solutions can leave behind chemical residues and odours. Whether you are using a small amount of spot-clean spray or a detergent in a carpet-shampooing machine, the basic ingredients are much the same.

Carpet shampoos typically contain water and a mixture of other ingredients like detergents and surfactants, petroleum-based solvents such as *butyl cellosolve* and preservatives. Some contain enzymes to remove protein stains, optical brighteners, soil-retardants such as *formaldehyde*, perfumes and deodorisers.

Upholstery cleaners are similar in their formulation to carpet cleaners and can produce the same toxic effects. All commercial carpet- and upholstery-cleaning solutions leave chemical residues on your carpet and soft furnishings. This residue is perhaps the greatest risk to young children who tend to: a) crawl around on carpets and soft furnishings; and b) stick their hands in their mouths a lot.

Spot removers are, at best, a short-term solution for stains and, at worst, a toxic hazard. Most of these are poisonous when ingested, highly irritating when inhaled and a cause of skin reactions in sensitive people. Typically, they contain *perchloroethylene*, *trichloroethylene*, *diethylene glycol*, ammonium hydroxide, naphthalene and *oxalic acid*.

▶ TRY THIS INSTEAD ...

Regular steam-cleaning is the best way to keep your carpet toxin-free. It may be expensive, but some may reason it is worth the money since the very hot water used in steam-cleaners kills dust mites, fleas, bacteria and mould as well as providing effective cleaning power.

Throw rugs should be laundered regularly, if possible. Non-washable rugs should be shaken outside or hung on a line and beaten with an old-fashioned rug beater or old tennis racket.

In between steam-cleans, you can help keep your fitted carpets clean by:

Removing shoes. Most dirt is tracked in on the bottom of shoes.

Vacuuming regularly. If possible, aim to vacuum weekly to keep the amount of dust and dirt you send into the air to a minimum.

Use a carpet sweeper in between vacuums. These are great for picking up spills and bits of unidentifiable stuff that falls to the floor.

Spot-clean carpets and upholstery with a solution of ½ cup borax in 1 litre of warm water. Use a stiff-bristle brush for carpets and a softer one (like a toothbrush) for upholstery stains. Vacuum well when dry.

Buy washable soft coverings (cushion covers, etc) and launder them regularly. If your sofas and chairs get a lot of wear, consider a washable throw for everyday protection.

CARPET DEODORISERS AND FABRIC FRESHENERS

Carpet fresheners or deodorisers are mostly heavy perfumes formulated to cover up odours. Most commercial carpet-deodorising powders are not all that sophisticated. Usually, they comprise a baking-soda base and a strong petrochemical-derived fragrance.

Fabric fresheners are similar to carpet deodorisers. These products are often marketed to smokers and pet-owners as a way of removing nasty smells from their soft furnishings. They are mostly made up of surfactant, which allows the chemicals to penetrate deeply into the fabric, and perfume. They don't remove smells. Like air fresheners, they contain chemicals that alter your sense of smell.

Given that some commonly used surfactants are contaminated with carcinogens like 1,4-*dioxane*, it hardly seems worth the risk. Prevention is still the best way to avoid carpet and upholstery smells.

▶ TRY THIS INSTEAD ...

Make your own You can make your own carpet deodorant by using plain baking soda fragranced with essential oils. Sprinkle this on your carpet and work it well into the pile. Leave it anywhere from 15 minutes to overnight, depending on the strength of the odour, and then vacuum. This is less expensive than buying commercial brands and just as effective.

Disinfect carpets with borax. Sprinkle it on your carpet, work it into the pile and wait for anywhere from 2 to 24 hours before vacuuming it up. Really mouldy or foul-smelling carpets may need more than one application. *Note*: Inhaling any powder can cause respiratory problems in some individuals, so make sure you use other rooms while these minerals are soaking in.

Open a window. It's still the best way to deodorise most things in your home.

■ DISH DETERGENTS

While not to the same degree as laundry detergents, washing-up liquids can still add to your total toxic load, especially if you use hot water and no protective gloves.

Because dishwashing detergents are generally made from anionic and non-ionic surfactants, they are less well absorbed than some other types of household cleaners and so are considered low in toxicity. Nevertheless, anionic and non-ionic detergents can still cause irritation to the skin, eyes and mucous membranes.

YOUR DISH DETERGENT IS LIKELY TO CONTAIN ...

Petroleum-based detergents such as *diethanolamine* and *sodium dodecylbenzenesulphonate*, preservatives, alcohols, petroleum distillates, ammonia, salts, colouring and perfume.

▶ TRY THIS INSTEAD ...

There are probably more urgent things to worry about than your dishwashing liquid and, in truth, there are few good alternatives. To make using dishwashing detergents safer for the environment:

Choose vegetable-based detergents. More and more supermarkets sell at least one or two good alternatives. Just be aware that some detergents that claim to be 'natural' can still contain other undesirable ingredients such as colourings and perfumes. If you are unsure about an ingredient, write, e-mail or call the manufacturer for clarification.

Use less. Adding a little borax to the water beforehand will make even the smallest amount of washing-up liquid more effective. This is because borax is an effective water softener.

Wear rubber gloves to prevent irritation of the skin and to prevent the absorption of contaminants in the water, including nitrosamines, dioxanes, dyes, colourings and perfumes.

Avoid ammonia. Some washing-up liquids contain small amounts of ammonia, so don't mix them with bleach or bleach-containing products as this combination will form a deadly chloramine gas.

Avoid products that are coloured or fragranced. This will help reduce the number of chemicals you are exposed to.

Dilute your regular brand. Most dishwashing liquids are very concentrated, and we all tend to use much too much to get the job done.

Diluting will not substantially affect the cleaning power of the product. So try mixing equal amounts of vegetable-based washing-up liquid and water. The mixture can be thickened with approximately 1 tbsp of salt. Store in a squirt-top bottle (any well-rinsed dishwashing detergent bottle will do). This will still foam and will still clean your dishes, but will expose you to fewer chemicals.

To make an even less toxic version of this recipe, replace conventional dish detergent with castile soap. Dr Bronner's scent-free liquid baby soap is a good choice. That way, you can add your own fragrance with essential oils if you wish.

As an alternative to dish detergent, wash your dishes in soap flakes with a dash of vinegar to cut through the grease. You will not get loads of bubbles, but your dishes will be clean. You can also wash your dishes effectively in washing soda or borax (always wear gloves when using these substances).

Rinse your dishes well before leaving them to dry. Soaping them up and then leaving them to drain means that chemical residues remain on the plate and are likely to get into the next serving of food you eat from that dish.

AUTOMATIC-DISHWASHER DETERGENTS

Most automatic-dishwasher detergents are either irritants or corrosives, depending on their composition, concentration and physical form. They are made using strong petroleum-based detergents and a strong alkali, giving them a pH value of between 10.5 and 12.0. Skin irritation or burns may result following exposure to dissolved detergents. Many also contain washing soda (sodium carbonate) and occasionally phosphates, which pollute waterways. They may also contain sodium silicate to prevent damage to the dishwasher, a surfactant to prevent waterspots and a fragrance.

Some of these detergents also contain dry chlorine, which becomes activated when mixed with the water in the dishwasher. This means that, when you open the dishwasher, chlorine fumes are released in the steam that leaks out. These can cause eye irritation and difficulty breathing, especially for those with respiratory problems.

The average individual is unlikely to have any prolonged contact with automatic-dishwasher detergents. However, if you have children in the house, you might like to consider using a powdered variety rather than the tablet or liquid varieties. Tablets have become a significant source of poisonings among children and animals, so if you choose these, be sure to store them carefully.

▶ TRY THIS INSTEAD ...

All automatic-dishwasher detergents will leave some chemical residues on your dishes. However, you can cut your exposure to these by trying the following:

Choose powdered brands which, generally speaking, contain fewer harmful ingredients than the liquid variety. Powders are also less likely to be mistakenly swallowed by young children.

Use less. The powder receptacles in dishwashers are larger than they need to be and encourage us to use more detergent than necessary in the machine. The average dishwasher only needs about 2 tbsp of detergent in the closed cup dispenser or 1 tbsp in the open dispenser to work well.

Use low or no phosphate brands. These are much kinder to the environment.

If commercial products are unacceptable, try using ½ tsp of pure soap powder (more will produce too many suds) mixed with 3 tbsp of baking soda.

For normally soiled dishes, use 2 tsp of borax predissolved in hot water, followed by vinegar in the rinse cycle.

For heavily soiled dishes, try washing with ¼ cup of sodium hexa-metaphosphate, a relative of trisodiumphosphate (TSP).

Sprinkle your dishes with baking soda before loading them in the dishwasher, then add detergent to the closed dispenser only. This will cut down on the amount of detergent used, but you will still have clean dishes (but don't put baking soda on your aluminium pans as it will discolour them).

■ FLOOR CLEANERS

Floor cleaners are generally made from either petroleum distillates and solvents or water-based detergents. The mixture makes a cocktail that is dangerous to inhale and possibly irritating to the skin. Of the two types, water-based cleaners are much less toxic. Those containing the solvent glycol monomethyl ether are much more hazardous: if accidentally swallowed, they can cause nausea and vomiting, stomach pain, bleeding and/or chemical pneumonia.

Those which use *pine oils* can cause convulsions, coma and even death if ingested. While this is unlikely because of their strong taste, parents of very young children might reason that, given good alternatives, it's just not worth the risk keeping such products in the house.

Of course, floor cleaners don't have to be swallowed to be toxic. If you have young children who tend to crawl about on the floor, they may well be picking these substances up on their hands and breathing in their fumes. Prolonged and repeated exposure of the skin and to the vapours from floor cleaners can affect the central nervous system, producing symptoms similar to drunkenness, and damage the kidneys.

You don't need anything special to clean your floors. The average household floor attracts average household grime and dust. Cleaning this off is a fairly simple task that can be made much easier if you make a habit of wiping up spills as they happen.

YOUR FLOOR CLEANER IS LIKELY TO CONTAIN ...

Petroleum-based detergents, *ammonia*, *bleach*, phosphates, *pine* or *citrus oil*, solvents such as *butyl cellosolve*, *phosphoric acid*, *potassium hydroxide*, colouring and perfume. Most contain undisclosed preservatives as well. If you use a floor polish on top of this, you will be adding plastics (possible hormone disrupters) that can damage vinyl tiles and turn them yellow over time, as well as petroleum distillates, *naphtha* and *nitrobenzene*.

▶ TRY THIS INSTEAD ...

As with all toxic cleaners, the best alternative is to use less. Most of these products are highly concentrated, and we all tend to overestimate how much we need to use. To make using conventional cleaners safer, always wear gloves and always open a window. Or consider these alternatives:

A simple floor cleaner can be made from hot water and vinegar. Add one cup of vinegar to a full bucket of water. If your floor is really dirty, mix a small amount of liquid soap or soap flakes in with the hot water. Rinse afterwards with a vinegar and water solution. This works well on ceramic, polyurethane-finished wood floors, and on linoleum and other vinyl tiles.

To disinfect mop the floor with ½ cup of borax in a bucketful of hot water. To make sure the borax dissolves thoroughly, put the borax in first and then add the water, stirring until it is dissolved.

To cut grease mix ½ cup of washing soda (sodium carbonate or sal soda) with 1 tbsp of liquid soap, ¼ cup of distilled white vinegar and ½ bucket of water. Washing soda is caustic, so use gloves and avoid splashing. Don't use on waxed floors as it will mottle the finish.

For wood floors use ¼ cup of liquid soap with ½ to 1 cup of distilled vinegar or lemon juice to a bucket of water. To improve the fragrance, use a cup of strong, freshly brewed herbal tea of your choice.

For linoleum combine 6 tbsp of cornstarch for every cup of water, mix together in a bucket and use it as you would any floor polish.

■ GLASS AND MIRRORS

Glass and mirrors show up smudges and fingerprints more readily than other surfaces because they reflect light. No one likes a smeared, smudgy window, but the products that we use to clean our windows and mirrors are still disproportionately strong, given that they generally have a simple job to do.

Once again, this is down to manufacturers responding to what they see as consumer demand for fast-acting products. But apart from paying a premium price for something that is mostly water, you are also exposing yourself to a number of chemical hazards. As window cleaners are inevitably sprays and because you work so close to the glass or mirror while cleaning it, you cannot help but inhale the mixture as you go, and this can be mildly irritating to the eyes, skin, nose and throat.

YOUR GLASS CLEANER IS LIKELY TO CONTAIN ...

Solvents such as *isopropyl alcohol* or *butyl cellosolve*, *ammonia*,

glycol ether, *silicon*, waxes, *formaldehyde* and, if it's an aerosol, propellants such as *isobutane* or *propane* and, sometimes, colourings and
perfumes.

▶ TRY THIS INSTEAD ...

If you are stuck on using conventional products, always use them in a
well-ventilated room, and choose pump sprays over aerosols.

For most glass and mirrors in the home, water is the best cleaner.
Consumer reports show that water cleans mirrors and windows better
than some 60 per cent of the products on the market. Likewise, most
homemade mixtures can equal and, in some cases, better the
commercially available products. What's more, they do it at a fraction
of the price of commercial brands.

Whatever you end up using to clean windows and mirrors will be
made more effective and easier with the right tools. Make sure you have
two lint-free cloths to do the job – one for cleaning and one for drying.
Most people just use paper towels, which are equally effective, but they
are also an expensive and wasteful way to clean. Some of the best and
least expensive cleaning cloths are those big muslin squares that are
commonly used as nappy liners. You can buy these in practically any
mother-and-baby shop. Or, if you want a bit of luxury, invest in the pure
linen scrims used by professional window cleaners.

Simple glass cleaner 1: Put some plain club soda in a spray bottle.
Many people swear by this cleaner, which appears to work because it
contains sodium citrate, which acts like a water softener and, thus, helps
the water to clean more effectively. It won't dry as quickly as conventional cleaners but, for lightly soiled glass and mirrors, this is a perfectly
adequate solution.

Simple glass cleaner 2: Mix equal amounts of water and distilled
vinegar in a spray bottle. The vinegar will help cut through greasy fingerprints and also acts as a room deodoriser.

Foaming glass cleaner is for you if you like some sort of foam to show you where you've sprayed, or your windows or mirrors are particularly greasy and dirty, you can make up a stronger mixture using:

½ tsp liquid soap
3 tbsp distilled white vinegar
2 cups water

Put the ingredients into a spray bottle and shake well. This works well inside the house (and is also an effective all-purpose cleaner for light cleaning), but can sometimes cause streaks on outside and car windows.

■ LAUNDRY PRODUCTS

Wearing clean clothes and sleeping on clean sheets is a pleasure. And in supermarkets nowadays, you can find just about everything you need to make sure that your clothes and household textiles are clean and bright. But, as with all cleaning products, there is a downside to having whites that are whiter than white.

Detergents were first developed as a result of the petroleum industry trying to find a way to make money from the toxic waste materials that they generated each year. One of these was propylene. Eventually, scientists found a way of mixing propylene with **benzene** to produce **sulphuric acid**. They then added **sodium hydroxide** to the mix to neutralise this harmful acid. A sodium salt somewhat like ordinary soap was the result, and the detergent industry was born. Today's detergents are still made largely from the waste materials generated by the petroleum industry.

Powders and liquids contain the same basic ingredients, although liquids include extra ingredients such as opacifiers to make them look nice. These give the liquid a rich, creamy opaque appearance, but do not clean your clothes. They also contain synthetic colours. Liquid detergents contain no filler at all and are more concentrated than powders. Other than that, there is no difference between types of laundry detergents. Liquid tablets and gel packs do not clean better, they don't get into the wash quicker and they don't penetrate fabrics more efficiently. Such claims are used to justify the high price of these novelties, which are invariably much more expensive to use per wash than regular powders.

To help boost the power of your laundry powder, there are a number of wash additives on the market, including:

Pretreatments and stain-removers. These are available in a variety of forms such as pump sprays, liquids, gels, solids or aerosols. They contain surfactants and solvents. Aerosol versions also use a variety of petroleum distillates and propellants. Most pretreatments are just liquid detergents under another name. Logic dictates that if you put detergent in a high concentration on a stain before you start to wash, you will have a better chance of getting the stain out.

Solid or stick formulas are probably best for ground-in stains because the action of rubbing them onto the fabric ensures that they are pushed deeply into the stain. They also have fewer chemicals in them. Frankly, you can substitute a liquid soap or detergent for most pretreatments as it will do exactly the same job.

Laundry boosters. Most laundry detergents include a small amount of added *bleach*, but not enough to handle really tough stains. This is why there are now separate bleaches that you can add to the wash to boost cleaning power. Laundry boosters used to be made with common bleach (*sodium hypochlorite*) – the same stuff used in swimming pools and drain cleaners.

However, as fabrics have become more colourful and sensitive to the effects of common bleach, manufacturers have come up with new colour-sparing bleaches based on sodium perborate or *sodium chloride.* Sodium perborate breaks down into hydrogen peroxide in the wash and liberates oxygen, which oxidises, or bleaches. Sodium chloride liberates *chlorine* gas to oxidise or bleach stains. Chlorine is the more powerful of the two types of bleaches; it is also more irritating to the skin, eyes and lungs. All bleaches are corrosive and harmful if swallowed.

YOUR LAUNDRY PRODUCTS ARE LIKELY TO CONTAIN ...

Petroleum-based detergents and surfactants, enzymes, bleaches, optical brighteners, builders/water softeners (pH adjusters) and processing aids, corrosion inhibitors, anti-redisposition agents and fragrances. Powdered varieties also contain fillers – inert substances that keep the

(continued, page 224)

Toxic softeners

Fabric softeners are made from mild detergents and cationic surfactants such as **quaternary ammonium compounds**. They work by magnetic attraction. A fabric softener has a strong positive charge that forms a uniform positively charged layer on the fabric surface, making it feel softer to the touch (an excess of negative charge on fabrics is responsible for a scratchy feeling after washing and for static cling). Cationic surfactants are also used in laundry products that boast fabric-softening properties.

Fabric-softening sheets release a special resin in the dryer that deposits a waxy coating on the clothes to make them feel softer.

Along with surfactants and resins, fabric softeners deposit a range of other chemicals onto your clothes as well. According to a report by the US Environmental Protection Agency, fabric softeners and dryer sheets contain an enormous number of potentially toxic chemicals. Among them are:

- **A-terpineal (Alpha-terpineol),** which is highly irritating to mucous membranes. It can also cause excitement, ataxia (loss of muscular coordination), hypothermia, CNS* and respiratory depression, and headache. Repeated or prolonged skin contact is not advised.

- **Benzyl acetate,** the vapours of which are irritating to eyes and respiratory passages, and may cause coughing. The chemical can be absorbed through the skin, causing system-wide effects. It is a carcinogen that has been linked to pancreatic cancer.

- **Benzyl alcohol,** which is irritating to the upper respiratory tract, and can cause headache, nausea, vomiting, dizziness, a drop in blood pressure, CNS* depression and, in rare cases, death due to respiratory failure.

- **Camphor,** which is on the EPA's hazardous-waste list. It is readily absorbed through body tissues; vapours and inhalation can irritate the eyes, nose and throat. It is a CNS* stimulant, and associated with dizziness, confusion, nausea, twitching muscles and convulsions.

▶

- **Chloroform,** which is also on the EPA's hazardous-waste list. A neurotoxin, anaesthetic and carcinogen, inhalation of its vapours can cause headache, nausea, vomiting, dizziness, drowsiness, irritation of the respiratory tract and loss of consciousness. Chronic effects of overexposure may include kidney and/or liver damage. Its use can aggravate disorders of the kidney, liver, heart and skin.

- **Ethyl acetate,** which is yet another on the EPA's hazardous-waste list. It can be irritating to the eyes and respiratory tract; it's a narcotic, and exposure may cause headache and narcosis (stupor). It has also been linked with anaemia, leucocytosis (an increase in white blood cells as an immune reaction), and damage to the liver and kidneys.

- **Limonene,** an irritant to the skin and eyes, and a possible cause of allergic reactions. It is also a carcinogen.

- **Linalool,** a narcotic shown to cause CNS* disorders. Animal tests have proven it to adversely affect mood, muscle coordination and spontaneous motor activity.
  Exposure can cause fatal respiratory disturbances. It even attracts bees (thereby posing a threat to people who are allergic to beestings).

- **Pentane,** which is irritating to the eyes and can cause skin rashes. Its vapours may cause headache, nausea, vomiting, dizziness, drowsiness, irritation to the respiratory tract and loss of consciousness. Prolonged and repeated inhalation of vapours may cause CNS* depression.

*CNS, central nervous system (the brain and spinal cord). CNS disorders include Alzheimer's disease, attention-deficit disorder (ADD or ADHD), dementia, multiple chemical sensitivity (MCS), multiple sclerosis (MS), Parkinson's disease, seizures, strokes and sudden infant death syndrome (SIDS). CNS symptoms include aphasia (loss of ability to speak or understand speech), blurred vision, disorientation, dizziness, headache, hunger, memory loss, numbness in the face, and pain in the neck and spine.

powder flowing freely. Some powders are as much as 50 per cent filler. Some contain disinfectants such as *pine oil*, which is highly irritating and may cause allergic reactions, as well as phenolics and *coal-tar* derivatives, which are carcinogenic.

▶ TRY THIS INSTEAD ...

Nearly all commercial brands of laundry detergent and fabric softener leave chemical residues on your clothes which can irritate the skin. While most are made to biodegrade within a matter of days, their manufacturing process is far from ecological. For a healthier environment, buy washing powders and liquids that use only vegetable-based detergents. Also, for everyday stains, non-biological detergents are perfectly adequate. Try to avoid fabric softeners altogether. Other laundry alternatives include:

Choose powders over liquids, tablets and gel packs and, as we all tend to use more detergent than necessary to wash clothes, use less of whichever type you buy.

Try pure soap flakes instead of detergent. Add ½ cup of borax or vinegar to the rinse to remove soapy residue. Vinegar has the advantage of acting like a fabric softener and mould inhibitor as well.

Go non-bio. Biological laundry detergents are formulated with enzymes to get the most common stains out. The enzymes are obtained from selected strains of bacteria. Products that have enzymes in them can be irritating to the skin, and a cause of allergic reactions such as asthma and dermatitis.

Although the addition of enzymes is promoted as the best way to remove 'protein' stains such as from grass, chocolate and blood, this is somewhat misleading. The most common clothing stains are not protein stains, but dirt and grease stains. When you use these specially formu-lated products, you are often paying for the money they have spent on advertising unnecessary additives to you on TV.

To remove heavy soiling add 1 tsp of trisodiumphosphate (TSP) to the wash. Borax and washing soda (sodium carbonate) can also remove heavy stains.

To remove perspiration and odours, pretreat with baking soda, white vinegar or borax dissolved in water. These ingredients can also be added to the wash to freshen the load.

Make use of a washing line if you have one. The sun's rays are the best bleaching agent in the world. Clothes that have been gently dried in the sun also tend to be naturally softer than those tumbled in the dryer.

Starches

Not many of us use starch in our laundry these days. Good thing, too. Laundry starches, while based on cornstarch formulas, contain a number of nasties such as *formaldehyde* – a carcinogen and irritant to the eyes, throat, skin and lungs; *phenols* – carcinogens which also cause CNS depression and severely affect the circulatory system, and are corrosive to skin; and *pentachlorophenol* – a reproductive toxin associated with foetal abnormalities and birth defects.

DRY-CLEANING

When you use a home dry-cleaning fluid or send your clothes out to be dry-cleaned, you are soaking your clothes in a mixture containing some of the most hazardous chemicals around. Not surprisingly, there is a large body of medical evidence showing that people who work in the dry-cleaning industry suffer from a wide range of health problems, including kidney and liver diseases, cancer of the larynx and oesophagus, optic neuritis (inflammation of the optic nerve resulting in vision loss) and memory impairment.

YOUR DRY-CLEANER TYPICALLY USES ...

Carbon tetrachloride, perchloroethylene, trichloroethane, naphthas, benzene and *toluene.* The ingredients in dry-cleaning fluids, whether for home or professional use, are basically the same.

▶ TRY THIS INSTEAD ...

Take a sniff of your clothes when they come back from the cleaners. Most dry-cleaning machines are built to recapture the chemicals used in the cleaning process so that they can be used over and over again. If you can still smell any chemicals at all on your clothes, it may be time to change dry-cleaners. To minimise the risk:

Buy clothes that don't need dry-cleaning. Dry-cleaning is a luxury that should be reserved for the most precious garments. Often, it is simply unnecessary, and manufacturers recommend dry-cleaning only to cover themselves against any potential damage done through careless washing.

Air out your clothes. When you bring clothes home from the cleaners, take the plastic bag off and allow them to air out near an open window before wearing.

Wear rubber gloves. If you are using a commercial household spot-remover, always wear rubber gloves and work so that the fumes are blowing away from you. Do not allow children or pets into the room while you are working. Keep the lid on the product while in use to avoid solvent being vapourised in the room. Always wash any splashes on the skin immediately with soap and plenty of water.

Never use dry-cleaning fluid in a washing machine or put articles that are damp with dry-cleaning fluid into the dryer as most dry-cleaning fluids are inflammable, and those that aren't will produce toxic gases in the dryer.

Look for dry-cleaners that use the Green Earth cleaning process, which is based on liquid silicone rather than volatile chemicals.

These days, you can buy special sheets that claim to freshen dry-cleanable clothes in the dryer. Approach these with caution. They contain powerful spot-removers similar to home dry-cleaning fluids, and strong surfactants and perfumes, both of which can cause allergic reactions.

■ OVEN AND DRAIN CLEANERS

Why do these products appear together, you might ask? Because both are made from the same strongly caustic ingredients.

There are two basic types of drain cleaners. Those used for maintenance are called buildup removers. They contain enzymes or cultured bacteria that produce enzymes, and are formulated to dissolve grease and soap scum.

The second type – drain openers – are highly corrosive and dangerous to use. This is because their main ingredients are **sodium hydroxide** (lye), a caustic that can burn the skin and cause blindness if it gets into the eyes, and **sulphuric acid**, a corrosive chemical that can also cause severe skin burns and blindness. Both types work by eating away at whatever is in their path. This includes your skin if you are unlucky enough to splash some on yourself. The vapours from commercial drain cleaners are also harmful.

The use of chemical drain cleaners as a preventative is not a good idea. If you have a septic tank, be aware that chemical drain openers can kill off all the beneficial bacteria necessary for the efficient working of the tank.

Even buildup removers which claim to be 'non-corrosive' or 'non-caustic' can contain chemicals that can be poisonous if inhaled or swallowed. Such products should clearly state their ingredients.

▶ TRY THIS INSTEAD ...

Regularly running boiling water down the drain is probably the best way to keep drains clear and running well. Since greasy deposits are a major cause of clogged drains, try not to pour grease down the drain if you can help it. In addition:

Make a foaming drain cleaner from 200 g (7 oz) of baking soda, 100 g (3½ oz) of table salt and 200 g (7 oz) of vinegar. When the alkali (baking soda) meets the acid (vinegar), they will bubble furiously, pushing the abrasive salt through the drain. All three ingredients will work to remove deposits from the drain and clear it out. After 20 minutes or so, pour boiling water down the drain to flush it clear.

Use a drain strainer. These little filters can be used in bathrooms and kitchens to keep large particles from going down the drain and forming blockages.

Use a plunger. This can be very effective for dislodging blockages. Once you have opened the drain, use boiling water or the foaming drain cleaner above to clear it out. Be warned though: do not use a plunger after using chemical drain openers as this invites hazardous splashback onto the skin and into the eyes.

Never mix commercial drain openers with anything else, not even natural alternatives. The combination could become reactive, and erupt out of the sink and onto you.

OVEN CLEANERS

Like drain cleaners, the main ingredients of most oven cleaners are *sodium hydroxide* (lye), a caustic that can cause burns to the skin and blindness if it gets into the eyes, and *sulphuric acid*, a corrosive chemical that can also cause severe skin burns and blindness. The reason why oven cleaners are made with lye is simple. When the lye mixes with grease in your oven, it makes a crude form of soap, which then facilitates cleaning.

The majority of oven cleaners are packaged as aerosols. This means that, in addition to lye and sulphuric acid, you are also being exposed to propellants. Strong alkalis can be used on cold ovens. However, there are newer types of oven cleaners that use fewer alkali chemicals. These only work in warm ovens to aid the removal of grease and grime. The vapours from both types are highly toxic.

▶ TRY THIS INSTEAD ...

Prevent messy grime from building up by lining the oven floor with a sheet of aluminium foil. This will catch most spills, and can be changed as often as necessary.

Use baking soda. This can be sprinkled into the oven while still warm to loosen grease, and then be wiped away with warm water. Or you can make a spray from 3 tbsp of baking soda dissolved in 500 ml (1 pint) of warm water. Spray it on, and wait 20 minutes before scrubbing it off with a fine wool pad if necessary. Baking soda is effective for light-to-medium soiled ovens. Heavily soiled ovens may require a different approach.

Use vinegar. Using the same principles for unclogging a drain, you can spray a solution of white vinegar into your warm oven. Sprinkle with baking soda, leave it to bubble and then scrub away.

POLISHES

Nothing says clean like a nice polish on your furniture, brass, copper and silverware as well as shoes and car. But to achieve that nice sheen, we use a mixture of dangerous solvents and waxes derived from petroleum.

FURNITURE POLISH

There are three basic types of commercial furniture polish, each of which uses a different type of chemical to aid the application of the wax or oil to the furniture surface. Solvent polishes use a chemical solvent to dissolve the oil or wax into a liquid. Emulsion polishes suspend the oil or wax in a liquid, usually water. Aerosol sprays are solvents or emulsions under pressure.

Caring for wood is simple. Often, it comes down to how you treat the wood in between cleans, rather than the polish that you buy. If you don't let hot or wet things stand on the surface of the wood, and protect it from hard knocks and sharp points like pens, your furniture should stand up to everything else that everyday life throws at it.

Although wood originally came from a living thing, wooden furniture is not alive. It doesn't need 'nourishing' or 'feeding'. The purpose of polish is mainly to make the wood look nice, and to keep any natural moisture from being released. If your furniture was varnished or polished in the factory, you only need to give it a good going-over once or twice a year. The rest of the time, a simple dusting is sufficient. Overuse of aerosol sprays, in particular, can leave a slight milky film on polished wood, which will be impossible to get out except by stripping and refinishing.

MOST FURNITURE POLISHES CONTAIN ...

Inflammable and hazardous ingredients such as solvents, *petroleum distillates*, volatile organic compounds (VOCs), *naphthas*, *nitrobenzene*, *phenol*, *ammonia formaldehyde* and *benzene*. The health dangers most often associated with polishes of all kinds are inhalation of fumes or vapours (especially from aerosols) and poisoning from ingestion. Polishes that look like strawberry soda or milk are especially tempting to children.

▶ TRY THIS INSTEAD ...

Unvarnished wood can be cleaned and polished easily and beautifully with very simple compounds. For instance, a dab of vinegar on a slightly damp cloth can be a very effective cleaner. A little light olive oil on a cloth will also polish and protect your wood. However, if you are feeling more ambitious, try making the following alternatives:

Simple furniture polish Fill a small bottle two-thirds of the way with oil (olive or walnut are good choices, or a mixture of one of these with linseed oil in a ratio of 2:1 works as well). Top up the bottle with white vinegar, then add 20–30 drops of essential oil (lemon or bergamot are good choices). Shake well before each use and apply sparingly with a soft cloth. Use a second clean cloth for buffing (this is an essential step to avoid a buildup of polish). The vinegar will help to clean your furniture while the oils will protect the wood.

Furniture wax Use this mixture occasionally to polish and protect wood:

2 tbsp beeswax
3 tbsp oil
1 tbsp white vinegar

Grate the beeswax (to help speed the melting process) into a small ceramic bowl or glass measuring cup. Add the oil and vinegar, and put the bowl into a shallow pan of boiling water. Stir it as it mixes and, when it has fully melted, leave it to cool a bit. While the mixture is still liquid, pour it into a small jar. Apply sparingly and leave to dry before buffing with a clean cloth.

METAL POLISH

Most metal polishes contain strong acids such as **phosphoric acid** and **oxalic acid**. They can also contain caustics such as ammonia hydroxide, and reproductive toxins and neurotoxins such as petroleum distillates, nitrobenzene, naphthalene and ethanol.

The most dangerous polishes contain **sulphuric acid** and hydrofluoric acid. The hydrofluoric acid found in some rust removers and aluminium polishes can eat right through the skin down to the bone. Less toxic polishes contain detergents, trisodium phosphates and **pine oils**, but these tend to be the least effective when it comes to removing tarnish.

Metal polishes are acidic because acid dissolves tarnish. Unfortunately, they can sometimes be so harsh that they damage the object you are trying to clean. They can eat through metal or metal plating. They can destroy the lacquer coatings commonly used on items such as brassware, and leave permanent stains on the surface of every type of metal. This is especially true of the 'quick-dip'-type polishes.

▶ TRY THIS INSTEAD ...

Combinations of natural acids like lemon juice or vinegar and salt make good metal cleaners. However, any chloride such as salt or washing soda can damage fine metals, so don't use these home-made polishes on family heirlooms. If an item is of particular value, always consider having it professionally cleaned.

For brass and copper Rub pans with a mixture of salt and vinegar or lemon juice (or lemon rind soaked in salt) and then wash. Heating the vinegar will aid the process since all acids are more active when hot. Give this time to work. The best way is to work the mixture all over the brass or copper item, and then let it sit for a while.

Alternatively, add 15 g (½ oz) of citric acid to ½ litre (1 pint) of water. (You may need to adjust the amount of acid by trial and error.) Swab this on your metal item and leave for a little while. Make sure you place the item on plenty of newspaper or other protective covering and leave a window open. This will remove tarnish and even rust, making polishing much easier.

For bronze Bronze should never be polished. It is easily damaged by water, and polishing will remove the patina that is part of its character. Brush very occasionally with a clean soft brush and use a cottonbud to remove dirt from cervices.

For pewter Likewise, pewter is easily damaged by metal polishes. The best way to protect it is to keep it dust-free with a clean dry cloth and, occasionally, rubbing the outside with a silver-cleaning cloth. Never rub polish on the inside of a pewter goblet or any other vessel intended to hold liquid. Pewter is absorbent, and this can make it unpleasant or even dangerous to drink from.

For silver Some experts believe that a bit of tarnish in the crevices brings out the character and design of the piece, so don't overpolish your silver. Intricate designs are best brushed with a soft brush to get the polish into the detail.

You can make your own simple silver dip by placing a plate-sized sheet of aluminium foil into a saucepan of water and a handful of washing soda. Heat this up and place the silver in the pan for a minute or two, until the tarnish and stains are just coming off. DO NOT leave for a long time and DO NOT use this method for cleaning silver-plated items. Buff with a soft clean cloth or long-term silver cloth.

To clean the inside of a silver teapot, fill it with boiling water and add 1 teaspoon of denture cleaner and leave overnight.

Silver-plated objects should only be polished when absolutely necessary. Try using a special silver-polishing cloth for this job and remember to wear gloves.

To make your own silver-polishing cloth, mix 4 tsp of whiting (a fine powder that can be purchased at most hardware stores) with 2 tbsp of household ammonia and 3 cups of water. Soak a soft absorbent cloth in this mixture, wring it out and allow it to only half-dry (preferably near an open window to avoid fumes filling your house), then store in a resealable plastic bag for use as needed.

For chrome Rather than a commercial mixture of ammonia and other chemicals, why not try straight ammonia and water. Put a dash of it in water and dip a soft cloth in the mix. Rub this on the chrome, rinse and then polish with a clean soft cloth. Make sure to wear protective gloves and try not to breathe in the fumes. If you are washing the car, be careful not to get the ammonia onto the paintwork. In the bathroom, chrome fixtures need only soap and water to clean them. Stubborn stains can be lifted by rubbing gently with a bit of bicarbonate of soda on a slightly damp soft cloth.

For stainless steel Even everyday stainless-steel pans, dishes and cutlery can be damaged by too much polishing and scratchy sponge cleaners. To clean stainless steel, you need hot water and a little detergent – that's all. If you really feel the need for a stronger mixture, use a dash of ammonia in hot water. Drying the items immediately will prevent annoying spots from forming.

SHOE POLISH

Most shoe polishes do not list their ingredients, yet many commercial shoe polishes contain a number of suspected human carcinogens that can be easily absorbed through your skin. Among them are *trichloroethylene*, *nitrobenzene* and *dichloromethane* (methylene chloride).

▶ TRY THIS INSTEAD ...

There is no doubt that your shoes will last longer and look better when they are properly taken care of. But sadly, there are very few good alternatives to conventional shoe polish. Nevertheless, while most of us would never think that there are safety issues involved with shoe polishing, there are. To protect yourself from the nasty chemicals which are found in shoe polish:

Wear gloves when polishing or cleaning shoes – the chemicals in the polish are easily absorbed into your skin.

Make sure shoes are dry before wearing. Many of the vapours emitted from shoe polish interact with alcohol. The presence of alcohol in the system, for instance, heightens the toxic effects of nitrobenzene. For this reason, it is wise not to wear shoes that are still wet with polish if you are going out (or staying in) drinking.

Keep shoe polish out of reach of children.

■ PAINTS AND DECORATING MATERIALS

When a building is overwhelmed with toxic chemicals, it is sometimes called a 'sick building'. When the people inhabiting such a building become sick from chemical exposures, this is known as 'sick building syndrome'. Studies show that, in many cases of sick building syndrome, the use of chemical paints was a key factor in the damage to health.

Not so long ago, our paint contained the heavy metals lead and mercury. Although this is no longer the case, many cases of sick building syndrome have been traced to the chemicals in interior paints. Most con-

---

Marble needs special care

Marble gives the impression of strength and grandeur, but it is really rather soft and easy to chip, break and stain. Marble surfaces in your home should never be cleaned with spirits or acids. Even water will eventually stain and weaken marble, so it is best dealt with by using a dry soft cloth. If you absolutely have to clean marble, try doing it with a little white spirit and a clean cloth. Family heirlooms should only be cleaned by experts. But there is no getting round cleaning marble floors, so try using water and a weak detergent solution. If possible, wash and then thoroughly dry the floor to prevent excess moisture from seeping into the stone.

ventional paints contain solvents and other volatile organic compounds (VOCs), and emit these toxic chemicals as gases for days, months and even years after they've been applied. These gases can cause headaches, and irritate the eyes, nose and throat; they are proven to increase allergies, asthma and respiratory problems and even to weaken immunity.

The chemicals in ordinary paints can also contaminate the environment. For every tonne of paint produced, the resulting waste can be anything up to 30 tonnes. This waste can be toxic and doesn't degrade naturally. Emulsions produce less waste than gloss or varnish, but can still cause damage. Harmful chemicals mean you shouldn't pour paint down the drain or throw it away with your rubbish. Your local authority can advise about paint disposal and recycling.

These days, paints sold in the EU require labels giving information as to their environmental effects – for example, whether the ingredients can damage the ozone layer. Paints should also be labelled if they can cause allergies. When choosing your paint, be sure to read the label. If the information you require is not there, always contact the manufacturer.

There are, however, alternatives. Some contain no chemical solvents, while others just contain fewer than conventional paints. Eco-friendly paints use ingredients such as turpentine or D-limonene as alternatives to white spirit. Instead of plastic binders, they may use linseed oil and casein, and chalk and clay may replace fillers such as titanium dioxide. Colours are often derived from natural earth and mineral pigments.

YOUR HOUSEHOLD PAINT IS LIKELY TO CONTAIN ...

Acetone, ammonia, benzene, ethylene acrylate, *ethylene glycol, formaldehyde, kerosene, methyl alcohol, phenol, propylene glycol, quaternary ammonium compounds, trichloroethylene* and *vinyl acetate/acrylic copolymer.*

▶ TRY THIS INSTEAD ...

Use latex (water-based) paint instead of oil-based paint and, if you can, choose low-odour paints or those based on natural ingredients and pigments – they are not only ecologically sound, but also safer for the immediate home environment. Paints based on natural ingredients have the advantage of allowing surfaces and materials to breathe more freely that chemical paints, which often create a totally impermeable film that encourages moulds and fungi to grow in homes, resulting in adverse effects on health. Most natural-paint manufacturers also openly declare all of the ingredients used in their products, which allows allergy sufferers to check out the particular products and avoid those that could cause a problem.

Polishing the car?

Car waxes typically are 75–85 per cent *naphtha* and 15–25 per cent wax. Naphtha is inflammable, and an irritant that can enter your system through inhalation, ingestion, and skin and eye contact. Chapped skin and sensitivity to light may develop with repeated and prolonged contact. When polishing the car, wear protective gloves. When the polish is not in use, make sure the top of the tin or bottle is securely closed and that the bottle is kept out of the reach of children.

Remember also that windscreen-wiper solution is more hazardous than most of us realise. Most types are anything from 37- to 100-per-cent solvent such as *ethylene glycol*, *isopropanol* and *methanol*, with the rest being made up of detergent and water. The most toxic windscreen-wiper solutions are 100-per-cent *methanol*.

Due to its hazardous nature, windscreen-wiper solutions should always have a child-proof safety cap. Needless to say, they should be stored away from children and pets. There are few real alternatives to their use, however, and when you're streaking along the highway on a murky, muddy, rainy day, the safety of a clean windscreen is certainly a top priority. So, try to choose solutions that are detergent-based. When topping up your car, wear gloves, and avoid skin contact and inhalation. Make sure the safety cap is replaced securely.

Dispose of any leftover paint with care You can avoid too much excess if you calculate the amount you need carefully before you buy. Many stores will help you do this, and some will take back unopened cans. Alternatively, consider donating any good leftover paint to a community organisation that can make use of it.

Consider these other useful tips:

Paintbrush cleaners Clean paintbrushes immediately after use. Wash away latex paint over a sink, not outside in the gutter. Work mechanic's 'waterless' hand cleaner into the brush, and wash with soap and water. Clean paintbrushes hardened with dried oil-based paint by soaking them in hot vinegar.

Paint thinners Avoid using oil-based paints, which require solvent thinners for cleaning up. If you do need to use a thinner, use it in a jar and pour off any clear thinner for reuse after the particles have settled. Wrap the particles in newspaper and throw into the rubbish bin.

Chemical paint strippers Avoid strippers containing *methylene chloride*, *trichloroethylene* (TCE) and *benzene* (all of which can cause cancer), 1,1,1-*trichloroethane* (TCA) (an irritant to eyes and tissues), *xylene* (toxic when drunk or breathed in) or *toluene* (known to cause birth defects). To strip away paint, use a heat gun, paint scraper or a sanding block with course sandpaper (wear safety goggles and a mask). Remember, stripping lead-based paint is dangerous and should be done by a professional. Inhaling the dust or vapours can cause lead poisoning. Safe and effective water-based paint strippers are now available. These are kinder to the environment as well as kinder to surfaces.

Spray paints Avoid using these. Aerosols make it more likely that the user will breathe in the paint, and the aerosol propellants contribute to air pollution.

Wood preservatives Do not use old products that contain *pentachlorophenol* (PCP) (causes cancer in laboratory animals), *creosote*, *tributyltin oxide* or *folpet*. Never burn wood treated with wood preservatives as this will release the chemicals into the air. Old treated scrapwood can be taken to a landfill for disposal. Water-based preservatives are available that can seal wood, and protect it from water rot and insects. A water sealer or polyurethane can prevent wood rot. Use types of wood (such as redwood and cedar) that are naturally resistant to insects and wood rot.

Wood stains and finishes Use finishes derived from natural sources such as shellac, tung oil, beeswax and linseed oil. Wherever you can, use water-based stains.

chapter **8**

home and garden pesticides

NO ONE LIKES THE THOUGHT of sharing their living space with 'pests'. While most of us have a clear idea of the kind of creepy crawlies we'd like to keep away – rodents, cockroaches and flies, for instance – a pest can be broadly defined as any plant, animal or otherwise that happens to be in the wrong place at the wrong time!

So, in addition to liberally treating our homes with commercial bug sprays, we spend billions each year trying to control the environment outdoors with a raft of garden pesticides, fungicides and weedkillers. Indeed, every year, in our obsessive bid to remove all traces of the humble dandelion from the earth's surface, we spray tonnes of toxic chemicals on home lawns, parks, playgrounds, golf courses and other recreation grounds – not because dandelions are inherently bad, but purely because this little plant has taken root somewhere inconvenient. Whatever pest you are trying to control, keeping it at bay with conventional pest-control products comes at a hefty cost.

While many of us worry about the pesticides that might be lingering in or on our food these days, few give more than a moment's thought before whipping out the bug spray whenever a wasp or troop of ants invades the house. This is why the vast majority of our pesticide exposure – some 80 per cent according to US data – actually happens in our homes, offices and schools, with measurable levels of up to 12 different pesticides found in the air of the average home.

In one 1995 survey, somewhere in the region of 85 per cent of American homes were found to have at least three to four different pesticide products in them, including pest strips, bait boxes, bug bombs, flea collars, pesticide-containing pet shampoos, aerosols, granules, liquids and dusts. Many household products such as disinfectants, cleansers and mildew removers also contain pesticides.

The picture is much the same in the UK. The British public spends around £50 million on pesticide products for their homes and gardens. According to the Pesticide Action Network (PAN) UK, British household-ers are dousing their homes and gardens with pesticides to the tune of 4306 tonnes of pesticides each year. Worse, as much as 20 per cent of these pes-ticides were disposed of by householders pouring them down the drain. Once in the water supply, these nasty chemicals become everyone's problem since most water-treatment facilities cannot adequately remove these chemicals from tapwater.

Of course, we don't just drink this water – we bathe and shower in it as well. It has been suggested that the amount of volatile chemicals inhaled during a 15-minute shower with contaminated water is equivalent to drink-ing about eight glasses of contaminated water. In addition, many industrial contaminants can easily pass through the skin into the body during showers, baths and dishwashing, more than doubling the amount of chem-icals that pass into your body.

Think pesticides, and the first thing that is likely to come to mind is insecticide, the stuff we use to kill ants, flies and cockroaches. But the term 'pesticide' is a blanket description for many other types of chemicals such as bacteriocides (which kill bacteria), herbicides (which target plants), fungicides (which kill fungi) and rodenticides (the poisons laid down to kill rodents). These days, a pesticide can also be an organism including, for example, a genetically modified crop.

Amazingly, given their widespread use, the pesticides that we use nowa-days didn't even exist before World War II. In fact, many of them were developed during the war for use as weapons. The organophosphate insec-ticides were first developed as nerve gases, and the phenoxy herbicides, including 2,4-D (one of the most commonly used herbicides in homes and the community), were created to eradicate the Japanese rice crop. Later, during the Vietnam War, it was included as a component of Agent Orange to defoliate large areas in jungle warfare.

After the war, the chemical manufacturers needed to find other uses for their products, which had been produced in massive quantities. And so they began to be applied as pesticides in agricultural production, for environmental spraying of neighbourhoods for mosquito eradication, and for individual home and garden use.

Although pesticides can be helpful in the short term around your home and garden, they can be dangerous if applied or stored carelessly – for instance, within the reach of children. It's worth remembering that pesticides are chemical weapons. They are designed to kill things. For this reason, they are not really 'safe' – even when used as directed. Regularly inhaling them, ingesting them or getting them on your skin constitutes a cumulative assault on your health. This is because most pesticides are poisonous and persistent chemicals – they don't biodegrade in your body or the environment, so the more you use them, the more they will accumulate around and inside you.

Pesticide products are made up of a mixture of active ingredients (the chemicals that kill specific organisms) and inactive, or inert, ingredients (the chemical base in which the active ingredients are mixed; see page 250 for more on inerts). Most pesticides on the market have not undergone a complete battery of tests to find out exactly how harmful their ingredients might be to humans. What's more, while some pesticides have been subjected to safety testing, as with all the other chemicals you will find in your home, they are tested one at a time. Yet, research from Duke University in North Carolina has shown that, when three pesticides (used at their 'safe' levels) are combined, their toxicity is increased by a factor of several hundred.

Our enthusiasm for pesticides in the home and garden is now such that US scientists have concluded that pesticide overexposure – once an occupational hazard of agricultural and factory workers – is now everybody's problem. Home use of pesticides rose 42 per cent between 1998 and 2001. In the garden, herbicides are applied more intensively for lawn care than they are on most farms, with application rates of between 3.2 to 9.8 pounds per acre for lawns, compared with agricultural averages of 2.7 pounds per acre.

As our use of home and garden pesticides increases, evidence is also accumulating of the health effects of this exposure in adults and children and, while it has long been assumed that you need to be exposed to high levels of pesticides to be damaged by them, emerging evidence says this isn't so. The weedkiller *atrazine*, for example, is an oestrogen mimic that has been shown to feminise male frogs at levels 10,000 to 30,000 times below the presumed 'safe' limits.

How we are exposed to pesticides

Pesticides get into our bodies in a variety of ways. We can ingest them with our food and water, and they can be inhaled or absorbed through the skin when we are using sprays or foggers. While agricultural use still accounts for the major use of pesticides in the world, their applications in other areas that intersect with our lives daily has become more widespread, moving from the field to the high street to the home, without much apparent enquiry into either appropriateness or safety or, more crucially, alternatives.

Sources of common household pesticides include bathroom- and kitchen-cleaning products, wallpaper pastes, paint, wooden furniture (especially if made from recycled railway sleepers), insecticides for wood (such as woodworm treatments) and woollens (mothballs), roach, fly and wasp sprays, pest strips, sprays for indoor plants, head-lice and intestinal-parasite treatments, swimming-pool and spa disinfectants and algaecides, and pest- and weedkillers used in the garden. Our irrational fear of 'bugs' has also led to soft furnishings, carpets and mattresses being pretreated with powerful pesticides such as *permethrin* (the same pesticide implicated in the debilitating symptoms of Gulf War syndrome).

But even if you don't use pesticides in your home, you cannot avoid being exposed. If your neighbour treats his home or lawn, chances are, you'll be breathing it in. If you are walking down a street where the local council has just sprayed, you will get it on your clothes and into your lungs. If you picnic in the park or play a few rounds of golf, you will be exposed.

Grocery stores, restaurants, hotels, hospital cafeterias, schools and many apartment buildings and nursing homes are routinely sprayed and fumigated. Wooden playground equipment, decking and picnic tables are treated with a variety of substances, including arsenic.

Know your pesticides

There are many different types of pesticides, each made from different starting materials and each with its own particular effects on the body.

A major 2004 review of the human health-effects of pesticide exposure by the Ontario College of Physicians concluded that, while there is a widely held perception that some pesticides are safer than others, this is not borne out by the evidence. They write: 'Exposure to all the commonly used pesticides – phenoxyherbicides, organophosphates, carbamates, and pyrethrins – has shown positive associations with adverse health effects. The literature does not support the concept that some pesticides are safer than others; it simply points to different health effects with different latency periods for the different classes.'

Below are some of the main classes of pesticides you will come into contact with in your home and garden, as well as in the wider community.

ORGANOCHLORINES

The main representatives of chlorinated pesticides are **aldrin**, **dieldrin**, **chlordane**, heptachlor, transnonachlor, **DDT** and its metabolites (**DDE**, DDD), endrin, hexachlorobenzene and **lindane** (alpha, beta, delta, BHC). This group of chemicals also includes **polychlorinated biphenyls** (PCBs), originally used as electrical coolants, but which have also been used to kill bugs. These have been used extensively in agriculture, in forestry and even in households over the last 20 years. Some organochlorines have been banned in Canada and the US due to their persistence in the environment. However, they are still manufactured in these countries and exported to developing countries for use in agriculture there. Chlorinated pesticides are hormone-disrupting and can cause various conditions in humans, including cancer. PCB exposure can result in neurological disorders, malignant melanoma and liver cancer.

▶

ORGANOPHOSPHATES

These have largely replaced organochlorines in agricultural pest control. They are often portrayed as safer than organochlorines because they break down more rapidly. Nevertheless, many organophosphates such as parathion, *malathion*, *diazinon*, phosmet and *chlorpyrifos* are highly toxic. They affect the central nervous system (CNS; the brain and spinal cord) and peripheral nervous system (nerves found outside the CNS). This particularly affects the muscles, glands and smooth muscles that are related to organ function, and has been found to cause delayed neurotoxicity involving the cerebral cortex, brainstem, spinal cord, peripheral nerves, muscles and eyes. Symptoms can appear 30 minutes after exposure and may last for up to 24 hours.

CARBAMATES

Including aldicarb, *bendiocarb*, *carbaryl*, *propoxur* and thio-phanate methyl, carbamates are used extensively in agriculture, forestry and gardening. The immediate effects of exposure include muscle weakness, altered perception, headache, nausea, vomiting, abdominal pain, visual problems and muscle twitches. Over the longer term, these compounds are associated with a higher risk of lung cancer, with reproductive effects including damage to testes, sperm and DNA, and behavioural effects.

PHENOXYS

In this group of toxic chemicals, the most well known are *2,4-D* and 2,4,5-T which, when proportionately mixed, constitute Agent Orange. Extensively used in the control of terrestrial broadleaved plants, they have been proven to cause leukopenia, and non-Hodgkin's lymphoma and lung cancer. Agent Orange exposure has recently been linked to the development of type 2 diabetes.

PYRETHRINS

Pyrethrins occur in nature in many plants, but today's pyrethrin pesticides are produced in the lab and known as synthetic pyrethrins (SPs). SPs interfere with the function of the insect's

▶

nervous system. They can be found in spray-on products, in flea, tick and head-lice treatments, and also imbedded into most soft furnishings. Examples include **allethrin**, syfluthrin, **cypermethrin**, **deltamethrin** and **resmethrin**. Exposure to pyrethrins is associated with chronic psychiatric effects, chromosomal aberrations, rashes in licensed pet groomers and intrauterine growth retardation, which is a major determinant of poor health in the first year of life.

THIOCARBAMATES

This group of fungicides includes the EBDCs (ethylene bis-dithio-carbamates) mancozeb, **maneb** and metiram. EBDC use is becoming more widespread. When these chemicals are used on stored produce and when such contaminated fruit and/or vegetables are cooked, EBDC's active ingredients break down into ethyl-enethiourea (ETU). ETU can cause goitres (enlargement of the thyroid gland), birth defects and cancer in exposed experimental animals. It has been classified by the US Environmental Protection Agency (EPA) as a probable human carcinogen.

Railway lines, waterways, embankments, city and suburban streets are regularly doused with bug-zapping chemicals. Even underground electric cables are treated with insecticides such as **aldrin** and **chlordane** to discourage any insects that may make the mistake of munching on them.

Most forms of public transport, such as buses and underground trains, make use of pesticides by being regularly fumigated. Airlines keen to get rid of insects looking for a free ride regularly fumigate their planes. This is particularly worrying since pesticides, while already dangerous on land, have the potential to be particularly harmful when used on planes as up to 50 per cent of the air inside the cabins is recycled. This means that passengers can sometimes find themselves sealed for hours at a stretch in a poorly ventilated chamber that has recently been gassed with no escape from the chemicals in the air. Interestingly, the symptoms of severe jet lag are very similar to pesticide poisoning.

How do pesticides work?

A pesticide is any substance or mixture of substances used to destroy, suppress or alter the lifecycle of any pest; it can be a naturally derived or synthetically produced substance. Most work by interfering with the normal life-sustaining processes of the organism. Pesticides have this effect on simple organisms such as bacteria and they also can do the same on more complex organisms like humans.

Disturbingly, the way most pesticides work is not fully understood, but most produce their toxic effects by:

- **Blocking photosynthesis.** In plants, the process of using sunlight energy to create carbohydrates from carbon dioxide and water is known as photosynthesis. Pesticides that disrupt photosynthesis prevent the plant from producing or storing energy which, ultimately, kills the plant.

- **Interfering with metabolism.** Metabolism is the transfer of energy within the cells of organisms, which is essential for the growth and survival of all living things. There are many inhibitory pesticides such as rotenone and cyanide in this category that disrupt respiratory function in animals, herbicides that inhibit seed germination or plant growth (especially at the root and shoot tips) and fungicides that inhibit germination of spores.

  Sometimes, a pesticide has to be metabolised (usually by being ingested) before it becomes toxic to the target pest.

- **Interfering with nerve function and signalling.** These pesticides affect mainly insects, nematodes and rodents. Some are narcotics such as some fumigant pesticides. Others, such as the organophosphate, carbamate and pyrethroid pesticides, disrupt the flow of nerve impulses.

- **Causing genetic damage.** Our chromosomes carry genes, and both are made up of DNA – the control centre of higher organisms. Chemicals that disrupt DNA can stop the organism from reproducing or alter the way it functions in important ways. Male insects can be made sterile with such pesticides. Interfering with DNA can disrupt the rate and timing of a range of cellular functions. When the cells don't function properly, neither does the organism.

Toxic timber treatments

Wood used for, among other things, playground equipment, climbing frames, patio decking, picnic tables, fencing and shelving is treated with preservatives to help keep wood-munching bugs at bay. Wood preservatives are pesticides and, because wood is porous, they can easily leach out of the wood and onto hands and feet, and into food. Exposure to wood treatments has been shown to raise the risk of several types of cancer:

* A 1998 occupational study on men involved in wood preservation suggested that *chlorophenol* exposure may increase the risk of soft tissue sarcoma.

* In 1997, scientists found an increased risk of non-Hodgkin's lymphoma associated with *chlorophenate* wood-preservative exposure among sawmill workers. Chlorophenate was widely used in British Columbia, Canada, as a fungicide starting from the 1940s and up to 1989, when its use was discontinued.

* Results from a 1995 study in Germany that investigated the adverse effects of wood preservatives used in daycare centres showed significantly reduced birthweights and body lengths in babies born to women exposed to organochlorines, pentachlorophenol (PCP) or *lindane*.

* Many outdoors wood products are pressure-treated with *chromated copper arsenate* (CCA). These products constitute our biggest exposure to the toxic element arsenic. CCA is poisonous to humans, and easily rubs off treated wood. Very young children, who are always putting their hands into their mouths, can ingest up to 2016 mcg (micrograms) of arsenic per day from just playing on treated wood. To put this dosage into perspective, the maximum safe amount of arsenic for an 11-kilogram (25-pound) child is 3.4 mcg/day. Arsenic is implicated in liver, lung, skin, bladder, kidney and prostate cancers. Low but chronic exposures can produce symptoms such as stomach ache, nausea, vomiting and diarrhoea.

During the lifetime of treated wood, especially if it's outdoors, the chemicals used to preserve wood can be washed away into

▶

the soil, eventually making their way into the water table. At the end of its lifecycle, treated wood may be chopped up for mulch or wood chippings, and 'recycled' back into our gardens, where it continues to pollute the soil and surrounding area for years to come.

Animals suffer from our use of timber treatments as well. In the UK, bat populations have declined sharply as a direct result of the chemical treatment of roof timbers against pests.

Chemical treatment of timber pests in homes or workplaces is always toxic, and there are strong arguments to support the theory that such chemical treatment is less effective, more expensive and more dangerous than alternative traditional methods.

The pests that attack timber in buildings belong to two main groups: wood-boring insects; and fungal rots. Pest problems arise where the environmental conditions are comfortable for them. Dry rot, wet rot and many wood-boring insects will only be found in damp timber.

So, solve your damp problem and you will have gone a long way towards solving your pest problem. Consider measures to manage the physical environment in terms of damp, ventilation and temperature, adequate damp-proofing, replacement of severely damaged timber, and use of materials and building techniques that reduce the risk of future pest attack.

- **Causing hormone disruption.** Hormones are biochemical messengers that control many of the biological functions of organisms, including the growth and reproductive cycles. Several pesticides simulate or otherwise interfere with reproductive hormones such as oestrogen and testosterone, and growth-regulating hormones such as thyroid hormones, to disrupt these cycles.

- **Causing protein synthesis and enzyme disruption.** Proteins are the basic building blocks of all cells. Enzymes are proteins that control many important cell functions, so many pesticides aim to disrupt enzyme processes or to denature proteins.

Some pesticides work in more than one way and fall into more than one of these categories. Some are physically toxic – in other words, they block the cellular processes of target organisms in a purely mechanical way. Examples include spray oils that clog the respiratory mechanisms of insects, petroleum oils that dissolve protective waxes on some insects and plants, or substances that destroy the membranes of plant cells, causing them to dry out and die. Some petroleum oils can deter feeding or egg-laying in some insects.

Inert ingredients

Some product labels, especially those on household cleaners and garden products, list only the 'active' ingredients. The rest of the ingredients are considered 'inert', or inactive, and therefore assumed to be harmless. But the average consumer should be aware that the word 'inert' on product labels is completely misleading. Far from being inactive or non-reactive, 'inert' ingredients in pesticide products may include highly toxic chemicals.

Among the 2300 inert ingredients used in pesticide formulations, over 1700 of them are of unknown toxicity, 209 are hazardous air and water pollutants, 21 are known or suspected carcinogens and 127 are listed as occupational hazards, according to a 1998 report by the Northwest Coalition for Alternatives to Pesticides.

Because so-called inert ingredients are considered harmless, they are not subjected to safety reviews. Interestingly, a chemical that is listed as inert in one product may be listed as an active ingredient in another.

The lack of disclosure of potentially toxic inert ingredients on product labels places consumers who wish to protect their health at a distinct disadvantage. This is especially true since inert ingredients can combine synergistically to create powerful toxins (see 'The Cocktail Effect', page 28).

When most of us think of the toxicity of pesticides, we tend to think of the active ingredients – the pesticide(s) that are included to kill bugs. But, in common with many pharmaceutical drugs, cosmetics, cleaners, soaps and perfumes, the active ingredients are usually present within a matrix of inactive or inert ingredients to improve storage, handling, application and effectiveness.

Inert ingredients are sometimes referred to as 'secret ingredients' because the recipe developed by formulation chemists to meet all the requirements of storage, handling, application, effectiveness and safety is considered a 'trade secret' and, as such, is protected by law. What is public knowledge is the list of EPA-approved substances that can be used in pesticide products.

For years, no one paid any attention to pesticide inactive ingredients until it began to emerge that some very harmful chemicals were being added to these formulations under the misnomer of 'inert' ingredients.

Even the notorious and harmful pesticide **DDT** has been used as an inert ingredient since its ban in most developed countries as an active ingredient. The EPA acknowledges that there is a complete lack of health-effect data on some 800 inerts used in pesticide formulations, and at least 160 inert ingredients are known toxic chemicals, including solvents such as chloroform, toluene and xylene.

The toxicity of inerts

The term 'inert' implies that a substance is non-toxic, but all inerts are toxic to some degree. So, these ingredients are tested to determine their toxicity, and only inert ingredients approved by the EPA are allowed in pesticide products. In addition, the EPA encourages pesticide registrants to use the least toxic inert ingredients in their products. As well as testing the toxicity of the active ingredient, the toxicity of pesticide products, including the inert ingredients, must be determined.

Inactive ingredient	Adverse effects
Carbon tetrachloride	Irritation of skin, eyes, nose, throat; dizziness, vomiting, abdominal pain; diarrhoea; damage to kidneys, liver; CNS depression; suspected carcinogen
Chlorobenzene	Eye and skin irritation, burns and inflammation; chest pain, slow heart rate, ECG irregularities; lung, liver and kidney damage; CNS depression; coma
Chloroform	Irritation to eyes and gastrointestinal tract; damage to liver and kidneys; CNS depression; nausea, dizziness, fatigue, respiratory distress; gonadal atrophy; foetal resorption; mutagen; coma and death by cardiac arrest; suspected carcinogen
Chloroethane	Irritation of eyes; abdominal cramps, nausea, vomiting; liver and kidney damage; neurological dysfunction; blood cell disorders; suspected carcinogen

Inactive ingredient	Adverse effects
Cresols	Skin irritation, burns and inflammation; irritation of eye, permanent eye damage and blindness; pneumonia; pancreatitis; CNS disorders; kidney failure
Dibutylphthalate	Irritation of eyes and throat; photophobia, conjunctivitis, nausea, dizziness
Diethylhexylphthalate	Eye, nose and throat irritation; liver damage; testicular damage; CNS depression; suspected carcinogen
Dimethylphthalate	Irritation of eyes, mouth, nose and throat; dizziness, abdominal pain, nausea, vomiting, diarrhoea; CNS depression; reduced respiratory rate; paralysis, coma
Epichlorohydrin	Skin and eye irritation, conjunctivitis, corneal clouding; nausea, vomiting, fatigue; liver and kidney damage; inflammation of lungs, chronic bronchitis; death by respiratory paralysis; mutagenic; foetotoxic
Ethylbenzene	Irritation of eyes, nose and throat; skin irritation, inflammation, blisters and burns; liver and kidney damage; CNS disorders; headache, sleepiness, difficulty in breathing; loss of consciousness and coma
Ethylene dichloride	Nausea, vomiting, diarrhoea; damage to liver and kidneys; CNS depression; death due to circulatory and respiratory failure
Isophorone	Irritation of skin, nose, throat and respiratory system; lung congestion and degeneration; CNS disorders; kidney and liver damage; suspected carcinogen
Methyl bromide	Eye and skin irritation; blurred vision, headache, dizziness, nausea, abdominal cramps; anorexia; bronchopneumonia, pulmonary oedema; brain damage, convulsions, coma; kidney and respiratory failure
o-Dichlorobenzene	Eye irritation and cataracts; skin irritation and lesions; headache, nausea, vomiting, drowsiness; respiratory depression; anaemia; kidney and liver damage; chromosomal breaks
p-Dichlorobenzene	Irritation of skin, eyes, respiratory system; headache, dizziness, hyperactivity, weakness, weight loss; liver and blood disorders; kidney damage; lung congestion, difficulty in breathing; mutagenic
Phenol	Irritation of eyes, nose, throat; headache, dizziness, fainting, abdominal pain, nausea, vomiting, diarrhoea; damage to liver, kidneys and heart; chromosomal aberrations and damage; mutagenic
Propylene dichloride	Eye and skin irritation; dizziness, disorientation, nausea, vomiting; liver and kidney damage; CNS damage; coma; haemolytic anaemia; suspected carcinogen

Inactive ingredient	Adverse effects
1,1,2-Trichloroethane	Gastrointestinal inflammation and congestion; liver and kidney damage; immune-function disorder; CNS depression; suspected carcinogen
Toluene	Skin, eye and respiratory irritation; abdominal pain, headache, nausea, dizziness, drowsiness, hallucinations; anaemia; liver disorders and enlargement; CNS dysfunction; coma and death
Trichloroethylene	Eye irritation, visual distortion; abdominal pain, nausea, diarrhoea; anorexia; liver and kidney damage; peripheral nerve damage, numbness and paralysis; blood disorders; cardiac arrhythmia; suspected carcinogen

CNS = central nervous system

The 'cide effects

Every year, millions of people worldwide (mostly in developing countries) suffer severe poisonings from pesticides. Many more are exposed to levels that are considered low, but are still dangerous to health. Regular pesticide use is also associated with neurological effects, decreased immunity, and reproductive and developmental abnormalities.

Pesticides are a significant and avoidable source of toxicity today. Unlike some forms of toxic exposure in the home, it is fairly easy to identify a cause and effect between pesticide use and ill health, and to track the adverse health effects from home and garden use. But there are other, equally worrying, effects. What's more, these effects are not new.

By the late 1950s, a number of commonly used pesticides, including *DDT* and arsenates, had been linked with disorders ranging from leukaemia to skin cancer. In 1955, rising rates of hepatitis in the US were being linked to the increasing use of DDT and other chlorinated pesticides.

As of 1990, 117 different pesticides still in use were identified as potential causes of chronic health problems; 27 of these show strong evidence of carcinogenicity (yet, only 6 of these require specific warnings on the label as to this health hazard). The other 90 pesticides cause problems such as birth defects and sterility.

There are, however, many who dispute the idea that pesticides kill people as well as bugs. They argue that daily exposure levels are low, that such products would not be on sale if they weren't safe. But such arguments fly in the face of mounting evidence that pesticide exposure is causing deep and lasting harm to our health.

Pesticides can affect the immune system and the central nervous system, and other bodily systems such as the endocrine (hormonal) system, as well as genes. Damage to genes may be inherited by the next generation, and then passed on to subsequent generations. These important non-cancer effects of pesticides have hardly been studied by government health authorities.

- **Acute 'ill-defined' symptoms** Typical symptoms that can occur following an acute exposure to pesticides include nausea, low energy levels, weakness, sleep problems, dizziness, headache, migraine, anxiety, depression, aching joints, mental disorientation, inability to concentrate, vomiting, convulsions, skin irritations/rashes, flu-like symptoms, allergic reactions and asthma-like problems.

- **Chronic health effects** These effects include cancer (children and adults); birth defects; genetic damage; neurological, psychological and behavioural effects; blood disorders; chemical sensitivities; reproductive effects; and abnormalities in liver, kidney and immune function. These chronic health effects can develop following either an acute poisoning or low-level exposure over an extended period of time.

The ill-defined symptoms of pesticide exposure can, of course, be the result of a number of different conditions or diseases. Nevertheless, according to a 2003 report issued by the Health Care Without Harm organisation, 'Pesticide poisonings are frequently misdiagnosed or unrecognised, largely because most health care providers receive minimal training in environmental illnesses and few people know when they have been exposed to a pesticide.'

Children at risk

Concern over children's increased risk from pesticide exposure is not new. In 1989, the US Natural Resources Defense Council (NRDC) alleged that as many as 6200 children might develop cancer later in life due to exposure to just eight pesticides during their preschool years. That same year, the EPA

Increasing our vulnerability

Many aspects of our lifestyles make us more or less vulnerable to health problems of pesticide exposure. Certainly, women and children are more vulnerable because they tend to be smaller and so, pound for pound, receive a higher exposure than most men.

In addition, specific health conditions or individual vulnerabilities that directly increase susceptibility to pesticide effects include:

- Alcoholism
- Autoimmune conditions (such as lupus)
- Blood disorders (such as anaemia)
- Chemical sensitivity
- Youth (aged 13 or under)
- Colitis
- Diabetes
- Elderly (aged 74 and over)
- Heart disease
- Homelessness
- Immune dysfunction
- Kidney disease
- Leukaemia
- Liver disease
- Lung disease (chronic)
- Malnourishment
- Neurological disease
- Previous pesticide exposure
- Pregnant and lactating women and their offspring
- Prescription medications
- Skin conditions (which increase dermal absorption)
- Smoking

Our prescription-drug culture complicates the picture further by introducing the risk of drug-pesticide reactions. About 10 per cent of all prescription drugs are known to increase the toxicity of pesticides. These include:

- Ambenonium
- Beta-blockers (for heart conditions)
- Chemotherapy

▶

- Cycrimine (for Parkinsonism)
- Demarcarium
- Digoxin
- Glaucoma medications
- Isoflurophate
- Myasthenia gravis medications
- Neostigmine
- Phenobarbitol
- Phenytoin
- Phospholine iodide (echothiophate)
- Physostigmine
- Pilocarpine
- Procaine (used in general anaesthesia)
- Propranolol (Inderol)
- Pyridostigmine
- Succinyl choline (used in general anaesthesia)
- Cimetidine (Tagamet)
- Methimazole (Tapozole)

released a preliminary report suggesting that between 15,000 and 50,000 infants and children in the US each day run the risk of getting sick from potatoes on which the insecticide aldicarb has been used. But, as always, it is the link between pesticide exposure and the development of childhood cancer that has grabbed most of the headlines.

Childhood cancer

In spite of the objections of major chemical companies, the evidence linking pesticide exposure to childhood cancer is firmly established, though not all studies show that it is the ingestion of pesticides that poses the greatest risk. Research has shown that pesticide use in the home – for instance, to get rid of termites, flies and wasps, and in the form of no-pest strips, flea collars, and garden insecticides and herbicides – resulted in a significant increase in childhood brain cancers.

Other reports and studies have linked pesticide exposure to a wide range of malignancies in children, including leukaemia, neuroblastoma, Wilms' tumour of the kidneys and non-Hodgkin's lymphoma as well as cancers of the brain, colorectum and testes.

In a 1987 National Cancer Institute study, the risk of childhood leukaemia increased nearly four times when pesticides were used within the home at least once a week, and increased by more than six times when garden pesticides were used at least once a month.

In another 1995 study involving 474 children, those living in homes where no-pest strips embedded with insecticides were used had up to a threefold greater risk of developing leukaemia than those living in homes without the strips. Even worse, children under 14 had four times the normal risk of tumours of connective tissue if their gardens at home were treated with pesticides or herbicides.

In the same study, pregnant women exposed to the pesticides used by professional exterminators in their homes were three times more likely to have a child with non-Hodgkin's lymphoma, and children directly exposed to pesticides by professional exterminators were more than twice as likely to develop the disease.

Otherwise rare cancers can also become more common with exposure to pesticides. One study at the University of Southern California found that children whose mothers used pesticides in the home once or twice a week were nearly two-and-a-half times as likely to develop non-Hodgkin's lymphoma. Those whose mothers used pesticides on a daily basis were seven times more likely to have the cancer.

Child development and intelligence

There is also ongoing concern regarding the toxic effects of pesticides on the developing brain and nervous system. In 1998, German researchers, for example, report that early exposure to *polychlorinated biphenyls* (PCBs), which are sometimes found in pesticides, can interfere with early childhood development.

The researchers looked at both the pre- and postnatal exposure of 171 otherwise healthy infants, and measured their development at 7, 18, 30 and 42 months. At all of these timepoints, there was evidence that PCB exposure could retard mental and motor development. The only good news in the study was the fact that, where the mother breastfed her infant for longer (even if her breastmilk was a source of PCBs) and in families where parents provided a stimulating home environment, the damage done by the PCBs was significantly less.

In another 1996 study published in the *New England Journal of Medicine*, children exposed to a variety of pesticides in an agricultural community in Mexico showed impaired stamina, coordination, memory and capacity to represent familiar subjects in simple drawings. Yet another study showed that children exposed to PCBs during foetal life had IQ deficits, and hyperactivity and attention deficits, when tested years later.

Adult exposures

Among adults exposed to pesticides, there are three major areas of concern: cancer; reproductive effects (ranging from sterility, infertility and subfertility to birth defects, stillbirths and miscarriage); and effects on the brain and central nervous system (neurotoxicity). It is highly likely that the link with adult diseases reflects a lifetime's exposure to pesticides beginning in childhood.

Generally speaking, ingested pesticides, like many other toxins, are stored in fatty tissue and released gradually into the bloodstream, especially during periods of stress. Also in common with many toxic exposures, the early signs and symptoms associated with chronic exposure to pesticides are often labelled 'idiopathic' (of unknown origin) or psychosomatic, a diagnosis that prevents the person from getting the help they need to get well again.

Adult cancers

Throughout the world, studies have shown that the risk of different cancers increases with increasing pesticide exposure. In adults, the use of chlorophenoxy acid herbicides (such as **2,4-D**) has been linked with an increased incidence of lung cancer, stomach cancer and leukaemia. Two studies have found a fivefold increased risk of Hodgkin's lymphoma, and other evidence suggests a five- to sixfold increased risk for non-Hodgkin's lymphoma.

In addition, many studies have shown a two- to sevenfold increased risk of soft-tissue sarcomas. One showed that farmers in the American state of Kansas using herbicides for as few as 20 days a year have six times the risk of developing lymphoma and soft-tissue sarcomas compared with non-exposed individuals. Those who mixed and applied herbicides, and were exposed for 20 or more days per year, were eight times as likely to develop non-Hodgkin's lymphoma.

In 1992, a Swedish investigation of 275 confirmed cases of multiple myeloma (cancer that starts in the bone marrow and spreads to various bones, especially the skull) among farmers found that exposure to chlorophenoxy acid herbicides and DDT were the most important risk factors for the disease.

Neurological disorders

Pesticide exposure is increasingly being linked to a number of neurological disorders now common in old age. While research in this area is still in its infancy, there is a good theoretical basis for the idea that pesticide exposure can lead to degenerative disorders such as Alzheimer's and Parkinson's diseases.

Many pesticides are designed specifically to attack and destroy the nervous systems of insects. Once disabled, the insect is not able to fly or move its legs; paralysed and unable to feed itself, it dies. It is likely that chronic exposure to some pesticides will do much the same to the human nervous system, though research into this area is sparse.

Nevertheless, there is some evidence to suggest that people who are frequently exposed to pesticides, such as farmers and gardeners, have a higher risk of developing mild cognitive dysfunction (MCD). MCD is a somewhat more subtle disorder than dementia, though the two share some common symptoms such as memory loss and confusion. In 2000, a study from the Netherlands found that adults exposed to pesticides on a regular basis – for instance, farmers and gardeners – had five or more times the usual risk of developing the subtle neurological impairments or learning problems considered common in MCD.

Osteoporosis

Other deleterious effects of pesticides have recently come to light. A 1999 analysis of bone density in agricultural workers published in the scientific journal *The Lancet* showed that exposure to pesticides can make bones significantly more porous.

The discovery was made when British researchers assessed agricultural workers seeking litigation for ill health caused by chronic exposure to organophosphates. The men had been exposed to this type of pesticide for between 3 and 20 years at some point in their lives. Bone biopsies showed significant erosion of the bones in the exposed men as well as much lower bone formation at tissue and cellular levels compared with non-exposed men.

Because of a lack of data, the researchers were unable to say categorically whether the damage to the bone was a direct or indirect result of exposure to organophosphates. While the pesticide can directly enter bone and cause damage, it can also produce other symptoms (such as lethargy, fatigue and depression) that may limit an individual's level of physical activity and, thus, have a further, indirect impact on bone health.

Diabetes

Recent research suggests that exposure to herbicides during the Vietnam War, especially Agent Orange (a mixture of the pesticides **2,4-D** and 2,4,5-T), may be associated with the development of diabetes later in life.

When published, the results of this study were treated as isolated and relevant only to Vietnam vets. But the use of 2,4-D is particularly widespread even today. It is commonly used by local authorities to inhibit weed growth on roads and right-of-ways. It can also be purchased at garden stores for home lawn care and is often used by commercial lawn-care companies.

No one understands exactly how pesticides can cause changes in glucose metabolism or lead to diabetes, but it may be the result of some sort of hormonal effects.

Lowered immunity

For years, nobody was sure whether pesticide exposure could damage immunity or not. Then, in 1996, scientists at the Washington, DC-based World Resources Institute (WRI) undertook a review of all reports of compromised immunity as a result of pesticide exposure. The conclusion was that many widely used pesticides are deeply damaging to human immune function.

Many of the studies reviewed by the WRI scientists came from the former Soviet Union, one of the few places where scientists have examined the impact of pesticides on human immunity. In one investigation of water and soil contamination in Kishinëv, in Moldova, high levels of pesticide residues on many local crops resulted in elevated rates of skin diseases, tuberculosis, tooth decay, ear infections and acute respiratory diseases among the local children. Rates of infection in adults were also higher than expected, and laboratory testing revealed that, as an individual's exposure to pesticides went up, so the levels of T cells (infection-fighting cells) went down.

The report also included data from studies of Inuit children in the northern Hudson Bay area of Canada. The children, nursed on human milk highly contaminated with organochlorine pollutants, not only suffered an increased risk of infections, but some had immune systems so depressed that they could not withstand a standard course of childhood vaccinations.

Pesticides may also interfere with thyroid function and this, in turn, may have a debilitating effect on immunity. The mechanisms by which pesticides might affect human thyroid function are not clear, though some have hypothesised that pesticides deplete the body's mineral stores, thereby resulting in thyroid disorders.

Chronic fatigue

In traditional Indian, or Ayurvedic, medicine, chronic fatigue syndrome (CFS) is the result of accumulated toxins in the body. Western medicine, too, is beginning to acknowledge the link between CFS and chemical poisoning. Pesticide poisoning, for example, can produce symptoms similar to CFS and fibromyalgia (widespread musculoskeletal pain, tenderness and fatigue), and patients suffering from chronic fatigue have been found to have, on average, twice the levels of pesticides in their blood compared with those not suffering from CFS.

Organophosphate pesticides and insecticides, in particular, are strongly associated with CFS – a condition identical to that suffered by farm workers who regularly work with sheep dips and insecticides.

Looking for more evidence of a connection, scientists in Glasgow studied a small group of individuals who had been experiencing neuro-behavioural symptoms for over a year, and who had been exposed to organophosphates – through sheep dip – for between two and five years.

Their symptoms included an acute flu-like condition followed by incapacitating fatigue. In all cases, there was a long delay between exposure to the pesticides and the onset of the condition – a problem seen with many toxic exposures and one that, for a doctor who knows nothing about environmental illness, makes diagnosis difficult.

Dealing with household pests naturally

Insect pests are an intimate part of every home. In the air or the cupboard, on the carpet or the counter, every home shares its resources with these tiny, often unseen invaders. But many pesticides now in use are simply not necessary. Opportunistic pests can be kept at bay with regular cleaning and attention to basic hygiene measures. Don't leave food out on countertops and, where possible, consider installing screens over windows to keep flying bugs out. The use of fungicides (for instance, in the bathroom) can be avoided by making sure rooms are well ventilated and humidity levels kept low. Save common household bug-busters like bleach for when they are really needed, as its overuse encourages stronger and more resistant species.

Pesticides are available for most common household insect pests, but these potent chemical compounds may be more harmful to you and the environment than the pests are.

Here are some natural, non-toxic ways to control household pests.

ANTS

According to a 2001 study by researchers at Stanford University, ants appear to invade kitchens and dining rooms to escape searing heat or excessive dampness – and there is little we can do to stop them. The study found that cold, wet conditions were those most likely to drive ants indoors, though hot dry weather also triggered small infestations.

Even if the weather is the main determinant of ant invasions, it can pay to remove the things that make life indoors cosy for ants: keep counters and floors free of crumbs and sticky spots; store food in sealed containers; and cut off water sources such as drips or dishes left soaking overnight, as these can attract ants.

COMMON ANT TREATMENTS INCLUDE ...

Allethrin, cypermethrin, bendiocarb, boric acid, carbaryl, chlorpyrifos, cypermethrin, deltamethrin, diazinon, fenitrothion, lindane, permethrin, D-phenothrin, pyrethrin, tetramethrin and **trichlorphon.**

▶ TRY THIS INSTEAD ...

Fill a spray-bottle with soapy water, and spray the ants.

Trace the ant column back to its point of entry. Set any of the following items at the entry area in a small line, which ants will not cross: cayenne pepper, citrus oil (can be soaked into a piece of string), lemon juice, cinnamon or coffee grounds.

Try creating a sticky barrier (you can buy these or just use petroleum jelly) which ants simply will not cross.

Create your own bait. Mix half a teaspoon each of honey, borax and aspartame (the artificial sweetener sold as Equal and NutraSweet) in small bottles, and place the bottles on their sides, with lids off, in areas of ant activity. Ants will carry the bait back to their colonies. Important: use indoors only; must be kept away from pets and children.

Encourage ants nesting in a plant pot to move to another home by flooding the pot.

Flooding with boiling or soapy water will effectively kill ants nesting beneath outdoor surfaces such as patios and paved areas.

DUST MITES

Microscopic dust mites are everywhere in the home – in our beds, clothing, furniture, book shelves and stuffed animals. For most of us, they are not a problem, but for people with allergies or asthma, dust mites can trigger sometimes severe reactions.

COMMON DUST-MITE TREATMENTS INCLUDE ...

Alpha cypermethrin, bioresmethrin, chlorpyrifos, chlorpyrifos methyl, *cypermethrin, D-phenothrin, fenitrothion, methoprene, permethrin, pirimiphosmethyl, propoxur, resmethrin,* S-bioallethrin and *tetramethrin.*

▶ TRY THIS INSTEAD ...

Vacuum mattresses and pillows regularly.

Wash bedding at 55° C or higher. Commercial laundry products have no effect on mites unless the water temperature is high.

Keep the bedroom mite-free. Books, stuffed animals, throw rugs and laundry hampers should be kept out of the bedroom of allergy sufferers. Wash stuffed animals occasionally in hot water.

Cover mattress and pillows with laminated covers that prevent penetration by dust mites. Avoid fabric-covered headboards.

Cover heating ducts with a filter that can trap tiny dust particles smaller than 10 microns.

Avoid using humidifiers. Dust mites thrive on warmth and humidity.

COCKROACHES

The best defence against cockroaches is a clean house. If roaches are a problem in your home, vacuum well and wash the area with a strong soap. Dispose of the vacuum-cleaner bag in a sealed container outside the house.

COMMON COCKROACH TREATMENTS INCLUDE ...

Alpha cypermethrin, azamethiphos, bendiocarb, bioallethrin and *D-allethrin, bioresmethrin, carbaryl, chlorpyrifos,* chlorpyrifos methyl, *cypermethrin, diazinon, dichlorvos, dimethoate, D-phenothrin, enitrothion, fenoxycarb, fipronil, flufenoxuron, hydramethylnon, hydroprene, iodofenphos, lambda cyhalothrin, lindane, methoprene, permethrin, pirimiphosmethyl, propoxur,* piriproxyfen, *resmethrin, S-bioallethrin* and *tetramethrin.*

▶ TRY THIS INSTEAD ...

Roaches like high places. If you put boric acid on top of your kitchen cabinets (not inside) – if space allows between ceiling and cabinets – the roaches will take the boric acid back to their nests, killing all of them. Boric acid is toxic if swallowed, so keep it away from children and pets.

Catnip can be used as a natural repellent to cockroaches. Its active ingredient is nepetalactone, which is non-toxic to humans and pets. As long as you don't have cats in your home, you can try leaving small sachets in areas of cockroach activity. Catnip can also be simmered in a small amount of water to make a 'catnip tea', which can be used as a spray along skirting boards and behind counters.

Keep a spray bottle of soapy water on hand. Spraying roaches directly with soapy water will kill them.

Non-toxic roach traps are commercially available. Remember to inspect these regularly.

MOSQUITOES

Mosquitoes can transmit serious, potentially fatal organisms causing such diseases as encephalitis, dengue fever, malaria and yellow fever. They are generally most active from April through October. The first line of defence against mosquitoes is to seal their point of entry. Mosquitoes are most active in the early morning and early evening. They seek areas of still air because their movements are hampered by breezes. Closing windows and doors is your first priority.

COMMON MOSQUITO TREATMENTS INCLUDE...

Bioallethrin, bioresmethrin, cypermethrin, D-allethrin, deltamethrin, dichlorvos, fenothrin, *permethrin, pyrethrins, S-bioallethrin, S-methoprene* and *tetramethrin.*

▶ TRY THIS INSTEAD ...

Remove standing water. The most important measure you can take is to remove standing water sources. Change the water in birdbaths, ponds and pets' water bowls twice a week. This will prevent mosquitoes using the water to breed.

Keep your gutters clean and clear of debris. that would stop them draining. Remove garden items that collect water.

Use essential oils. Making and using a spray with eucalyptus oil at a 30 per cent concentration (that is, 3 parts oil to 10 parts water) can keep mosquitoes from biting for up to two hours (the eucalyptus oil must have a minimum of 70 per cent cineole content, the active therapeutic ingredient). Studies have shown this is more effective than a similar concentration of citronella oil.

Try neem oil. Neem oil is a natural vegetable oil extracted from the neem tree, which grows in India. The leaves, seeds and seed oil all contain sallanin, a compound that has effective mosquito-repelling properties. You can make your own repellent using neem oil or buy neem oil-based sprays.

Throw a bit of sage or rosemary on the barbeque coals. The scent will help to repel mosquitoes while you are cooking and eating outdoors.

Plant marigolds around the garden – they work as a natural bug repellent because the flowers give off a fragrance bugs and flying insects do not like.

HOUSEFLIES

Houseflies have evolved in close association with people and their environment. While houseflies are plentiful and annoying, of greater importance is their role in the possible transmission of organisms that cause diseases and illnesses such as typhoid, cholera, dysentery and diarrhoea. As with mosquitoes, the best defence is, if at all possible, not to let them into your home.

COMMON HOUSEFLY TREATMENTS INCLUDE ...

Bioallethrin, *bioresmethrin*, *cypermethrin*, *D-allethrin*, *deltamethrin*, *dichlorvos*, fenothrin, *permethrin*, *pyrethrins*, *S-bioallethrin*, *S-methoprene* and *tetramethrin.*

▶ TRY THIS INSTEAD ...

Make your own flypaper with this simple recipe: mix ¼ cup water, 1 tbsp granulated sugar and 1 tbsp brown sugar in a small bowl. Cut strips of brown craft paper and soak in this mixture. Let dry overnight. To hang, poke a small hole at the top of each strip and hang with string or thread.

Use a fly swatter. It's an inexpensive and effective way to kill the odd fly that invades your home.

Try small sachets of crushed mint. They can be placed around the home to discourage flies.

Bay leaves, cloves and eucalyptus wrapped in small cheesecloth squares can be hung by open windows or doors.

Place a small, open container of sweet basil and clover near pet food or any open food in the house.

A few drops of eucalyptus oil on a scrap of absorbent cloth will deter flies. Leave in areas where flies are a problem.

WASPS

Solitary wasps in the home are more of a nuisance than a threat. Daily sightings of wasps in the home may indicate indoor nest building, in which case more attention to the problem is required. Avoid swatting and squashing individual wasps; when a wasp is squashed, a pheromone is released that attracts other nearby wasps and encourages them to behave aggressively. It's best to walk away from a hovering wasp.

COMMON WASP TREATMENTS INCLUDE ...

Bendiocarb, carbaryl, chlorpyrifos, dichlorvos, D-phenothrin, enitrothion, iodofenphos, permethrin, pirimiphosmethyl, pyrethrins, resmethrin, rotenone, S-bioallethrin and *tetramethrin*.

▶ TRY THIS INSTEAD ...

Seal any entry points – it is the best line of defence. Check your house for unsealed vents, torn screens, cracks around windows and door frames, and open dampers. Observe the flight path of a wasp, especially in the morning, which may reveal the entry/exit point.

Remove food sources. In the spring and early summer, wasps are attracted to protein foods. Any food left outdoors such as pet food, picnic scraps, open garbage containers or uncovered compost piles should be removed or covered. Wasps imprint food sources, and will continue to search an area for some time after the food has been removed.

Cover open food and drink containers. In late summer and early fall, the wasps' food preference turns to the sweet. Their behaviour is also more aggressive. Open cans of soda, fruit juice, fallen apples beneath fruit trees and other sweet food sources will attract them. Be sure to cover drinks and open food containers, keep a lid on the compost and avoid walking barefoot near fruit trees. Pick up and dispose of any fallen fruit rotting on the ground.

Minimise use of perfumes and other strong scents. In the later part of the summer, wasps (and bees) are attracted to sweet smells.

Try these alternatives for other common household pests:

Moths

- Cedar chips in a cheesecloth square or cedar oil in an absorbent cloth will repel moths. The cedar should be 'aromatic cedar', also referred to as 'juniper' in some places.
- Homemade moth-repelling sachets can also be made with lavender, rosemary, vetiver and rose petals.
- Dried lemon peel is also a natural moth deterrent; simply toss it into your clothes chest, or tie a handful in cheesecloth or old tights and hang it up in the closet.

Earwigs

- Diatomaceous earth is a safe and effective way to control earwigs in the home. One application in key spots (bathroom, skirting boards, windowframes) can be a long-term repellent.
- To trap earwigs, spray a newspaper lightly with water, roll it up loosely and secure with a string or rubber band. Place on the ground near earwig activity. The next morning, discard the paper in a sealed container.
- Another way to trap earwigs is to take a shallow, straight-sided container and fill it halfway with vegetable oil. Clean the trap daily; the oil can be reused.

Silverfish

- Silverfish prefer damp, warm conditions such as those found around kitchen and bathroom plumbing. Start by vacuuming the area to remove food particles and insect eggs. Silverfish can be easily trapped in small glass containers. Wrap the outside with tape so they can climb up and fall in. They will be trapped inside because they cannot climb smooth surfaces. Drown them in soapy water. The best preventive control is to remedy the damp conditions.

MICE

House mice are 'commensals', which means that they prefer to live in structures provided by humans or close to human residences rather than outside. Any house or apartment, old or new, cat or no cat, can be a 'mouse house', so care must be taken to ensure that they don't get too comfortable in your home – if they do, they can be hard to get rid of.

Older techniques of controlling mice, such as trapping and poisoning, can also endanger companion animals and children. Live traps can be used to humanely trap and relocate mice, but unless you mouseproof your house, you will have a continual problem.

Mice and rats can be very persistent in their efforts to invade your home and, often, our feeble attempts at rodent-proofing only bring frustration and failure. The most common chemical weapons in the battle against rodents are anticoagulant rodenticides such as **difenacoum** and **bromadiolone**, which prevent blood-clotting and cause death from internal bleeding. These rodenticides are usually incorporated in a bait of attractive food. Care needs to be taken not to place these chemical baits in areas where children, pets or other non-target animals can gain access as these pesticides are designed to kill mammals.

▶ TRY THIS INSTEAD ...

Mice like your house because you offer food, water and shelter. Eliminate access to these things and your problems will be over. Mouseproofing your house may take some time though.

Remove the food source. Grains, sugar, sweets, pastas, nuts and dry pet foods, for example, should be stored in lidded glass or metal jars, not in plastic bags and containers. Keep your bread in a breadbox, not on the counter. Dribbles around the mouths of syrup, honey and jam jars should be washed off before the containers are put away. Fruit with broken skin should be refrigerated as should potatoes and onions, unless you can keep them in a mouseproof cupboard. Drawers are virtually impossible to mouseproof, so don't keep edibles in them.

Remove access. A mouse can squeeze through any pencil-sized opening. Inspect your upper cupboards for pencil-sized cracks. Rats and mice can also run along or climb electrical wires, ropes, cables, vines, shrubs and trees. Knowing this, you should trim the vegetation from around your home. Try to leave a couple of feet between your house and the vegetation. You should also check any wires or cables that enter your home. Remember, a pencil-sized opening around a cable or wire is sufficient for mouse entry. The cupboard under your kitchen sink is probably the most mouse-vulnerable one in your house. Check for openings around pipes. Seal any small openings with tin or lath, as mice can chew through caulking. Shove bits of steel wool into any other cracks you find. Mouseproofing your kitchen will probably solve most of your mouse problems. If they can't find anything good to eat, they'll move out pretty quickly.

Be humane. Most good hardware shops will stock live mouse and rat traps, or will order them for you from their suppliers.

Tending your garden naturally

Whether you are growing vegetables or flowers, whether you have a large plot of land or just a few window boxes, chances are, you have lavished a lot of care on your little patch of green. The last thing you want spoiling it are opportunistic insects, fungi and other pests.

While the environmental problems of the world may seem beyond your control, you can make a difference right in your own backyard by adopting a more natural approach to gardening.

Pesticides can be an effective way of controlling garden pests in the short term, but they are toxic, encourage resistance among fungi and adaptable insects, and spell disaster for the environment.

Remember, the more of these products you use in your home and garden, the greater the risks. For example, in 2002, it was found that expo-sure to a mixture of three herbicides commonly used to kill household weeds – **2,4-D**, **MCCP** (mecoprop) and **dicamba** – increased the risk of miscarriage and reduced fertility in an animal experiment.

The levels used in this study were very low – as low as 39 parts per billion (ppb), or comparable to one drop of pesticide in 500 bathtubsful of water. This level is seven times less than the established 'safe' level for drinking water. Nevertheless, among the exposed animals, there was a 20 per cent increase in failed pregnancy.

In many cases, there are alternatives that are often more effective in the long run, and less harmful to the environment and the applicator, than the quick and dirty method of commercial pest control.

Gardeners have been battling pests for centuries. Begin by learning good gardening strategies, many of which will result in fewer pest problems, then learn how to use less harmful methods for managing insect pests, weeds and diseases in your garden before reaching for chemical controls.

COMMON GARDEN PESTICIDES INCLUDE ...

The insecticides *acephate, carbaryl, chlorpyrifos, dichlorvos (DDVP), malathion, trichlorphon*; the herbicides *atrazine, benfluralin* (Benefin), *bensulide, 2,4-D, DSMA* (disodium methanearsonate), *dacthal* (DCPA), *dicamba, endothall, glyphosate, isoxaben, MCPP* (mecoprop), *MSMA, pendimethalin, pronamide, siduron, triclopyr* and *trifluralin*; and the fungicides *chlorothalonil, maneb, pentachloronitrobenzene* (PCNB; quintozene), sulphur, *triadimefon* and *ziram*.

According to the US group Beyond Pesticides, of these commonly used garden pesticides, 19 have studies pointing towards carcinogenic effects, 13 are linked with birth defects, 21 with reproductive effects, 15 with neurotoxicity, 26 with liver or kidney damage, 27 are sensitisers and/or irritants and 11 have the potential to disrupt the endocrine (hormonal) system.

▶ TRY THIS INSTEAD ...

A full discussion of how to manage a natural garden is beyond the scope of this book, but there are a number of simple things you can do in your garden to keep it beautiful while also making it healthy and safe for your family, pets and the environment.

First of all, be realistic

- Keep your garden as natural as possible by using less grass, and more trees, ground covers, flowers and mulches.
- Choose plants that are native to the region. These plants are heartier and more resistant to pests and diseases than exotic varieties.
- Use plants that are well suited to your garden's habitat. Consider drainage, sun exposure and soil type when making your choices.
- On sloped areas, plant ground covers instead of grass to alleviate mowing and control erosion.

Healthy soil makes healthy plants

- Test your soil for pH and nutrients. A soil test kit can be picked up at the garden centre. Add what is needed based on results.
- Add compost and organic fertiliser to your garden each year.
- For lawns, aerate soil, overseed and top-dress with compost.

Maintain the health of your plants and lawn

- Prune plants to optimally utilise the plants' energy sources.
- Shear off dead or diseased portions as they may attract pests.
- Mow no more than a third of a grass blade and leave clippings on the lawn.
- Water deeply, but less frequently.
- Use only slow-release fertilisers.

When pests become a problem

- Use physical controls to exclude pests such as mulch, compost, bark, grass clippings, traps, sticky wraps, pheromone bags, barriers/screens, floating row covers, seedling collars and cheesecloth.
- Practise cultural controls such as handpicking weeds and tilling soil in areas of weeds rather than applying herbicides.
- Practise landscape diversity. A pest that likes a certain type of plant is less likely to spread if other species are planted in between.
- A simple soap spray is one of the oldest non-toxic pesticides you can use. It can be made by mixing 1–2 tbsp of mild liquid soap (such as washing-up liquid) to 1 litre of water. Transfer this mix to a sprayer and use as needed.

Use natural pest control products, usually found at local garden centres or DIY stores. These include:

- **Horticultural oils.** A safe alternative that has been used since before the pesticide revolution. It is popular for controlling pests on ornamental plants.
- **Insecticidal soap,** which can be purchased at garden centres, is a safe treatment for aphid, mite and whitefly control, and used by many greenhouses. It works by impairing the waxy layer of the insect's exoskeleton and eventually kills the insect.
- **Neem seed extract** discourages all types of fungi, moulds and even ants, and acts as a growth regulator.
- **Diatomaceous earth**, derived from the fossil remains of one-celled algae, can be used for insect and mite management.
- **Boric acid or borax** will kill ants and even cockroaches. Since most ants like sweets, try mixing a bit of honey or other sugar with boric acid to make a paste. Spread this on small cardboard squares and put these in the ant trail so that the ants will eat the mixture and take some back to their nest (you can also find pesticide-free fly and wasp traps at most garden centres).

chapter **9**

pet supplies

PETS ARE EXPOSED TO THE SAME CHEMICALS in their diet and grooming supplies that people are. As consumers have become increasingly attracted to, and comfortable with, the use of natural and organic products themselves, they are becoming equally receptive to the use of natural products, including pest control and herbal supplements, for their pets. Indeed, a 1999 study led by one source, US Business Research, found that 22 per cent of pet owners had used some form of alternative therapy on their pet.

The petcare industry is big business. In the US, pet owners spend around $16 billion (£8.8 billion) a year on pet products. In Europe, they spend $18 billion (£10 billion). Pet food accounts for about 80 per cent of what we spend on our pets, but sales of a whole range of petcare items – cat litter, flea and tick products, dietary supplements, toys, pet homes (from cages to kennels or fish tanks), baskets, feeding bowls, collars, leads, clothing, brushes and shampoos – are all increasing.

So, we spend a lot of money, but are we really making our pets' lives better?

Surveys show that overall pet health is declining almost as rapidly as human health. As with humans, this is a relatively recent phenomenon that began shortly after World War II.

Cats and dogs, which make up the majority of companion pets in the world, are now developing a vast list of degenerative diseases, including: autoimmune diseases, allergies, heart disease, diabetes, joint and arthritic problems, and cancer. By the age of three, some three-quarters of dogs will have developed gum disease, eye problems, ear problems, untreatable infestations of fleas and other parasites; thyroid imbalances, personality disorders and birth defects are all becoming commonplace among our pets.

The problem is so acute that a relatively new phenomenon – pet insurance – has been invented to help pet owners cope with spiralling vet bills. While once, visits to the vet were rare and were usually reserved for emergencies, today they are common and our pets are being subjected to the same arsenal of modern drugs – vaccines, antibiotics, steroids, painkillers, insulin and even antidepressants – that humans are.

The adverse effects from these drugs are as common in animals as they are in humans. Dogs given non-steroidal anti-inflammatory drugs (NSAIDs), for example, can develop ulcers from them just as humans do.

As with humans, a pet's diet is the basis of good health. Yet, recent studies have shown processed foods to be a factor in increasing numbers of pets suffering from cancer, arthritis, obesity, dental disease and heart disease. Dull or unhealthy coats and skin problems are a common problem with cats and dogs.

Modern dogs, cats and other animals live for years on convenience foods that come out of bags, cans and boxes, and a growing number of vets believe that this highly processed pet food is the main cause of illness and premature death in the modern dog and cat.

There is some research to back this up. In December 1995, the *British Journal of Small Animal Practice* published a paper contending that processed pet food suppresses the immune system, and leads to liver, kidney, heart and other diseases. The study found that, when young animals were fed cooked and processed foods, they initially appeared to be healthy. However, as the animals reached adulthood, they began to age more quickly than normal and also developed chronic degenerative disease symptoms. A control group of animals raised on raw foods aged less quickly and were free of degenerative disease.

Food is the basis of good pet health, but other factors are also influential. Everyday hygiene items such as flea and tick collars are also a major source of poisonings and illness among pets. Flea collars emit continuous, undetected pesticide vapours into the home, car, and around the pet. These vapours are highly toxic to the animal's skin, eyes, nose, lungs, blood, heart, liver and kidneys. They are also harmful for the adults – and especially children – who hug, handle, pet or otherwise enjoy the pleasure of being in close proximity to their furry friends.

Given the vast number of pet companions kept by people, it is astonishing how little relevant research there is to show how pet lifestyles, diets and environmental exposures can contribute to illness. Such studies that have been done are usually funded by major petcare product manufacturers and often exonerate pet products of any ill effects. However, the question of funding raises the spectre of the same kind of unacceptable bias that regularly turns up in medical trials sponsored by drug manufacturers.

Humans are meant to be caretakers for pets but, clearly, we are failing in our duties.

■ PET FOOD

Pet food has quite literally become a dog-eat-dog business – cat-eat-cat, too.

According to a startling 2001 report from the US Animal Protection Institute (API), commercial pet foods contain mostly grain wastes and meat byproducts, which can include everything from euthanised shelter animals to cancer-ridden livestock, road kill, downer animals (those unable to walk), mouldy grains and rancid restaurant grease. Feeding these low-in-nutrition packaged 'scraps' to pets greatly increases their chances of developing cancer and other degenerative diseases.

According to the API, more than 95 per cent of companion animals in the US derive their nutrition from processed pet foods. The group's report found that, in slaughterhouses, 'whatever remains of the carcass [after choice cuts for human food have been removed] – bones, blood, pus, intestines, bowels, ligaments, fat, hooves, horns and beaks' – is what ends up in the can. The motive for this unhealthy practice is profit, not health. Many pet food companies are branches of human food conglomerates, keen to turn waste products from one business into sales for another.

There are several problems with using rendered animal parts in processed animal foods. Using what are known as '4D animals' – dead, diseased, dying or disabled – means that whatever made the animal sick and whatever treatment was given to it before its death – for instance, medicines like antibiotics – remain in the food chain, passed on to your pet.

Commercial pet foods have other problems that are not immediately apparent from the labelling or the advertising spin. Many manufacturers cut costs by using the cheapest ingredients available at the time a food is made. As costs rise and fall, some manufacturers vary ingredients from batch to batch, resulting in changed nutrient values for each batch and possible digestive illness. Here's what's in conventional pet foods:

- **Substandard protein** Soya bean meal, wheat, corn glutens, corn meal, whole corn, crushed corn and ground corn are commonly used for their protein content in many pet foods. These ingredients are generally poor sources of protein compared with meat.

- **Rancid fats** Restaurant grease has become a major component of feed-grade animal fat over the last 15 years. Often held in 50-gallon drums for weeks or months in extreme temperatures, this rancid grease is then picked up by fat blenders, who mix the animal and vegetable fats together, stabilise them with powerful antioxidants to prevent further spoilage and then sell the blended products to pet food companies. Rancid, heavily preserved fats are extremely difficult to digest, and can lead to a host of animal-health problems, including digestive upsets, diarrhoea, gas and bad breath.

- **Salt** The high salt content in some pet foods can cause animals to become unnaturally high strung and nervous. The salt content of many products can be up to 1000 times more than your pet needs in one day. The excess salt can cause high blood pressure and heart disease in animals. Epilepsy is now more common in dogs than in humans.

- **Sugar** Semi-moist pet food usually contains as much as 25 per cent sugar, which can come in many forms such as sucrose, corn syrup, beet pulp and caramel, to name but a few.

- **Humectants** Used to keep the food moist, some can contain up to 10 per cent *propylene glycol*. Both sugar and propylene glycol are linked to obesity, allergies, tooth decay and other problems like cancer. Propylene glycol is used in the making of antifreeze – and yet, it's in the food we feed our pets. Once again, our own foods, like common salad dressings, contain propylene glycol also (just read the label). Alarmingly, a US Food and Drug Administration (FDA) report in 1994 noted that propylene glycol 'reduces red blood cell survival time, renders red blood cells more susceptible to oxidative damage and has other adverse effects in cats consuming the substance at levels found in semi-moist food'. In January 2001, the FDA together with the Center for Veterinary Medicine (CVM) finally banned propylene glycol in semi-moist catfood, but it is still used in products for dogs.

- **Synthetic preservatives** *Butylated hydroxyanisole* (BHA) and the related compound **butylated hydroxytoluene** (BHT) are used to prevent the fats and oils added to animal food from going off. BHA and BHT have been shown to affect the nervous systems of animals, in particular, the neurological development of young animals. Sometimes, these preservatives will be listed on the label as 'EU permitted antioxidants' without identifying them by name. A newer antioxidant is *ethoxyquin*. A component of this additive – quinoline – is regarded by some in the scientific community as the ultimate carcinogen.

  Ethoxyquin is made by GM (genetic modification) giant and pesticide manufacturer Monsanto, and was originally created as a rubber hardener. It has also been used as a pesticide The FDA has received reports that it causes allergic reactions, major organ failure, behavioural problems, skin problems and even cancer. One study commissioned by Monsanto found evidence of liver pigmentation changes and elevated liver enzymes.

- **Artificial colours** Food colourings are still commonly used in pet foods today, despite the fact that they are not necessary and that some have been linked to medical problems.

- **Other additives** Pet foods can contain the same mind-boggling array of potentially harmful additives that human foods have, including flavour enhancers, and anticaking, curing and drying agents, as well as emulsifiers, sweeteners, solvents, stabilisers, thickeners and texturisers.

IMPROVING YOUR PET'S DIET

Dogs and cats were designed to handle raw, uncooked foods. Owners can easily mix fresh cuts of meat (not ground) with wholegrains and vegetables for a balanced diet.

The meat contained in canned pet food is cooked, devoid of 'real' nutrients and usually full of many potentially harmful preservatives, colourings and additives. Dry and processed tinned food also lacks the natural teeth-cleaning properties of fresh raw meat. Without the natural cleansing action of the meat on the teeth, unhealthy bacteria build up in the mouth, causing infection and foul-smelling breath.

Animals require the enzymes, amino acids and other nutrients in raw meat to stay healthy. Many skin and coat problems are a direct result of a lack of raw animal fat in the diet – fat that humans often believe is bad for their pet. Animals need a diet of at least 30 per cent raw fat, and their systems are not designed to handle cooked meat or cooked fat.

Cats need care

Cats' nutritional needs are much the same as dogs, but the way their bodies process nutrients is very different. Both cats and dogs are natural predators and both are natural meat-eaters. But dogs' bodies have evolved to be omnivorous. In the wild, they will survive on a varied diet of plants and meat. Cats, however, are 'obligate carnivores' – they die if they don't eat meat. Cats also find it difficult to process plant materials and, with the exception of vitamin C, which cats can make themselves, felines must obtain all their nutrients – especially the amino acids arginine and taurine – from the food they eat.

In comparison to dogs, cats require three times as much protein to stay healthy, but only negligible amounts of carbohydrates. Contrary to popular belief, cats were originally desert-dwelling animals so, while we tend to associate cats with fish, seafood is not their natural diet and a steady diet of things like canned tuna can actually promote severe nutritional deficiencies in cats, especially of vitamins E and A. In the wild, cats will eat the whole of the animal – skin, bones and flesh – and from this totality obtain all the nutrients necessary to remain healthy.

There is very little difference between the meat byproducts that are included in catfood and those that are regularly found in

▶

dogfood. As with dogs, vets are concerned that tinned catfood may lie at the root of a range of immune diseases such as allergies, digestive upsets, thyroid problems, adrenal and pancreatic dysfunction, tooth and gum decay, arthritis, and kidney and liver failure. A recent study of 25 brands of catfood found that all bar one also contained cancer-causing amines – fuelling speculation that a diet of processed food might well be the reason for the increasing incidence of cancer among cats.

Dry catfoods have been blamed for a range of health problems, including kidney disease, cystitis, diabetes, inflammatory bowel disease, obesity, dental problems and autoimmune disorders. Many of these problems are related to the lack of water and the high carbohydrate levels of dry cat kibble. Cats' natural prey – for instance, a mouse or other small animal – would comprise around 70 per cent water.

Our knowledge of cats' nutritional needs is relatively sketchy, but most experts in holistic petcare believe that supplementing or replacing your cat's diet of tinned food with raw or lightly cooked meat will greatly improve its overall diet. To make sure your cat gets all it needs, make sure you provide a variety of meats – for example, organs, tripe and muscle meat.

■ FLEA AND TICK CONTROL

Fleas usually gain free entry to your home through your pet or visitors' pets. Remember, for every flea on your pet, there may be as many as 30 more in its environment.

Fleas and ticks are a profitable business for the chemical/pesticide industry, responsible for billions in sales every year. Pet owners are seduced into believing that these products are safe and effective, but read the warning label on conventional flea and tick products. Shampoos and dips, foggers and collars – in fact, all conventional flea and tick treatments – caution users to wear gloves, and to keep the product away from skin and mucous membranes. And yet, these chemicals are being applied in some cases all over your pet, where they can be easily absorbed, inhaled or licked off by the pet. In addition, foggers release a great deal of toxic chemicals into the air that will then settle on carpets, furniture and curtains.

These regular pesticide exposures are highly toxic and further weaken the overall health of your pet. Based on the very limited data available, it appears that hundreds and probably thousands of pets have been injured or killed through exposure to pet products containing pesticides. As with small children, pets cannot report when they're being poisoned at low doses.

Chronic low-dose exposures to these toxins may not kill pets or humans with the initial exposure, or even after several exposures. Exposed in this way, it takes longer for the negative effects to accumulate and disable

---

Pet grooming

Most mass-produced pet-grooming supplies contain the same contentious chemicals that you will find in human toiletries, including petroleum-based detergents, preservatives, artificial colours and synthetic perfumes. These ingredients can cause the same kinds of skin reactions in pets as they can in humans.

Pet owners are also bamboozled by the same marketing jargon for pet supplies as found on toiletries for people such as 'all-natural', 'organic', 'pure', 'hypoallergenic' and 'aromatherapy-derived' – and should use the same common sense when faced with such claims. Indeed, many 'natural' pet products are made from a raft of synthetic chemicals, with a small number of natural extracts thrown in for good measure.

If your pet is sensitive or allergy-prone, you may want to check the label of your grooming products for the following potentially irritating ingredients:

- **Sodium lauryl sulphate (SLS).** Tests show that sodium lauryl sulphate can damage eyes, and be absorbed into systemic tissues such as the brain, heart and liver. SLS is also an irritant, and can cause eye irritation, skin rashes, hair loss, scalp scurf similar to dandruff and allergic reactions.

▶

- **DEA and MEA.** These hormone-disrupting chemicals are used as foam-boosters, stabilisers and viscosity builders/modifiers in shampoos, hand soaps and bath products. Examples include *cocamide DEA* or *MEA*, and *lauramide DEA*. When mixed with formaldehyde-forming ingredients such as *2-bromo-2-nitro-propane-1,3-diol* (bronopol), quaternium-15, *DMDM hydantoin* and *imidazolidinyl urea*, they can form cancer-causing nitrosamines (see also page 111).

- *Mineral oil.* Also known as *paraffinum liquidum*, this coats the skin and stops it from 'breathing'. Skin is the largest body organ and needs to release toxins freely, but mineral oil blocks this process. Mineral oil also acts like a solvent, breaking down the skin's natural oils. With every application, it will dry your pet's skin even more.

- *Talc.* Dry pet 'shampoos' are often based around *talc*, which is carcinogenic when inhaled.

There's no magic in choosing safe pet products – just take the same care when choosing pet shampoos and other treatments as you would in choosing products for yourself.

the immune system. Because of this, the pesticide industry continues to mislead the public and the government regulatory agencies by insisting that there is no scientific proof showing a definite cause-and-effect link between pesticide exposure and illness in either pets or humans. When industry representatives have been asked by environmental and health advocates to conduct new studies on the relationship of pesticides to cancer, respiratory and neurological disorders, their default reply is that there is no need for such studies.

But, in November 2000, a report issued by the US Natural Resources Defense Council (NRDC) found that pest-control products can expose adults and children to toxic pesticides at concentrations that exceed – by as much as 500 times – the safe levels established by the US Environmental Protection Agency (EPA). The result: possible acute poisoning of pets and humans, and possible long-term problems for children, too. The risks include acute poisoning and longer-term problems like brain dysfunction or cancer.

The report found that the riskiest pet products contain a family of pesticides known as organophosphates (OPs) and carbamates. OP pesticides, which are derived from nerve gas, interfere with nerve-signal transmission. Since the neurological process they attack is common to insects, humans, dogs and cats, these pesticides can harm more than just fleas and ticks. Carbamates disrupt the same neurological processes as OPs, and so are potentially just as harmful.

The chemical industry claims that no scientific studies have demonstrated a conclusive relationship between chemical exposure and disease, and then refuses to initiate new studies on the basis that they are not needed, even though many small studies have indicated otherwise. The carbaryl class of chemicals, for instance, is associated with increased frequencies of diarrhoea, coughing, breathing difficulties and congestion. OPs can produce symptoms of headache, dizziness, nausea, fatigue and dermatitis.

Millions of dollars spent on toxic flea control have not bought consumer satisfaction or healthy pest-free pets. This is because fleas and ticks can develop resistance to pesticides in the same way that bacteria become resistant to antibiotics. Survival of the fittest, a short lifespan and rapid replication (multiple generations every year) have created superbugs. In fact, fleas and lice now have a longer lifecycle than they did 50 years ago. They breed more easily and even survive bouts of cold weather. As a result, it has become necessary to use stronger poisons in higher doses.

COMMON FLEA TREATMENTS INCLUDE ...

Amitraz (amidine), **carbaryl**, **chlorpyrifos**, coumaphos, cythioate, **diazinon**, **dichlorvos**, **fenitrothion**, fenthion, **fipronil** (phenyl pyrazole), flumethrin, imidacloprid, **iodofenphos**, **lufenuron** (benzoylurea), **malathion**, naled, **permethrin**, phenothrin, phosmet, **piperonyl butoxide**, **propoxur**, **pyrethrin/pyrethrum**, **S-methoprene** and tetrachlorvinphos.

▶ TRY THIS INSTEAD ...

To keep your family safe, remember that you should avoid all organophosphate-based products. This is particularly important for pregnant women and families with children. Don't let children 'help' apply flea shampoos, dusts, dips or other products containing OPs or carbamates to their pets.

In many cases, fleas and ticks can be controlled with simple physical measures such as brushing pets regularly with a flea comb while inspecting for fleas, and vacuuming and mowing frequently in areas where pets spend the most time outdoors.

A chronic flea infestation can serve as an early-warning sign of immune deficiency caused or exacerbated by a nutrient-poor diet. To strengthen an animal's compromised immune system, make sure your pet is getting the right vitamins and minerals to help protect against fleas and ticks. The B vitamins, particularly B1 (thiamine) and B6 (pyridoxine), are natural flea and tick repellents. Brewer's yeast and rice bran contain high levels of all of the B vitamins. As a first line of therapy, try adding brewer's yeast and garlic or apple-cider vinegar to your pet's food. (Note: It is not advisable to use raw garlic as a food supplement for cats.)

You can also try these natural alternatives:

Bathe and comb your pet regularly. Use natural vegetable-based soap or shampoo, not insecticides. If you find fleas on your pet's brush or comb, dip it in a glass of soapy water to remove them.

Frequent vacuuming of floors, carpets, furniture, crevices and cracks in the area where pets sleep and spend time is advised, along with weekly washing of pet bedding. During heavy infestations, daily vacuuming may be necessary. Dispose of the sealed bag properly outside the home or by incinerating it.

Cedar shampoo, cedar oil and cedar-filled sleeping mats are commercially available. Cedar repels many insects, including fleas.

Make a herbal flea collar. Make up a mixture of ½ tsp alcohol with one drop each of the following essential oils: cedar wood, lavender, citronella and thyme. Add the contents of four garlic capsules. Buy a soft flea collar (untreated), and soak the collar in this mixture until it has absorbed enough of it to be thoroughly soaked through, then leave it to dry completely. This will be effective for about a month.

Add a few drops of tea tree oil to a herbal pet shampoo to repel fleas and help heal flea-bitten skin. You can also try mixing a teaspoon of tea tree oil in 250 ml (8 fl oz) of water and spraying this on the animal's fur. This is recommended for pets that dislike baths, which includes most cats. It is also practical for in-between baths.

■ CAT LITTER

For litter-box-trained animals, holistic vets recommend avoiding conventional clay litters as they are laden with silica dust, a known carcinogen. Many 'scoopable' clay litters have also been found to cause intestinal blockages in cats and kittens when inadvertently consumed while grooming.

Is your home killing your pets?

Veterinarians are treating more and more cases of cancer in animals as well as increased numbers of behavioural problems and poisonings. Cats, in particular, have difficulty eliminating toxic chemicals because their systems aren't efficient at metabolising foreign intruders. Without question, the incidence of feline leukaemia is reaching epidemic proportions among cats.

Household cleaners can be extremely toxic to pets, as can common bug sprays and garden pesticides. Although modern energy-efficient construction provides superior insulation, these 'improvements' prevent proper ventilation in your home. However, this energy cost-saver may also result in a buildup of chemical fumes within the home. And, as many pets now spend most of their time indoors, they may also develop serious health problems. Furthermore, pets inhale higher concentrations of these toxins based on their given body weight, so that many symptoms attributed to toxic fumes may appear in our pets before they appear in us.

Aerosol sprays are also a hazard to a pet's health, especially if the pet already has respiratory problems. And many cleaning products

▶

are inherently petrochemicals, especially air fresheners and polishes, and use volatile organic chemicals (VOCs) that permeate
the indoor environment. These fumes may linger in the home for
long periods of time, particularly when the windows are closed
during the heating and air-conditioning seasons.

The actual symptom of cleaning-product poisoning that the
animal exhibits depends on the type of agent, but there are some
general symptoms of which dog and cat owners should be aware,
such as:

- Anxiety
- Burns on the mouth and oesophagus
- Colic
- Corneal damage
- Cough
- Excessive salivation
- Foaming at the mouth
- Muscle weakness
- Restlessness
- Seizures
- Shallow breathing
- Skin ulcers
- Slow respiration
- Vomiting

Once upon a time, cat litter boxes were homemade affairs, filled with
anything at hand that the cat might dig into and use. Sand was popular if it
could be easily sourced; garden dirt was another natural choice, since most
cats were indoors-outdoors, and that is where they usually 'did their business'. Shredded newspaper and ashes were also common.

Then, in the late 1940s, absorbent 'Kitty Litter' based on fuller's earth
appeared on the market. For a long time, this was the standard for cat owners.
Then, in the 1980s, 'scoopable' clay litters containing sodium bentonite came
onto the market and became an instant success. Sodium bentonite, a naturally swelling clay, is often added as an extremely effective clumping agent.
When liquid is added, bentonite swells to approximately 15 times its original
volume. Traditional clay litters had to be replaced frequently; with

scoopable litter, only the solids and the clumps of urine need to be scooped out, then a small amount of fresh litter added. The box would last up to a month without completely replacing the used litter.

Scoopable clay litters are convenient and cost-effective for owners, but they have several downsides that can impact on the health of your cat:

- The dust in clay is silica dust, a known carcinogen, which is easily inhaled into both feline and human lungs.

- Cats can ingest the clay while cleaning their feet, and kittens sometimes eat litter. The powerful clumping abilities of sodium bentonite cause the ingested clay dust and particles, when combined with natural and ingested liquid, to form a solid mass in the animal's intestines. This lump can draw fluid out of the body, causing dehydration and, possibly, consequential urinary tract problems.

- Ingested clay dust coats the digestive tract, attracting the collection of old faecal material, increasing toxicity and bacteria growth, and prohibiting proper assimilation of digested food. This can lead to stress on the immune system, leaving the animal susceptible to viral, bacterial, parasitic and yeast infections.

- These problems can also extend to dogs that occasionally eat 'litter box snacks'.

Apart from the problems already mentioned, clumping clay kitty litters have been linked to a wide variety of seemingly unrelated cat health problems, including diarrhoea, frothy yellow vomiting, mega-bowel syndrome, irritable bowel syndrome, kidney problems, respiratory problems, general failure to thrive, anaemia, lethargy and even death.

▶ TRY THIS INSTEAD ...

A good alternative to conventional kitty litter is wheat-based litter that is scoopable, biodegradable and flushable. Some natural kitty litters make use of recycled and 'pelletised' paper. A third option is litter made from recycled pinewood waste.

chemicals: a to z

THE NUMBER OF CHEMICALS we encounter each day is staggering, and it would take several full volumes just to list them all. However, some chemicals turn up in our homes more frequently than others, and this A to Z provides a snapshot of their potential effects.

Not everyone will experience the reactions listed here. Indeed, that is the frustrating thing about chemical research. We know so little about who is likely to react, and why and to what extent. For this reason, this A to Z tries to be as comprehensive as possible in terms of recognising adverse reactions.

Some background information may help you to understand what you read here. For instance, hazardous chemicals can be absorbed into the body through:

- the respiratory tract via inhalation

- the skin via dermal contact

- the digestive tract via ingestion. (Ingestion can occur if a chemical is deliberately put into food, or because of eating or smoking with contaminated hands or in contaminated work areas.)

A chemical may have serious effects by one route of exposure and minimal effects by another.

In addition, chemicals can produce both local and systemic (widespread) effects. With a local effect, the chemical does not need to be absorbed to produce an effect. Instead, it takes place at the point of contact, which may be skin, mucous membranes, the respiratory tract, gastrointestinal system or the eyes. Such chemicals are known as irritants because they can cause inflammation of the skin and the mucous membranes in the eyes, nose or respiratory tract.

A systemic effect is an adverse health effect that takes place at a site distant from the body's initial point of chemical contact due to the chemical being absorbed into the body. Substances with systemic effects often have 'target organs' in which they accumulate and exert their toxic effect such as the kidneys, liver or heart. Some substances that cause systemic effects are cumulative poisons. These substances tend to build up in the body as a result of numerous chronic exposures. Chemicals that cause systemic effects can further be classified as:

- **Reproductive toxins**, which cause impotence or sterility in men and women.

- **Carcinogens**, substances that can cause cancer.

- **Mutagens**, anything that causes a change in the genetic material of a living cell. Many mutagens are also carcinogens.

- **Teratogens**, any agent that interferes with the developing embryo and can cause birth defects on exposure during pregnancy.

- **Neurotoxins**, which affect the nervous system, including diseases associated with nervous system damage such as multiple sclerosis, Parkinson's disease, Alzheimer's disease and sudden infant death syndrome (SIDS).

When exposure involves several substances simultaneously, the resultant systemic toxic effect may be significantly greater with the combination than with the cumulative toxic effect of each substance alone. This is called 'synergy'. Good examples of this include exposure to alcohol and chlorinated solvents, or smoking together with asbestos.

ACEPHATE

An insecticide found in a variety of commercial garden products, in common with other organophosphates, this can cause a host of symptoms, including changes in heart rate, central nervous system impairment, blurred vision, gastrointestinal problems (cramps, heartburn, hyperperistalsis) and breathing difficulties. With long-term use, it is a foetal toxin and hormone disrupter.

ACESULFAME K

E950, acesulfame potassium, Sunette, Sweet One

An artificial sweetener used in foods and medicines, acesulfame K is about 200 times sweeter than sugar. It has a bitter aftertaste, so is usually combined with sugar or the other popular sweetener **Aspartame** to mask its bitterness. Each of these chemicals carries its own health risks and it is possible that the combination may be more damaging than if taken individually. Acesulfame K has been shown to cause cancer in animals, which means that it may also pose a cancer risk in humans.

ACETAMIDE MEA

N-2-hydroxyethylacetamide

A wetting agent/humectant used in cosmetics such as lipsticks and cream blushers to retain moisture, in the short term, acetamide can cause mild skin irritation. No studies are available on the effects of long-term exposure in humans but, in animals, chronic ingestion has produced benign and malignant liver tumours in rats, and an increased incidence of malignant lymphomas in mice. It may be contaminated with harmful impurities linked to cancer and other health disorders (*see* **Monoethanolamine**).

ACETONE

Dimethyl ketone, methyl ketone

An industrial denaturant and solvent used in the manufacture of waxes, plastics, varnishes, aerosol paints, explosives and chloroform, it is also found in a staggering number of domestic products, including furniture polish and cleaners, surface cleaners, laundry presoaks and starches, shoe polish, garden insecticides, pet flea and tick products, premoistened wipes, nail-polish remover and perfumes. Used to extract flavours, aromas and perfumes from herbs, spices and flowers, it can also be found in the marking inks used on meats, and is used in some skin-cleaning formulas for its ability to dissolve fats and grease.

Used on the skin, it can produce skin rashes, dryness and irritation. Inhaling acetone even for short periods can provoke nose, throat, lung and eye irritation, headaches, lightheadedness and fatigue. Chronic exposure can damage the kidneys and liver.

ACRYLATES

These are film-formers, emulsifiers and surfactants that help cosmetics and body-care products stick to the skin and can make it feel softer. Their safety has not been thoroughly investigated. Although they are presumed non-toxic, they can be irritating to skin and eyes.

ALCOHOL, DENATURED

Ethanol, ethyl alcohol

A solvent used extensively in the manufacture of varnishes, artificial flavourings, perfumes and inks, it is a fuel and petrol additive and, medicinally, it is used as an antiseptic. But it can also be found in pizza crusts in the US, where it is used to extend handling and storage time. The starting material for denatured alcohol is ethyl alcohol (ethanol), the alcohol commonly found in beer, wine and spirits; denatured, or industrial, alcohol is ethanol to which poisonous or nauseating substances have been added to prevent its use as a beverage. It's clear and colourless, and highly inflammable. Used on the skin, it can cause dryness and irritation over time. Ingestion of small amounts of denatured alcohol can cause behavioural changes and impaired vision; large amounts can cause nausea, vomiting, coma and death.

ALDRIN

An organochlorine insecticide, aldrin breaks down to a related compound, *Dieldrin*, in the body and in the environment. Those who are chronically or occupationally exposed to moderate levels of this compound can experience headaches, dizziness, irritability, vomiting and uncontrolled muscle movements. Aldrin builds up in the body after years of exposure, and is toxic to the nervous system as well as a suspected carcinogen and hormone disrupter. Aldrin is banned or restricted in around 50 countries, including the UK and US, though it is still used in some countries for termite control.

ALLETHRIN

D-allethrin

Used almost exclusively in homes and gardens for control of flies and mosquitoes, and in combination with other pesticides to control flying or crawling insects, it is also used to control lice in humans and animals. Allethrin is a synthetic *Pyrethrin*, a botanical insecticide extracted from chrysanthemum flowers. It is harmful if swallowed, its vapours can worsen chronic respiratory diseases such as asthma and skin contact can cause dermatitis. It is a suspected mutagen and immunotoxin, and harmful to birds, fish, crustaceans and aquatic insects.

ALKYL COMPOUNDS

Alkyl compounds are used as surfactants and detergents found in cosmetics, toiletries, household goods and pesticides. They are problematic in many ways. One common type, the alkyl benzyl sulphonates (ABS), include linear alkyl benzene sulphonates (LAS) and linear alkyl sodium sulphonates, both of which are slow to biodegrade. LAS are the most common surfactants used in household products.

Another type, *Alkylphenols*, are hormone disrupters. One member of this family of chemicals is the spermicide nonoxynyl (used on condoms, and in spermicidal foams and gels), which may give some idea of their powerful biological toxicity.

ALKYLPHENOLS

Nonylphenol, nonylphenoxy ethoxylates, alkylphenol polyglycol,
poylethylene glycol, alkyl aryl ethers

These surfactants and detergents are found in household cleaners, laundry detergents, cosmetics, pesticides, paints and varnishes. Although still used in commercial products in the US, they are confined to industrial detergents in the UK. They can easily get into the water supply and food chain, and are hormone disrupters believed to be contributing to reproductive problems in men such as low sperm counts, damaged sperm and testicular cancer. Many alkylphenols are toxic to aquatic organisms and are implicated in the feminisation of male fish.

ALPHA CYPERMETHRIN

A pyrethroid insecticide used against a wide range of insects, including ants, roaches, spiders and crickets, it is also used in agriculture on cereals, vegetables and fruit, and on foods during storage. It can be irritating to the skin and eyes. Longer-term exposure can cause headache, dizziness, nausea, vomiting, diarrhoea, excessive salivation and fatigue. It is a suspected hormone disrupter.

ALPHA-HYDROXY ACIDS

Alpha-hydroxy acids or AHAs come from a variety of sources, including citrus fruits such as grapefruit and papaya. *Lactic acid* is also an AHA.

In their more concentrated form, AHAs are used by dermatologists to remove the top layers of the skin, usually as a treatment for skin disorders and wrinkles. Patients like to call such procedures 'facial peels', but dermatologists call them 'chemical burns'. While not used in skin products at anywhere near such concentrations, AHAs still burn the skin slightly. The 'glow' you get from products containing AHAs is actually a mild irritation caused by the chemical burning. Some people react more to this burning than others, and AHAs are reported to be a major cause of adverse reactions to soaps, shampoos and moisturisers.

ALUM

Potassium alum

Alum usually refers to synthetic *Aluminium*-containing crystals produced in the lab for commercial use as natural deodorants. A powdered form is used as an astringent to prevent bleeding from small shaving cuts. The styptic pencils sold for this purpose contain aluminium sulphate or potassium aluminium sulphate. Similar products are also used on animals to prevent bleeding after nail-clipping.

ALUMINA

Aluminium oxide
　　See Aluminium

ALUMINIUM

E173

One of the most abundant minerals on the planet, aluminium has many uses in household products. It is a colour additive in cosmetics (especially eyeshadows) and in foods. It is also a common ingredient in antacids, and in deodorants and antiperspirants (most commonly as aluminium chlorohydrate, aluminium zirconium, aluminium chloride, alumina, aluminium sulphate and aluminium phenosulphate).

The human body has no dietary requirement for aluminium and, if ingested in large doses, it is considered toxic, carcinogenic and mutagenic. Applied to the skin (for instance, in deodorants), it is an irritant and, with a lifetime's use, has been associated with an increased risk of Alzheimer's disease (a common form of dementia). Products containing aluminium zirconium compounds have been shown to cause granulomas (small nodules of chronically inflamed tissue) under the arms with prolonged use.

ALUMINIUM CHLORIDE

An industrial fungicide that is a suspected neurotoxin and reproductive toxin.

ALUMINIUM CHLOROHYDRATE
See Aluminium

ALUMINIUM PHENOSULPHATE
See Aluminium

ALUMINIUM SULPHATE
See Aluminium

ALUMINIUM ZIRCONIUM TETRACHLOROHYDREX GLY
See Aluminium

4-AMINO-2-NITROPHENOL
p-Aminonitrophenol

Used as an oxidising agent in permanent and semi-permanent hair dyes, it has also been linked to bladder cancer in animal and human studies.

AMINOMETHYL PROPANOL
2-amino-2-methylpropanol

A thickener and gelling agent used in cosmetics, this is a skin irritant, and can also be contaminated with harmful impurities. As an amine, it can mix with other chemicals in the product, on the skin or in the body after absorption to form carcinogenic nitrosamine compounds (see also Chapter 6).

AMMONIA
Ammonia, anhydrous

A cleaning and bleaching agent commonly found in glass cleaners, all-purpose cleaners, disinfectants, floor cleaners, furniture and metal polishes, drain cleaners, oven cleaners and toilet-bowl cleaners, ammonia is toxic by all routes of exposure. Its fumes, even at the low levels contained in most household products, are irritating and, in some cases, damaging to the eyes, nose and lungs. On contact with the skin, it can cause redness and even burns. Ammonia must never be mixed with *Bleach*, as the combination results in toxic chloramine gas.

AMMONIUM LAURETH SULPHATE
This surfactant is found in shampoos and foaming bath products. Although considered mild, it can be irritating to sensitive skin. Laureth compounds can be contaminated with 1,4-**dioxane**, a known carcinogen. Since consumers have no way of knowing which laureth compounds are contaminated, avoidance is the safest option.

AMMONIUM LAURYL SULPHATE
Ammonium dodecyl sulphate

A surfactant found in shampoos and foaming bath products, it can be mildly irritating to the skin.

AROMA
Added to foods and tobacco products, an aroma is just flavouring by another name (and

flavourings are simply perfumes by another name). Health effects of aroma include allergic reactions – some of these may mimic common dental problems such as bleeding gums, mouth ulcers and gingivitis. Like fragrances, aromas can affect the central nervous system to produce headaches, mood swings, fatigue, dizziness and nausea, among other symptoms. Aromas are generally petroleum derivatives and can be contaminated with cancer-causing substances.

AROMATIC HYDROCARBONS

A family of petroleum-derived chemicals often used as solvents, common aromatics include *Toluene, Xylene, Coal tar, Naphthas*, styrene and *Benzene*. Widely used in cosmetics, perfumes and household cleaners, they are also used in printing, fibreglass-reinforced products, glues and veneers. Aromatic hydrocarbons derive their name from the pleasant, slightly sweet odour attributed to many of them.

However, they are powerful neurotoxins, and symptoms of overexposure include fatigue, confusion, dermatitis and chemical pneumonia. Aromatic hydrocarbons are readily absorbed through the skin and subsequently affect the lungs, skin, blood, eyes, kidneys and nervous system. Some are associated with reproductive hazards. Benzene, for instance, suppresses production of blood cells and can cause leukaemia. See also *Polycyclic aromatic hydrocarbons*.

ARSENIC

A pesticide primarily found in treated wood in the form of chromated copper arsenate, it is used for picnic tables, decking and playground equipment. Because wood is porous, the arsenic can easily be transferred onto hands and from there into mouths, especially with children. Ingesting small amounts of arsenic can cause nausea and vomiting, decreased production of red and white blood cells, abnormal heart rhythm, damage to blood vessels, and a sensation of 'pins and needles' in hands and feet. Ingesting high levels can result in death. Exposure to arsenic can increase the risk of lung, skin, bladder, liver, kidney and prostate cancers.

ASPARTAME

E951, NutraSweet, Equal, Benevia

An artificial sweetener made from the amino acids aspartic acid and phenylalanine, and methyl alcohol, since its discovery in 1969, it has become a staple ingredient in breakfast cereals, chewing gum, colas and other sodas, yoghurt, breath mints, juice and manufactured desserts.

All regulatory authorities believe aspartame is safe. Nevertheless, it has been dogged by health concerns from the outset. During storage and when heated, it quickly breaks down into its component parts, each of which is considered toxic. Aspartame's two major constituents, phenylalanine and aspartic acid, can cause brain damage in very high doses. Even at the low levels permitted in foods, aspartame can be toxic to people who suffer from phenylketonuria (PKU). Relatives of those who have PKU may also be genetically sensitive to aspartame.

However, neurotoxicity is the major concern and, indeed, is cited as the number-one problem in a recent lawsuit against the manufacturer. According to the US Food and Drug Administration (FDA), aspartame is associated with headache, dizziness, loss of balance, mood swings, nausea, memory loss, muscle weakness, blurred vision, fatigue, weakness, skin rashes, and joint and musculoskeletal pain, even when consumed in only moderate amounts. Aspartame is believed to cause or worsen epileptic seizures, fibromyalgia, multiple sclerosis (MS), lupus, attention-deficit disorder (ADD), diabetes, thyroid problems, Alzheimer's disease, chronic fatigue, depression and eye conditions such as macular degeneration, diabetic blindness and glaucoma.

The most recent evidence suggests that regular consumption of aspartame at levels considered safe considerably raises the risk of rare tumours known as lymphomas.

A-TERPINEOL
Alpha-terpineol

A synthetic fragrance found in perfumes, colognes, laundry detergents, fabric softeners, air fresheners, aftershaves, hairsprays and deodorants, it is highly irritating to mucous membranes. Inhalation can cause excitement, loss of muscle coordination, hypothermia, central nervous system and respiratory depression, and headache.

ATRAZINE

Among the most widely used industrial herbicides in the world, this is the one most commonly found as a residue on foods and in the water supply. It is also used for weed control on non-crop land such as railways, roadsides and industrial areas. Atrazine can cause irritation to skin and eyes. Over the long term, it is a hormone disrupter, carcinogen and reproductive toxin. In the environment, atrazine has been shown to feminise male frogs at doses well below the accepted 'safe' levels.

AVOBENZONE
Butyl methoxy-dibenzoylmethane

A broad-spectrum synthetic sunscreen ingredient that can protect against the entire range of the sun's UVA rays, studies suggest that it is a potential hormone disrupter.

AZAMETHIPHOS

An organophosphate insecticide used to control cockroaches, beetles, spiders and flies, symptoms of exposure include headache, dizziness, nausea, vomiting, abdominal cramps, diarrhoea, blurred vision and muscle twitches.

AZO DYES

A large category of dyes used in foods and cosmetics as well as for dyeing textiles such as cotton, silk, wool, viscose and synthetic fibres, these are considered easy to use, relatively cheap and able to provide clear, strong colours. There are approximately 2000 azo dyes on the market.

The majority of these dyes are water-soluble and are, therefore, easy for the body to absorb. Absorption takes place through inhalation and swallowing of dust as well as through skin contact. In humans, azo dyes can cause allergic reactions such as hives. Many are considered neurotoxic and carcinogenic. Azo dyes can cause 'cross-reactivity' with the **Phenylenediamine** colourants used in hair dyes. This means that if you are sensitive to one type of dye, you can, over time, develop sensitivity to the other. Azo dyes, which frequently are washed down the drain, may also be toxic to aquatic organisms and cause long-term damage to aquatic environments.

BENDIOCARB
Carbamic acid, methyl-,2,3-(dimethylmethylenedioxy) phenyl ester

A carbamate insecticide used to control mosquitoes, flies, wasps, ants, fleas, cockroaches, silverfish, ticks and other pests in homes, industrial plants and food storage sites, this is highly toxic, especially to the central nervous system, if it is ingested or absorbed through the skin. Symptoms of bendiocarb poisoning include weakness, blurred vision, headache, nausea, abdominal cramps, chest discomfort, pupil constriction, sweating, muscle tremors and decreased pulse. Persons with asthma, diabetes or cardiovascular disease are at special risk with any kind of exposure.

BENFLURALIN
Benefin

A herbicide used primarily on turf, including lawns and golf courses to control grasses and other weeds, it is a skin-sensitiser, and can be irritating to skin and eyes. In animal studies, it affects the circulation and the liver.

BENSULIDE
Phosphorodithioic acid

An organophosphate herbicide used on vegetable crops such as carrots, cucumbers, peppers and melons, in cotton, and on turf to control annual grasses such as bluegrass, crabgrass and broadleaf weeds, it is a central nervous system disrupter that can provoke chest tightness, nausea, abdominal cramps, diarrhoea, headache, dizziness, weakness, blurring and teary eyes, loss of muscle coordination and face muscle twitches.

BENZALDEHYDE

Various benzaldehyde compounds are used as synthetic fragrances; 4-methoxy benzaldehyde, for instance, has a sharp, bitter almond-cherry fragrance while 4-hydroxy-3-methoxy benzaldehyde (or vanillan) has a vanilla fragrance. Benzaldehydes can be irritating to the mouth, throat, eyes, skin, lungs and gastrointestinal tract, causing nausea and abdominal pain. In laboratory studies, they have been linked to kidney damage, cellular mutations and central nervous system disruption.

BENZALKONIUM CHLORIDE
Alkyl benzyl dimethylammonium chloride

A ***Quaternary Ammonium Compound*** used typically as a disinfectant and preservative, this is found in disinfecting hand soaps, mouthwashes and aftershave preparations, as well as in dishwashing detergents, disinfectants and cleaners. It can be an irritant to the eyes and skin if used in high concentrations. Its wide use is causing new strains of resistant bacteria. Laboratory studies suggest it may cause reproductive defects and act as a mutagen.

BENZENE

A carcinogenic solvent derived from petroleum, this is found in lacquers, varnishes, oven cleaners, detergents, furniture polish, air fresheners, spot removers, nail-polish remover and perfumes. Irritating to mucous membranes and poisonous when ingested, harmful amounts may also be absorbed through the skin through the use of everyday products. It may cause sensitivity to light as well as skin rashes and swelling. Benzene is a carcinogen as well as a powerful bone-marrow poison, destroying the marrow's ability to produce blood cells.

BENZOATES

A large family of naturally occurring and synthetic chemicals used as preservatives in foodstuffs and cosmetics, they are commonly encountered as *Sodium benzoate*, *Benzoic acid*, *Benzoyl peroxide* and *Parabens* (see individual listings). Benzoates are universally associated with allergic reactions, especially in those suffering from asthma. They often cause gastric irritation, numbing of the mouth and urticaria (nettle rash or hives).

BENZOIC ACID

E210, carboxybenzene

A food and cosmetic preservative and member of the larger family of *Benzoates*, this is used to inhibit the growth of mould, yeast and some bacteria. It is also used as a pesticide. Although it occurs naturally in many plants, most commercial benzoic acid is synthetic. People who suffer from asthma, rhinitis or urticaria may find their symptoms get worse after consuming benzoates.

BENZOPHENONES

Used as fixatives in perfumes, some benzophenones such as dioxybenzone, oxybenzone, sulisobenzone and benzophenone-3 absorb ultraviolet light and are therefore used as a sunscreening agent, especially for UVA protection. In sensitive individuals, they can provoke allergic reactions and photosensitivity.

BENZOYL PEROXIDE

Found in products to treat acne, benzoyl peroxide loosens and removes the top layer of skin and kills bacteria on the skin. It can cause contact dermatitis and sensitisation, and is not to be used in cases of acne rosacea. Animal studies suggest that, when applied topically, it can promote the formation of skin tumours in animals. In foods, it is used as a bleaching agent for flours, and in blue cheeses such as gorgonzola, and milk.

BENZYL ACETATE

A synthetic fragrance with a floral, fruity aroma, this is found in perfumes and air fresheners and in a range of fragranced household products, including dryer sheets. Also used as a flavouring and aroma in foods and beverages, its vapours are irritating to eyes and respiratory passages, and may cause coughing. It can be absorbed through the skin, thus causing systemic effects. Long-term use has been linked to pancreatic cancer.

BENZYL ALCOHOL

Benzenemethanol

A solvent and synthetic fragrance found in a wide variety of fragranced household products, including perfumes and air fresheners and as well as foods, when applied topically, it is irritating to skin and mucous membranes. Inhaled, it is irritating to the upper respiratory tract and can cause headache, nausea, vomiting, dizziness, a drop in blood pressure, central nervous system depression and, in rare cases, death due to respiratory failure. Consumption of large doses may cause vomiting, diarrhoea and central nervous system depression. This is also a potential carcinogen.

BENZYL CINNAMATE

See Cinnamates

BENZYL SALICYLATE

See Salicylates

BETA-HYDROXY ACIDS

BHAs

Derived from many natural sources, BHAs like *Salicylic acid* are often found in anti-ageing creams and other types of cosmetics where they are used to burn off the top layers of skin. BHAs are similar to *Alpha-hydroxy acids*, but are thought to be marginally less irritating to the skin.

BIOALLETHRIN

See Allethrin

BIORESMETHRIN

A member of the synthetic pyrethroid family, this is a broad-spectrum insecticide that is effective against flies, mosquitoes and other flying pests in households, and is also widely used in commercial, industrial, food-storage and public-sector settings. In household aerosols and sprays, it is usually formulated in combination with *Pyrethrum*, *Bioallethrin*, *Tetramethrin* and *Piperonyl butoxide*. It is a hormone disrupter, and highly toxic to fish and bees, and aquatic invertebrates.

BISPHENOL-A

A ubiquitous plasticiser that is the building block for polycarbonate plastic (used to make food and beverage containers and babies' bottles), but also in the manufacture of epoxy resins and other plastics, it is also used as an inert ingredient in pesticides (although not in the US), and as a fungicide, antioxidant and flame retardant. Bisphenol-A is a hormone disrupter that mimics the effects of oestrogen in the body. Studies link regular exposure to this chemical to insulin resistance, miscarriage and diseases of the prostate, including cancer.

BLEACH

See Sodium hypochlorite

BORAX

Sodium borate

This mild alkali agent is used in cosmetics and toiletries as a water softener, preservative and texturiser. Mildly irritating when used externally, it should not be applied to broken skin. If ingested, it can produce symptoms such as nausea, persistent vomiting, abdominal pain and diarrhoea.

BORIC ACID

E284

An antimicrobial, preservative and pesticide commonly used to control fungus on citrus fruits, this is highly poisonous. Regular exposure has been linked to foetal malformations. Severe poisonings have occurred from topical use and ingestion. For instance, used externally, it can be absorbed through wounds or grazes and, at the low doses sometimes used in mouthwashes, it can result in chronic intoxication, leading to confusion, lethargy, anorexia and hair loss.

BROMADIOLONE

The active ingredient in certain rodenticides, this is an anticoagulant that causes the animal to bleed to death internally once ingested. This is toxic to all animals, including humans.

BROMINATED VEGETABLE OILS

443

These are vegetable oils to which bromine – a heavy volatile, corrosive, non-metallic liquid element – has been added. These are used in soft drinks, citrus-flavoured beverages, ice creams and baked goods. Blending these high-density oils and other low-density oils (used as flavourings) makes the finished product easier to cook with and improves the texture of prepackaged foods. Adding them to fruit juices gives a slightly cloudy look that makes them appear natural. Animal studies suggest these oils accumulate in the body, producing fatty deposits in the liver, heart and kidneys. The spleen, pancreas, lung, aorta and skeletal muscle may also be affected. Growth retardation and impaired metabolism have also been reported and, worse, all attempts to remove brominated vegetable oils from the bodies of animals once it has been stored have proved impossible. They are in your body for life. Banned in Belgium, Sweden and Britain, they are still allowed and used in the US and Canada.

BROMONITRODIOXANE

Used as a disinfectant in household cleaners, and as a biocide in shampoos and other hair products, this *Formaldehyde* releaser can cause allergic contact dermatitis, and mix with other chemicals in the product to produce carcinogenic nitrosamines (see also Chapter 6).

2-BROMO-2-NITROPROPANE-1,3-DIOL

Bronopol

A preservative found in toiletries, cosmetics and household cleaners, it is a *Formaldehyde-* forming chemical which can react with nitrosating ingredients in the mix to form carcinogenic nitrosamines (see also Chapter 6).

BRONOPOL

See 2-bromo-2-nitropropane-1,3-diol

1,3-BUTADIENE

A plasticiser found in containers for foods and cosmetics, this is also a common toxin in car exhausts, and an occasional contaminant in cosmetic ingredients such as *Acrylates* and *Isobutane*. Breathing in low levels of 1,3-butadiene can irritate the eyes, nose and throat. Inhaling high levels for a short time can cause central nervous system damage, blurred vision, nausea, fatigue, headache, decreased blood pressure and pulse rate, and unconsciousness. Long-term exposure is carcinogenic. Animal studies suggest that inhalation can cause birth defects, and liver and kidney damage.

BUTANE

E943a

A propellant used in foods, cosmetics and household and garden sprays; chronic exposure can produce a range of central nervous system symptoms such as headache, breathing difficulties, mood swings, nausea, vomiting and dizziness, and symptoms mimicking drunkenness. Butane is a highly inflammable volatile organic chemical (VOC) popular with solvent abusers because they produce a quick 'high'. However, it can also produce convulsions, coma and a quick death. VOCs also accumulate in human breastmilk. While butane doesn't damage the earth's ozone shield, it does contribute to the formation of ground-level ozone, or smog, which can cause serious breathing problems. See also *Isobutane* and *Propane*.

BUTYLBENZYL PHTHALATE
BBP

A widely used plasticiser that humans are most likely to come in contact with through food-packaging materials, BBP has been associated with adverse effects on the central nervous system in humans and is classified by the US Environmental Protection Agency (EPA) as a possible human carcinogen, based on limited evidence that it produces leukaemia in female rats. It is also a suspected oestrogen mimic.

BUTYL CELLOSOLVE
Butoxyethanol, 2-butoxy-1-ethanol

A solvent and grease cutter commonly found in heavy-duty all-purpose cleaners, degreasers and window cleaners, inhalation of this chemical can cause headaches and nausea. However, it is also easily absorbed through the skin into the bloodstream and can damage internal tissues as well as the liver, kidneys and central nervous system.

BUTYLATED HYDROXYANISOLE
E320, BHA

An antioxidant added to foods to keep fats from becoming rancid, this is also used as a yeast defoaming agent. BHA is found in butter, meats, cereals, chewing gum, baked goods, snack foods, dehydrated potatoes and beer. It is also found in animal feeds, food-packaging, cosmetics, rubber and petroleum products. Studies show it can provoke an allergic reaction in some people and may trigger hyperactivity. There are serious concerns over its potential carcinogenicity and oestrogenic effects.

BUTYLATED HYDROXYTOLUENE
E321, BHT

Although commonly used in toiletries and prepackaged foods, BHT is most widely used as an antioxidant in rubber and plastic, and in liquid-petroleum products such as gasoline and motor oil. Exposure through the skin or through ingestion can trigger contact allergies and dermatitis. Some evidence suggests BHT is a potential carcinogen and reproductive toxin. Once in the bloodstream, BHT can accelerate the breakdown of vitamin D (necessary to maintain immunity, and healthy bones and teeth).

BUTYLENE GLYCOL

Used in cosmetics as a humectant, solvent and fragrance fixative (keeps the scent strong), this can also be used as a preservative. It has a similar toxicity to *Ethylene glycol* which, when ingested, may cause depression, vomiting, drowsiness, coma, respiratory failure, convulsions, renal damage, kidney failure and death. It is a *Formaldehyde*-former and penetration enhancer. It is widely used even though it has not been granted GRAS (generally recognised as safe) status because of concerns (based on animal data) of reproductive and mutagenic effects.

BUTYLPARABEN
See Parabens

C13-14 ISOPARAFFIN

A solvent and lubricating agent derived from petrochemicals, this is a relative of mineral oil used to make the product go on smoothly. However, it may cause skin irritation and increase photosensitivity of the skin.

CALCIUM BENZOATE

See Benzoic acid

CALCIUM HYPOCHLORITE

See Sodium hypochlorite

CALCIUM SULPHITE

See Sulphites

CALCIUM THIOGLYCOLATE

Calcium mercaptoacetate

This depilatory (hair-removing) chemical has never been fully assessed for safety by any relevant group or association.

CAMPHOR OIL

Japanese white oil, camphor tree

Used as a flavouring for beverages, baked goods and condiments, it is also used in embalming fluid, and in the manufacture of explosives and lacquers, and as a moth repellent and fragrance in household products. Readily absorbed into the bloodstream through all routes of administration, this was banned for topical use as a liniment for sore muscles and colds in the US in 1980 because of reports of poisonings through skin absorption and accidental ingestion. Vapours and inhalation can irritate the eyes, nose and throat. On the US EPA hazardous waste list, it is a central nervous system stimulant that is associated with dizziness, confusion, nausea, twitching muscles and convulsions.

CAPRYLIC/CAPRIC TRIGLYCERIDE

Fractionated coconut oil

An emollient and solvent derived from plants, vegetable oils and dairy fats, this is commonly used in soaps and skincare formulas. It is also sometimes used as synthetic flavouring in foods. There are no known safety concerns.

CARBARYL

A carbamate insecticide used mostly against caterpillar pests on apples, but also on citrus fruit, mangoes, bananas, strawberries, nuts, vines, olives, soya beans, cotton, rice, tobacco and grains, it is also used to treat lice in humans and livestock. Inhalation or ingestion at high doses can be toxic to the nervous and respiratory systems, resulting in nausea, stomach cramps, diarrhoea and excessive salivation, sweating, blurring of vision, and lack of coordination and convulsions. Over the long term, carbaryl is considered a reproductive toxin and potential human carcinogen.

CARBOLIC ACID

See Phenol

CARBOMER

A gelling agent, this is a synthetic polymer (a plastic-like material) used to thicken, stabilise and promote the shelf life of cosmetic products. No adverse effects are known; however, this agent is poorly studied.

CARBON TETRACHLORIDE

A toxic solvent that produces cellular destruction throughout the body, especially in the liver, kidney and central nervous system, this is toxic by all routes of exposure: inhalation, absorption, skin contact and oral ingestion. In 1970, the US Food and Drug Administration (FDA) classified carbon tetrachloride as a substance so hazardous that no warning label could be devised that would adequately protect the householder. It was subsequently banned from use in household products, although it remains in use in industry, and as a fumigant and dry-cleaning solution.

CARBOXYMETHYLCELLULOSE

A synthetic gum used in creams and lotions as an emulsifier and stabiliser, this has been shown to cause cancer in animals when ingested. Its toxicity with topical applications is unknown.

CARRAGEENAN

E407, chondrus extract, Irish moss

Used as a thickener and emulsifier in a wide variety of foods and also in toothpastes, carrageenan is part of a naturally occurring family of carbohydrates extracted from red seaweed. Because it can contain traces of **monosodium glutamate**, it has the potential to trigger allergic reactions. Ingestion has been associated with stomach aches.

Most recently, there have been concerns that it is a carcinogen. This could be because inferior products can be contaminated with **Ethylene oxide**. However, it can also be because of the way some high-molecular-weight carrageenans break down in the body into more dangerous low-molecular-weight carrageenans and poligeenans. In animals, carrageenan has been associated with cancer of the gastrointestinal tract, and laboratory studies using human breast cancer cells suggest that it can act as a trigger for breast cancer.

CETEARYL ALCOHOL

Cetyl stearyl alcohol, emulsifying wax

An emollient, moisturiser and emulsifier that can be animal, vegetable or petrochemical in origin, it closely resembles human sebum (the waxy substance that protects the skin). Although it is largely non-toxic, in sensitive individuals, it can cause contact dermatitis, hives and skin sensitisation.

CHLORDANE

Although now widely banned, chlordane is a persistent organochlorine insecticide that continues to contaminate soil and water. Used primarily to control termites and as a broad insecticide on a range of crops, chlordane affects the nervous, digestive and immune systems, and damages the liver. Headaches, irritability, confusion, weakness, vision problems, vomiting, stomach cramps, diarrhoea and jaundice have occurred in people who breathed air containing high concentrations of chlordane or accidentally swallowed small amounts of this chemical. Tests show it can kill birds and fish.

CHLORINE

E925, sodium hypochlorite, chlorine dioxide, hydrochloric acid

Used in the processing of fish, vegetables and fruits, and as a flour-bleaching agent, this is also used as a bleach and disinfectant in a wide range of household cleaners, including laundry bleach, dishwasher detergent and tile cleaners.

Chlorine in food destroys nutrients and yet, in some areas, is routinely added to tap water to make it 'safer' to drink – even though there is growing evidence that chlorinated drinking water causes bladder and rectal cancers. In addition to its direct toxic effects on living organisms, chlorine also reacts with organic materials in the environment to create other hazardous and carcinogenic toxins, including trihalomethanes (THMs) and *chloroform*, and organochlorines, an extremely dangerous class of compounds that cause reproductive, endocrine and immune system disorders.

THMs can be removed from tap water with an adequate home-filtration system that uses activated carbon to filter the water. As a household cleaner, chlorine vapours are powerfully irritating to the eyes and respiratory tract. Chlorine and its related compounds are also environmentally damaging, break down slowly in the ecosystem and are stored in the fatty tissues of wild animals (*see also Sodium hypochlorite*).

CHLOROBENZENE

Benzene chloride, chlorobenzol

A solvent used in dyes, pesticides and perfumes, this is also used for degreasing vehicle parts. It is harmful if swallowed, inhaled or absorbed through skin. In the short term, it is a skin irritant; over the longer term, it is considered a possible carcinogen.

CHLOROETHANE

Ethyl chloride

A chlorinated solvent used for cleaning and degreasing, it is also used in the production of cellulose, dyes and medicinal drugs, as well as to numb skin prior to medical procedures such as ear-piercing and skin biopsies, and in the treatment of sports injuries. Toxic to the nervous, cardiovascular, gastrointestinal and musculoskeletal systems, this is a recognised carcinogen and suspected reproductive toxin.

CHLOROFLUOROCARBONS

CFCs

These are aerosol propellants such as trichloromethane and dichlorodifluoromethane used to disperse cleaning solvents and degreasers, paints, pesticides and cosmetics. Once in the atmosphere, CFCs stay there for a long time (several decades) and are the main cause of stratospheric ozone depletion and, therefore, important contributors to the phenomenon of global warming.

CHLOROFORM

Used as a solvent for fats, oils, waxes and resins, and as a cleaning ingredient, exposure may cause respiratory irritation and skin allergies. Chloroform is a neurotoxin, anaesthetic and carcinogen. Inhalation of vapours may cause headache, nausea, vomiting, dizziness, drowsiness, irritation of the respiratory tract and loss of consciousness. Chronic exposure to chloroform can aggravate some medical conditions such as kidney disorders, liver disorders, heart disorders and skin disorders. Studies have shown it to causes liver and kidney cancer in animals.

CHLORHEXIDINE

This is an antimicrobial used in mouthwashes, sprays and dental gels to prevent and treat the redness, swelling and bleeding gums associated with gingivitis. It is considered effective but, with regular use, it can discolour teeth and is implicated in rising rates of resistant bacteria.

CHLOROPHENATE

A fungicide and wood preservative not widely used today, but still present in older woods, evidence suggests that exposure increases the risk of non-Hodgkin's lymphoma.

CHLOROPHENOLS

Because of their broad-spectrum antimicrobial properties, chlorophenols have been used as preservative agents for wood, paints, vegetable fibres and leather, and as disinfectants. In addition, they are used as herbicides, fungicides and insecticides, and as intermediates in the production of pharmaceuticals and dyes. Chlorophenol exposure is irritating to skin and eyes. Prolonged exposure is toxic to the liver and immune system, and is a suspected trigger for cancer.

4-CHLORO-m-PHENYLENEDIAMINE

See Phenylenediamines

CHLOROTHALONIL

Chlorothalonil is a broad-spectrum organochlorine fungicide used to control fungi that threaten vegetables, trees, small fruits and grass. Exposure can cause severe eye and skin irritation. Very high doses may cause a range of symptoms, including loss of muscle coordination, rapid breathing, nosebleeds, vomiting, hyperactivity and death. In animal studies, female mice developed tumours in the fore-stomach area (attributed to irritation by the compound), and males developed both cancerous and benign kidney tumours. No studies on humans have been performed to date.

CHLORPYRIFOS

Dursban

A broad-spectrum organophosphate insecticide, this was originally used primarily to kill mosquitoes, although it is no longer registered for that use. Chlorpyrifos is effective in controlling cockroaches, grubs, flies, termites, fire ants and lice. It is also a skin and eye irritant. Short- and long-term exposure may affect the cardiovascular, respiratory and central nervous systems.

CHROMATED COPPER ARSENTATE

CCA

See Arsenic

CINNAMATES

A family of sunscreening agents that includes octocrylene, octyl methoxycinnamate and cinoxate, cinnamates are derivatives of cinnamon and are chemically related to balsam of Peru, tolu balsam, coca leaves, cinnamic aldehyde and cinnamic oil. People with sensitivities to these chemicals may have an allergic reaction to sunscreens containing them. The cinnamates are much less potent than many other chemical sunscreens and require the addition other UVB absorbers to achieve higher SPFs. Laboratory studies suggest that some cinnamates may act like oestrogens in the body.

CINNAMYL ALCOHOL

A synthetic fragrance with a sweet balsam, hyacinth odour, this is a common skin and eye irritant.

CINOXATE

See Cinnamates

CITRAL

A synthetic lemon fragrance used in perfumes, household cleaners and air fresheners, and in foods, citral is an allergen and irritant; it has oestrogenic effects and has been found to cause enlargement of the prostate gland in animals.

CITRIC ACID

E330

A food acid naturally derived from citrus fruit, and used in foods and cosmetics; as a flavouring, it is found in sodas and soft drinks, ice creams and ices, sweets, baked goods and chewing gum. It is also used as a pH (acid to alkaline) adjuster in beverages, as a preservative in cured meats and colour preserver in tinned vegetables. Prolonged exposure damages tooth enamel. Citric acid may interact with any protein in the food to which it is added, freeing up glutamic acid, which can trigger allergies in some people (see *Monosodium glutamate*). In cosmetics, it is a preservative and also an *Alpha-hydroxy acid*, used to strip off the top layers of the skin (supposedly revealing 'younger' skin underneath). Like all AHAs, citric acid can cause irritation. As AHAs become more popular in cosmetics like soaps, shampoos and moisturisers, they have also become a major cause of adverse skin reactions.

CITRONELLOL

A synthetic fragrance and flavouring, in perfumes it provides a sweet, rose-like odour. As an artificial flavouring in foods, it is used in berry, citrus, cola, fruit, rose and floral flavours for beverages, ice creams, sweets, baked goods, chewing gum and gelatine deserts. It is also used as a pesticide to combat mosquitoes and other flying insects. Applied topically, it can be a severe skin irritant.

COAL TAR

The black residue obtained by the distillation of coal, this is often found in antidandruff treatments and in products used to treat seborrhoeic dermatitis and psoriasis. It is found in some bath soaps, and may cause photosensitivity in some and, with prolonged use, also make itching worse. The US EPA classifies coal tar as a human carcinogen.

COCAMIDE DEA

Cocamide diethanolamine

Found in dishwashing liquids, shampoos and cosmetics, cocamide DEA is a strong detergent, foam stabiliser and thickener. It can irritate the skin. It also belongs to a family of fatty acids called alkanolamines, which are considered hormone-disrupting chemicals. While not carcinogenic on its own, it has the potential to form carcinogenic nitrosamines when mixed with *Formaldehyde*-forming ingredients (see also Chapter 6).

COCAMIDE MEA

See cocamide DEA

COCAMIDOPROPYL BETAINE

A detergent that is a strong allergen, and skin and eye irritant, this is also a penetration enhancer – allowing other chemicals in the mix to be more easily absorbed through the skin. It can be contaminated with *Diethanolamine* (DEA) which, when combined with *Formaldehyde* (released by other ingredients during storage), produces carcinogenic nitrosamines (see also Chapter 6).

COUMARIN

A naturally derived fragrance, coumarin is a common skin sensitiser. Several types of coumarin have already been banned in the European Union because of their potential to cause serious skin reactions and photosensitisation. In animals, it causes lung and liver cancers, and is damaging to the kidneys. According to the International Agency for Research on Cancer (IARC), coumarin is 'rapidly and extensively absorbed after topical or oral administration to human subjects'. Human data show it to be liver toxic. It may also cause central nervous system disruption.

CREOSOTE

Used in medicines to treat skin diseases such as psoriasis, and also used as animal and bird repellents, insecticides, restricted pesticides, animal dips and fungicides, creosote is a widely used wood preservative. As an antimicrobial agent, it can be found in heavy-duty household cleaners and disinfectants.

Once made by distilling tar extracted from beechwood, it is now largely derived from *Coal tar*. The US Environmental Protection Agency (EPA) has determined that coal tar-derived creosote is a probable carcinogen.

CRESOL

2-methoxy-4-methylphenol

A disinfectant (and relative of *Phenol*) that attacks the central nervous system, respiratory system, liver, kidneys, pancreas, spleen, skin and eyes, it can enter the body via the lungs or the skin. Repeated or prolonged exposure to low concentrations of cresol can produce chronic systemic poisoning. The symptoms of poisoning include vomiting, difficulty in swallowing, diarrhoea, loss of appetite, headache, fainting, dizziness, mental disturbance and skin rash.

CRYSTALLINE SILICA

Also known as silicon dioxide (SiO_2), it is the basic component of sand, quartz and granite rock. An abrasive mineral-based powder found in highly popular brands of all-purpose cleaners, when inhaled, it is an eye, skin and lung irritant. Crystalline silica has been classified as a human lung carcinogen. Additionally, breathing crystalline silica dust can cause silicosis, a fibrotic lung disease (producing scar tissue in the lungs) which can be progressive and disabling and, in severe cases, fatal (see also *Silica*).

CYCLAMATE
E952, Natreen, Cologran

An artificial sweetener 35 times sweeter than sugar with a sweet-sour taste, in tabletop sweeteners, cyclamate is often found blended with **Saccharin**. It is allowed in the EU, where it's widely used in 'budget' squash drinks and so is mainly consumed by children. In the US, the FDA banned it in 1969 after evidence emerged linking it to bladder cancer in animals. The ban is still in force. However, it is still widely used in Europe, Australia and New Zealand, though the noose has been gradually tightening around cyclamate as a food additive. The UK's Food Standards Agency (FSA), for instance, now advises parents to drastically limit children's exposure to this chemical.

CYCLOHEXASILOXANE
See Silicones

CYCLOMETHICONE
See Silicones

CYCLOPENTASILOXANE
See Silicones

CYPERMETHRIN

A pyrethroid insecticide that has wide uses in cotton, cereals, vegetables and fruit, and for food storage, cypermethrin is a skin and eye irritant, and central nervous system toxin. Symptoms of poisoning include abnormal facial sensations, dizziness, headache, nausea, anorexia and fatigue, vomiting and increased stomach secretion. The US Environmental Protection Agency (EPA) classifies it as a possible carcinogen. It may also suppress immune function.

2,4-D
2,4-dichlorophenoxy acetic acid

A herbicide used in agriculture, industry and household garden products, exposure to this phenoxy compound can cause eye and skin irritation. One single application to grass that is tracked indoors can be expected to linger in carpet for up to a year. Studies have linked 2,4-D to non-Hodgkin's lymphoma, childhood leukaemia and childhood brain cancer. Recently, exposure to lawns treated with 2,4-D has been associated with cancer in dogs.

D-ALLETHRIN
See Allethrin

D-LIMONENE
See Limonene

D-PHENOTHRIN

This synthetic pyrethroid insecticide, used to control bedbugs, flies, gnats, mosquitoes, cockroaches and lice, is also a skin, eye and respiratory tract irritant. With prolonged exposure, headache, dizziness, anorexia and hypersalivation can occur. It is toxic to fish and bees.

DACTHAL
DCPA, dimethyl tetrachloroterephthalate
Chlorinated herbicide used in agriculture (on fruits and vegetables), and in public and domestic settings, this is often found in home weed and feed preparations. It is also poorly studied for its effects on humans or the environment in spite of the fact that, in the US, DCPA and its breakdown products became the most commonly detected pesticide residues in an Environmental Protection Agency survey of drinking-water wells conducted during 1988–1990.

DDE
1,1-dichloro-2,2-bis(p-dichlorodiphenyl)ethylene
DDE is a breakdown product of DDT present in the environment and in the body. Exposure can cause headache, dizziness, nausea, vomiting, incoordination, tremor, mental confusion, anxiety and a sensation of tingling or crawling on the skin. It is a carcinogen and hormone disrupter.

DDT
Dichlorodiphenyltrichloroethane
DDT is an organochlorine insecticide. Its once widespread use on crops has been halted due to its extreme toxicity to humans and wildlife. However, it is still used widely to control mosquito-borne malaria. DDT is a persistent neurotoxin, and traces of it regularly turn up in foods grown in DDT-contaminated soils. Chronic exposure damages the nervous system, liver, kidneys and immune system in experimental animals. It is a reproductive toxin, hormone disrupter and carcinogen.

DEA-OLETH-3 PHOSPHATE
This surfactant, found in cosmetics and toiletries, is a relative of **Polyethylene glycol** (PEG). It can be carcinogenic in itself as well as contaminated with the carcinogen 1,4-**dioxane** (see also **Diethanolamine**).

DEA CETYL PHOSPHATE
See Diethanolamine

DEET
N,N-diethyl-m-toluamide
An insecticide found in a variety of commercial products used on clothing, household pets and furnishings, it is the active ingredient in most mosquito repellents and unusual in that it is licensed to be applied directly to human skin. It is, however, an irritant that can produce a variety of skin reactions, including rashes, blisters and mucous membrane irritation, and numb or burning sensations of the lips. DEET is also a neurotoxin that can produce insomnia, mood disturbances and impaired cognitive function and seizures. In addition, several cases of toxic encephalopathy in children have been linked to the use of this agent. Symptoms of toxic encephalopathy include agitation, weakness, disorientation, ataxia, seizures, coma and death.

DELTAMETHRIN
A pyrethroid insecticide found in a variety of commercial garden products as well as indoor-use products to control mosquitoes, flies, fleas and cockroaches, this is considered

the most powerful of the synthetic pyrethroids. Like all pyrethroids, it can produce a variety of symptoms linked to disruption of the central nervous system including headache, dizziness, sweating, rapid heart beat, tingling skin and hypersalivation; it is irritating to the skin, eyes and respiratory tract. It is also highly toxic to fish, bees and other beneficial insects.

DIAMINOBENZENES

Colour developers found in permanent and semi-permanent hair dyes, they work by a process of oxidation and, if absorbed, can be powerful mutagens. See also **Phenylenediamines**, which belong to this family of chemicals.

DIAMINOPHENOL

Oxidising colouring agent for general use hair dyes, this can cause allergic reactions and should never be used to dye eyelashes or eyebrows.

DIAMINOTOLUENES

Intermediates in the synthesis of dyes used for textiles, furs, leathers, spirit varnishes and wood stains and pigments, these were once widely used in hair dyes, but were removed from use by many countries after they were found to cause liver cancer in rats.

DIAMMONIUM EDTA

Diammonium ethylenediaminetetra acetate

A stabiliser used in cosmetics and household cleaners, laundry products and pesticides to prevent the ingredients from binding with trace elements (particularly minerals and metal impurities) which change the texture, odour and consistency of the product. The technical term for such ingredients is a 'chelating agent'. If ingested or absorbed into the body, chelating agents can concentrate these impurities in the body. (In the environment, they concentrate heavy metals and other contaminants in soil and the water supply.) Diammonium EDTA can be irritating to the mucous membranes and skin, leading to allergies, asthma and skin rashes.

DIAZINON

An organophosphate insecticide used to control cockroaches, silverfish, ants and fleas in the home and on pets, it is often found in formulations mixed with other pesticides such as pyrethrins, **Lindane** and disulphoton.

Symptoms associated with high-level exposure to this chemical include weakness, headaches, tightness in the chest, blurred vision, excess salivation, sweating, nausea, vomiting, diarrhoea, abdominal cramps and slurred speech. Diazinon is also known to be toxic to birds and fish.

DIAZOLIDINYL UREA

A broad-spectrum antibacterial preservative used in cosmetics and personal-care products, this has particularly good activity against *Pseudomonas* species. It is a **Formaldehyde**-releasing preservative that can form carcinogenic nitrosamines when mixed with nitrosating agents in the product (see also Chapter 6). It is also a sensitising agent that can provoke contact dermatitis.

DIBUTYLPHTHALATE

See Phthalates

DICAMBA

A **Benzoic acid** herbicide found in weed-control products, this chemical can cause irritation to the lungs, eyes and skin in humans. Acute exposures can produce symptoms such as vomiting, muscle weakness, slowed heart rate, shortness of breath, mood swings, incontinence, cyanosis (bluing of the skin and gums), muscle spasms and exhaustion. Long-term exposure can cause damage to the liver.

1,2-DICHLOROETHANE

Ethylene dichloride

An industrial-strength solvent found in paint, varnish and finish removers, and degreasers, this is also a skin irritant, a narcotic, and is toxic to the liver and kidneys as well as to the nervous and immune systems. A probable human carcinogen and mutagen, it may cause systemic effects, and is regarded as a priority pollutant (one which regulatory authorities urgently need to study to fully understand its toxicity) in many countries.

DICHLOROETHANE

See 1,2-dichloroethane

DICHLOROMETHANE

Methylene chloride, methylene dichloride

Powerful industrial solvent mainly used as a paint-stripper and a degreaser. In the food industry, it is used to decaffeinate coffee, and to prepare extracts of hops and other flavourings. It is also used as a fumigant pesticide for stored strawberries and grains. Chronic exposure may be carcinogenic, as it has been linked to cancer of the lungs, liver and pancreas in laboratory animals. It is a mutagen and teratogen, causing birth defects if exposure occurs during pregnancy.

DICHLORVOS

DDVP

Organophosphate insecticide used in household and garden pesticide products and in dog flea-collars, this is also given to dogs to kill intestinal worms. Exposure can quickly produce symptoms of tightness of the chest, wheezing, blurred vision, tearing, runny nose, headache, sweating, twitching, nausea, vomiting, abdominal cramps and diarrhoea.

DIELDRIN

This organochlorine insecticide is no longer used in most countries because of its toxicity, although some countries do still use it for termite control. Surveys of dairy products, meat products, fish, oils and fats and certain vegetables, such as root vegetables, regularly reveal traces of dieldrin in our food.

Dieldrin can form as a breakdown product of another pesticide, **Aldrin**, and because of its extreme persistence, it can be found everywhere in the environment. Symptoms of exposure to the two substances are basically the same and include headaches, dizziness, irritability, vomiting and uncontrolled muscle movements. Dieldrin is toxic to the nervous system and a suspected carcinogen and hormone disrupter.

DIETHANOLAMINE

DEA

A solvent, emulsifying agent, detergent, dispersing agent and humectant found in cosmetics and body-care products, this is irritating to skin and mucous membranes. DEA is used in relatively few products, but DEA-containing compounds, including *cocamide DEA*, cocamide MEA, DEA cetyl phosphate, *DEA-oleth-3 phosphate*, DEA lauryl sulphate, lauramide DEA, myristamide DEA and oleamide DEA are very widely used.

While DEA by itself is not harmful, it can react with other ingredients known as *Formaldehyde*-formers in the product to form a potent carcinogen called nitrosodiethanolamine (NDEA). NDEA is readily absorbed through the skin, and has been linked with health problems such as stomach, oesophageal, liver and bladder cancers. Related compounds such as TEA lauryl sulphate and *Triethanolamine* can also mix with other ingredients to form NDEA in cosmetics (see also Chapter 6).

DIETHYLENE GLYCOL

A solvent belonging to a family of chemicals called dioxanes (not to be confused with the pesticide *Dioxin*), this is commonly found in glass cleaners. Diethylene glycol has not been fully assessed by any relevant body or group; however, *Dioxanes* are thought to be carcinogenic, and research suggests that they are immune-system suppressants.

DIETHYL PHTHALATE

See Phthalates

DIETHYLHEXYL PHTHALATE

See Phthalates

DIFENACOUM

A rodenticide that works by preventing the animal's blood from clotting, it kills the animal by causing internal haemorrhage. It is acutely toxic to humans and other animals, causing the same kind of effects as it does in rodents.

DIGALLOYL TRIOLEATE

This sunscreening agent is poorly studied in humans or animals, so its potential toxicity is not clear.

DIMETHICONE

A film-forming, antifoaming agent and skin conditioner, based on silicone and found in toiletries and cosmetics, this chemical makes the product more spreadable and can make the skin feel smoother, but it also traps other substances (including other ingredients in the product) beneath it. Because film-formers do not allow the skin to breathe, properly they may exacerbate skin irritation caused by sweat or other substances in the product. See also *Silicones*.

DIMETHICONE COPOLYOL

A more waterproof form of *Dimethicone* that sticks to skin and hair better, this is a polymer based on silicone that is used as a conditioner in haircare products and as a skin protectant. It is not considered toxic but, with prolonged use, it can make the skin look dull. See also *Silicones*.

DIMETHOATE

An organophosphate insecticide used to control mites and other insects, repeated exposure can cause impaired memory and concentration, disorientation, severe depression, irritability, confusion, headache, speech difficulties, delayed reaction times, nightmares, sleepwalking, drowsiness or insomnia and flu-like symptoms. This is also a potential carcinogen and reproductive toxin.

DIMETHYL ETHER

Dimethyl oxide, wood ether, methyl ether

Found in hairsprays and other toiletries in pressurised containers, this is a relative of **Propylene glycol**, and is a solvent that it is easily absorbed through the skin. Once in the body, it can bioaccumulate and is known to be a reproductive toxin. It is also a solvent and a fuel used in welding, and finds use as a refrigerant. It has an anaesthetic effect in high concentrations.

5-DIMETHYLDANTOIN

A caustic found in toilet-bowl cleaners, it forms hypochlorite in water, which is corrosive to skin and mucous membranes.

DIMETHYLPHTHALATE

See Phthalates

DIMETHYLPOLYSILOXANE

See Silicones

DIOCTYL ADIPATE

Adipic acid

A plasticiser and solvent found in bath oils, eyeshadows, foundations, colognes, blushers, nail-polish removers, perfumes, moisturisers and fake-tan preparations, this is also an element in the plastic wraps used for prepackaged foods, especially meats. Studies show it can migrate from the wrapping material into food. Applied topically, it can be irritating to skin and eyes. With regular ingestion, it is considered a possible human carcinogen, based on animal studies that show an increased incidence of liver tumours.

DIOXANE

Diethylene dioxide, diethylene ether, diethylene oxide

Found primarily as a contaminant in toiletries and household products, dioxane is a hazardous air pollutant and carcinogen. It is often a contaminant in ethoxylated surfactants, detergents, foaming agents, emulsifiers and solvents. These ingredients are identifiable by the prefix 'PEG' or words like 'polyethylene', 'polyethylene glycol' and 'polyoxyethylene', or syllables such as '-eth-' or '-oxynol-'.

DIOXINS

Polychlorinated dibenzo-p-dioxins (PCDDs)

Dioxins are the toxic byproducts of several types of industry: during incineration of organic waste containing chlorine (i.e. plastics); and during manufacture of paper, wood preservatives and chlorinated aromatics such as 2,4,5-trichlorophenol (an intermediate in the manufacture of the herbicide 2,4,5-T). Found in bleached paper products, including disposable nappies, tampons, panty liners, toilet paper, milk and juice cartons, and paper containers for microwaveable food, they are also used in some pesticides and herbicides. However, more than 90 per cent of all human exposure to dioxins comes from food, mainly from animal fat.

Tetrachlorodibenzo-*p*-dioxin (TCDD) is the most well-researched dioxin and arguably the most toxic. When scientists refer to the toxic effects of dioxins, they usually mean TCDD. Many PCDDs are known to be toxic, hormone disrupting and carcinogenic.

DIOXYBENZONE

A chemical used in sunscreen to block UVB, it is a derivative of ***Benzophenone***.

DISODIUM EDTA

E386, disodium ethylenediaminetetra acetate

A preservative and antioxidant used in foods, cosmetics and household cleaners. In foods, it promotes colour retention in tinned vegetables, and is found in cereals, fruit pie-fillings and salad dressings. In cosmetics and other formulations, its purpose is to prevent the ingredients in a given formula from binding with trace elements (particularly minerals and metal impurities) and thereby changing the texture, odour and consistency of the product.

The technical term for such ingredients is 'chelating agent'. If ingested or absorbed into the body, chelating agents can concentrate these impurities in the body. In the environment, they concentrate heavy metals and other contaminants in soil and the water supply. Applied topically, Disodium EDTA is irritating to eyes and skin, and acts as a penetration enhancer, allowing other active ingredients, and more harmful chemicals, to penetrate deeper into the skin and eventually reach the bloodstream.

DMDM HYDANTOIN

Diemethylol dimethyl hydantoin

A water-soluble preservative used in cosmetics, this can act as a ***Formaldehyde***-releasing agent. This should not be combined with DEA or DEA-containing compounds as this can cause the carcinogenic substance NDELA to form. See also ***Diethanolamine***.

DSMA

Disodium methanearsonate

An ***Arsenic***-based weed-killer. Fatal if swallowed.

EDTA

Ethylenediamine tetraacetic acid, ethylene-diaminotetra acetate

A preservative that stabilises the bleach and foaming agents in detergent products, preventing them from becoming active before they are immersed in water. It is also used as a water softener. Unfortunately, it binds with toxic metals in the environment and carries them back into our drinking-water supply and into foods, especially fish and shellfish. EDTA can be irritating to skin and mucous membranes, and may cause allergic reactions. Liquid detergents are more prone to contamination and therefore use more of this preservative than the powdered variety.

ENZYMES

Enzymes are living organisms that are added to a diverse spectrum of consumer products such as laundry detergents. Most laundry detergents are formulated with enzymes that act as stain removers. These products are called 'biological' detergents. Enzymes are obtained from selected strains of bacteria. Products that have enzymes in them can be irritating to the skin, and cause allergic reactions such as asthma and dermatitis.

Enzymes are also added to prepackaged foods to improve flavour, texture and digestibility. Although enzymes occur naturally in foods, the ones used in commercial food production are synthesised in the lab and often genetically engineered. To date, there have been no reports of consumer allergies to enzyme residues in food, but then, there has been little formal research into adverse effects. Like all proteins, enzymes can cause allergic reactions when people have been sensitised through exposure to large quantities. Those that have been genetically engineered may be more likely to provoke allergic reactions. Use the table below to identify added enzymes in foods.

Some enzymes used in food production

Market	Enzyme	Purpose/function
Dairy	Rennet* (protease)	Coagulant in cheese production
	Lactase	Hydrolysis of lactose to give lactose-free milk products
	Protease	Hydrolysis of whey proteins
	Catalases*	Removal of hydrogen peroxide
Brewing	Cellulases, beta-glucanases, alpha amylases*, proteases*, maltogenic amylases*	For liquefaction, clarification and to supplement malt enzymes
Alcohol production	Amyloglucosidase	Conversion of starch to sugar
Baking	Alpha-amylases*	Breakdown of starch, maltose production
	Amyloglycosidases	Saccharification
	Maltogen amylase (Novamyl)	Delays process by which bread becomes stale
	Protease*	Breakdown of proteins
	Pentosanase	Breakdown of pentosan, leading to reduced gluten production
	Glucose oxidase	Stability of dough
Wine and fruit juice	Pectinase	Increase of yield and juice clarification
	Glucose oxidase*	Oxygen removal
	Beta-glucanases*	
Meat	Protease*	Meat tenderising
	Papain	
Protein	Proteases, trypsin, aminopeptidases	Breakdown of various components

Market	Enzyme	Purpose/function
Starch	Alpha amylase*, glucoamylases, hemicellulases*, maltogenic amylases*, glucose isomerases*, dextranases, beta-glucanases*	Modification and conversion (e.g. to dextrose or high fructose syrups)
Inulin	Inulinases	Production of fructose syrups

Enzymes marked with an asterisk (*) are produced using GM technology. Other genetically engineered enzymes in food production include alpha-acetolactate decarboxylase (brewing), chymosin (cheese), alpha-glucanotransferase (starch), lipase (fats, oils), phytase (starch), pullulanase (brewing, starch) and xylanase (baking, starch).

ENDOSULPHAN

The use of this chlorinated hydrocarbon insecticide is widely restricted. It is poisonous to a wide variety of insects and mites, and can be used as a wood preservative as well as on a wide variety of food crops, including tea, coffee, fruits, vegetables, rice and grains. It is a nervous system stimulant that can produce symptoms of lack of coordination, imbalance, difficulty breathing, gagging, vomiting, diarrhoea, agitation, temporary blindness, convulsions and loss of consciousness. Toxic to the liver and kidneys with long-term use, it is a suspected mutagen and reproductive toxin. It is poisonous to birds, fish and bees.

ENDOTHALL

A dicarboxylic acid herbicide used to control weeds on land and in water, this agent is very irritating to the eyes, skin and mucous membranes. In humans, ingestion can damage the lungs and gastrointestinal tract.

EPICHLOROHYDRIN

A major raw material used in the manufacture of epoxy and phenoxy resins, it is also used as an insecticide and fungicide. Skin contact can cause burns, and contact with eyes may cause permanent damage. It is a carcinogen, and a reproductive and central nervous system toxin; long-term exposure may, in addition, lead to liver or kidney damage.

ETHYL ACETATE

This solvent, flavouring and fragrance is found in foods, toiletries and household products. In foods, it is used to flavour beverages, ice creams, baked goods, chewing gums and desserts. It is also used in the decaffeination of green coffee beans and tea leaves. In the home, it can be found in air fresheners and dryer sheets. It is a mild skin and respiratory-tract irritant, and central nervous system depressant. Its vapours damage the lungs, liver, heart and central nervous system. It can have narcotic effects and has also been linked with anaemia and leucocytosis (an increase in the number of white blood cells, an immune-system reaction), and with damage to liver and kidneys.

ETHYL ACRYLATE

This solvent and synthetic flavouring is used in foods and as a fragrance ingredient (though this latter use is restricted in many countries). It is also used in the manufacture of water-based latex paints and adhesives, textile and paper coatings, leather finish resins and in the production of acrylic fibres. Highly irritating to eyes, skin and the mucous membranes, ethyl acrylate is a potential human carcinogen, and toxic to the liver and kidneys as well as the immune and gastrointestinal systems.

ETHYL ALCOHOL

Ethanol
> See Alcohol

ETHYL DIHYDROXYPROPYL PABA

> See PABA

ETHYL LINALOOL

> See Linalool

ETHYLBENZENE

A solvent found in natural products such as **Coal tar** and petroleum, this is also found in manufactured products such as inks, insecticides and paints. People exposed to high levels of ethylbenzene in air can experience dizziness, throat irritation, tightening of the chest and a burning sensation in the eyes. Animal studies have shown effects on the nervous system, liver, kidneys and eyes on exposure to fumes.

ETHYLENE DICHLORIDE

EDC, 1,2-dichloroethane, glycol dichloride
A solvent and an intermediate in the manufacture of **Trichloroethane** and fluorocarbons, it is also found in paint varnish and finish removers, and pesticides. In foods, it is used in the production of spices.

It is highly toxic whether taken into the body by ingestion, inhalation or skin absorption. In laboratory tests, exposure has led to stomach, breast and skin cancers in animals. Chronic (long-term) exposure to ethylene-dichloride vapours produced effects on the liver and kidneys in animals. Men occupationally exposed to EDC have been rendered sterile.

ETHYLENE GLYCOL

A solvent and humectant often found in windscreen-wiper solutions, this chemical can cause damage to the internal organs, especially the kidneys, heart and nervous system through skin absorption; inhalation can cause dizziness, drowsiness and respiratory failure.

ETHYLENE OXIDE

This industrial chemical is an intermediate in the production of **ethylene glycol** and other chemicals. Ethylene oxide is a common indoor pollutant that is toxic by inhalation and ingestion. Symptoms of overexposure include headache and dizziness, progressing with increasing exposure to convulsions, seizure and coma. It is also an irritant to skin and the respiratory tract, and inhaling the vapours may cause the lungs to fill with fluid several hours after exposure.

Laboratory animals exposed to ethylene oxide throughout their lives have had a higher incidence of liver cancer.

ETHYLHEXYL P-METHOXYCINNAMATE
See Cinnamates

ETHYLHEXYL SALICYLATE
Octyl salicylate
   See Salicylates

ETHYLPARABEN
See Parabens

EUGENOL
A synthetic flavouring in foods and a fragrance in cosmetics, it is also used as a fungicide and insecticide. A skin irritant and allergen in cosmetics, if ingested, it may cause vomiting and gastric irritation. It is poorly studied with regard to human safety, but is known to cause tumours in rats.

FARNESOL
Used both as a pesticide and perfume, this agent may cause skin and eye irritation. Little data are available on its toxicity in humans.

FENITROTHION
An organophosphate insecticide used to control a variety of boring insects such as beetles, as well as flies, mosquitoes and cockroaches, it is irritating to the eyes. Symptoms of longer-term exposure in humans include general malaise, fatigue, headache, loss of memory and ability to concentrate, anorexia, nausea, thirst, loss of weight, cramps, muscular weakness and tremors. It is a carcinogen, and an immune system and reproductive toxin.

FENOXYCARB
A carbamate insecticide used to control fire ants, fleas, mosquitoes and cockroaches, long-term animal studies suggest it is toxic to the liver. But, overall, this pesticide is poorly studied with regard to its effects on human health.

FIPRONIL
A phenyl pyrazole insecticide used for ant and cockroach control as well as in flea and tick products, pets treated with fipronil have experienced skin irritation and hair loss; dogs appear to be more prone to these effects than cats. In other animal studies, this chemical has proven carcinogenic and, on this basis, it is classified as a possible human carcinogen.

FLUFENOXURON
A benzoylurea insecticide that is irritating to eyes, skin and mucous membranes, long-term exposure can cause nausea, vomiting, diarrhoea, headache, confusion and electrolyte depletion.

FLUORIDE
Sodium fluoride, sodium monofluorophosphate
   Added to toothpastes and to water to prevent dental caries, in chemical tables, fluoride

falls somewhere between arsenic and lead in terms of its toxicity. When containers of fluoride arrive at the doors of toothpaste manufacturers, they come with a skull and crossbones on the front. Fluoride is a systemic poison and there is enough of this substance in half a tube of family toothpaste to kill a small child.

Fluoride works best applied topically, but toothpaste rarely stays on the teeth long enough to be totally effective. Its benefits are highly contested and continually overstated. Ten years ago, fluoride was touted as reducing the incidence of dental caries by 40–60 per cent; today, the revised figure is 18–25 per cent. Levels of caries tend to be lowest in nonfluoridated areas, and better diets and conscientious brushing are likely to be the major factors in improved dental health.

While there is very little concrete evidence that fluoride genuinely protects teeth, there is plenty of evidence to show that regular exposure can cause harm.

Studies have shown a clear relationship between oral cancers and fluoride intake in both animals and humans. Benign squamous papilloma, for instance, which appears as a white patch on the inside of the mouth and is the precursor of squamous cell carcinoma, can be triggered by fluoride exposure.

Fluoride can cause sensitivity/allergic-type reactions and is now suspected in a host of illnesses, including gastroesophageal reflux disease (GERD), bone problems, diabetes, thyroid malfunction and mental impairment. Fluoride exposure from toothpaste, supplements and water before the age of six is also an important risk factor for dental fluorosis, which mottles and discolours teeth.

FOLPET

A carboximide fungicide found in many commercial garden products, this is irritating to the skin, eyes and mucous membranes. Animal studies suggest that long-term exposure can trigger cancer in the duodenum.

FORMALDEHYDE

E240, paraformaldehyde

This disinfectant, germicide, fungicide, defoamer and preservative is not used in foods, but can be used to disinfect containers, pipes and vessels in the food industry. It is widely used in personal care and household products such as deodorisers, disinfectants, furniture polishes, detergents, personal-care products (including shampoo) and cosmetics (including nail polish and hardeners). Formaldehyde vapours are common indoor pollutants, and are suspected human carcinogens that also alter your sense of smell and can cause respiratory irritation. Anyone with asthma, lung infections or similar ailments can be severely affected by exposure to formaldehyde. It can also cause stuffy nose and itchy or watery eyes, nausea, headache and fatigue. Some preservatives used in cosmetics and household products break down into formaldehyde during storage. Examples include *2-Bromo-2-nitropropane-1,3-diol*, *Diazolidinyl urea*, *DMDM hydantoin*, *Imidazolidinyl urea* and quaternium-15.

G-METHYLIONONE

This synthetic fragrance is a known contact allergen that is commonly found in household cleaners, laundry detergents and dishwashing liquids as well as cosmetics.

G-TERPINENE

A synthetic fragrance commonly found in cologne, perfume, soap, shaving cream, deodorant, air freshener, it can trigger asthma. As a central nervous system disrupter, it can cause symptoms such as headache, mood swings, depression, incoordination and lethargy.

GERANIOL

This synthetic fragrance is found in cosmetics, soaps, detergents, creams, lotions and air fresheners. It is also used as a synthetic flavouring agent in beverages, ice creams and sweets, and is sometimes found in 'natural' pesticides to repel mosquitoes, flies, cockroaches, ants, gnats and ticks. It is irritating to skin and eyes, and a sensitiser and neurotoxin.

GLUTARAL

Glutaric dialdehyde, glutaraldehye

An antimicrobial, bactericide, fungicide and virucide sometimes found in household and garden products, this agent is also used as a preservative in cosmetics. Inhalation can damage mucous membranes, act as a sensitiser and trigger allergic reactions. It is harmful if absorbed through the skin.

GLYCERIDES

Formed from a mixture of fatty acids and glycerol, glycerides have a variety of uses. In cosmetics, they are often used as emulsifiers and emollients in soaps and detergents as well as moisturisers. In foods, they also act as emulsifiers and defoaming agents. They can be added to bakery products to improve softness, and are found in beverages, spreads, shortening and desserts. Generally presumed to be safe, full safety data are lacking.

GLYCERIN

E422, glycerol

A form of alcohol used as a solvent, humectant (water magnet) and lubricant in cosmetics, glycerin can be processed from plants or animals. Prolonged contact can dry the skin (in common with other humectants such as **PEG**s) as glycerin draws moisture from the closest, most abundant source. If you live and/or work in a dry environment, the nearest source of moisture will be your skin. In foods, glycerin is used to keep soft foods such as bakery goods, confections, chewing gums and sauces moist. It is generally considered safe.

GLYCERYL PABA

See PABA

GLYCERYL STEARATE

An emulsifying wax made from hardened vegetable oil and *glycerin*, with the addition of vegetable stearic acid, this is generally considered safe, although it can provoke allergic reactions or contact dermatitis in some individuals.

GLYCOL ETHERS

Widely used industrial solvents, these can be used alone or, in combination, they can be found in products such as paints, varnishes, dyes, stains, inks, cleaners (for degreasing, dry cleaning), perfumes and cosmetics as well as jet fuel, de-icing additives and brake fluids. Glycol ethers enter your body when they evaporate into the air you breathe, and are rapidly absorbed into your body if the liquid contacts your skin. Overexposure can cause anaemia, intoxication similar to the effects of alcohol and irritation to the eyes, nose, or skin, and they can damage the kidneys, liver and central nervous system. In laboratory animals, low-level exposure to certain glycol ethers has caused birth defects and infertility in males. There is evidence that workplace exposure can reduce human sperm counts. Common glycol ethers include:

- Ethylene glycol monomethyl ether
- Ethylene glycol monomethyl ether acetate
- Ethylene glycol monoethyl ether
- Ethylene glycol monoethyl ether acetate
- Ethylene glycol monopropyl ether
- Ethylene glycol monobutyl ether
- Ethylene glycol dimethyl ether
- Ethylene glycol diethyl ether
- Diethylene glycol
- Diethylene glycol monomethyl ether
- Glycol monoethyl ether
- Diethylene glycol monobutyl ether
- Diethylene glycol dimethyl ether
- Triethylene glycol dimethyl ether
- Propylene glycol monomethyl ether
- Propylene glycol monomethyl ether acetate
- Dipropylene glycol
- Dipropylene glycol monomethyl ether

GLYCOLIC ACID

See Alpha-hydroxy acids

GLYPHOSATE

An organophosphate herbicide found in a variety of commercial garden products, it has a generally low toxicity, but chronic exposure in animals to high doses of glyphosate has led to birth defects, and damage to blood and the pancreas.

HEXYL LAURATE

Dodecanoic acid, lauric acid

This synthetic flavouring and fragrance remains largely unevaluated for its effects on humans.

HEXYLCINNAMALDEHYDE

See Cinnamates

HEXYLENE GLYCOL

Used as a humectant, plasticiser, solvent and emulsifier in cosmetics, this can cause skin irritation in some individuals. Vapours can be irritating to the eyes and lungs. In animals, repeated ingestion or skin applications have been shown to affect the kidneys and liver.

HOMOSALATE

See Salicylates

HYALURONIC ACID
Hyaluronan

Used in skincare products as a moisturiser and humectant, hyaluronic acid occurs naturally throughout the body and is an important component of connective tissue. The synthetic nature-identical version used in cosmetics provides little more than a temporary boost to ageing skin. It appears to be safe, although it has not been fully evaluated for safety in humans.

HYDRAMETHYLNON

An insecticide used to kill insects both indoors and outdoors, this is a skin and eye irritant. Long-term exposure in animals has produced liver damage and accumulation of the chemical in the testicles. It is also highly toxic to fish.

HYDRATED SILICA
Amorphous silica

A silica gel comprising **Crystalline silica** in a watery matrix, hydramethylnon is used in pharmaceutical and personal-care products as a carrier for active ingredients, a dispersant for colours and dyes, and as an anticaking agent. It is also used as an abrasive and stain remover in toothpastes and in some household cleaning products.

While it's the crystalline form of silica that is considered carcinogenic when inhaled, wet formulations contain these same particles. Used on teeth, it can weaken tooth enamel and damage gums. In rare cases, the silica can build up under the gum margins, causing inflammation that mimics gingivitis. The safety of ingested silica has not been adequately proven, and some observers have linked it with Crohn's disease, although this claim remains unsubstantiated (see also **Silica**).

HYDROCHLORIC ACID
E507

A caustic and acidity regulator commonly found in toilet-bowl cleaners, metal polishes, bathroom cleaners, and limescale and rust removers, in foods, it is used as a solvent, as a modifier for starch, and in the manufacture of **Monosodium glutamate** and gelatine. In cosmetics, it is used in hair bleaches to speed up oxidation and remove colour. Fumes are irritating to eyes, nose and throat, and it can cause side-effects such as wheezing, sneezing and a feeling of being suffocated. It can dissolve and destroy skin tissue, so splashes and spills can result in burns, permanent scarring and, if in contact with the eyes, blindness.

HYDROFLUORIC ACID

Commonly found in rust removers and aluminium cleaners, this agent easily penetrates the skin and body tissues – and may even reach the bone. This is a dangerous acid that, due to its anaesthetic effects, causes no warning signs of pain.

HYDROFLUOROCARBONS
HFCs

Used as refrigerants, cleaning solvents and propellants, HFCs are promoted by industry as replacements for CFCs and **HCFC**s (see below)/ While they pose no direct threat to the ozone layer, they are still very powerful global warming gases as well as being environmentally destructive chemicals.

HYDROCHLOROFLUOROCARBONS
HCFCs

These synthetic industrial gases, primarily used in refrigeration and semiconductor man-ufacturing, are also found in household products where they are used as propellants. Although introduced primarily as substitutes for ozone-depleting *Chlorofluorocarbons* (CFCs), HCFCs remain in the atmosphere for decades to centuries, and are themselves damaging greenhouse gases that are hastening the phenomenon of global climate change.

HYDROGEN CHLORIDE
See Chlorine

HYDROGEN PEROXIDE

A disinfectant, bleaching and oxidising agent found in toiletries (such as hair dyes) and household cleaners, it irritates the eyes, skin and mucous membranes, is carcinogenic in animals and mutagenic in laboratory tests.

HYDROGENATED CASTOR OIL

This is castor oil that has been thickened with the addition of hydrogen atoms. It improves the feel of cosmetic products such as body lotions, but can be a contact allergen.

HYDROGENATED VEGETABLE OIL

This is vegetable oil to which hydrogen has been added to thicken it. Widely used in mar-garines and spreads, and in snack foods such as crisps and baked goods, hydrogenation is a process that can promote the formation of free radicals in oils. Free radicals are highly reactive molecules that can damage and age the skin and body tissues. Hydrogenated oils are also high in unhealthy trans fats, the consumption of which is linked to a higher risk of heart disease, high cholesterol, pre-eclampsia and ulcerative colitis. Complete hydro-genation converts unsaturated fatty acids to saturated ones. In practice, the process is not usually carried to completion, which is why this type of oil is often listed on the label as 'partially hydrogenated vegetable oil'. Since there is no 'safe' level of trans fats, partially hydrogenated fats are no healthier than hydrogenated ones.

HYDROPRENE

An insecticide used to control cockroaches, beetles and moths, it is a hormone-disrupting chemical. Although animal studies suggest it is generally low in toxicity, the data are both incomplete and poor, and no human studies have been conducted on this chemical to rule out harmful effects due to long-term exposure.

HYDROQUINONE

This agent inhibits melanin production when applied to the skin, and so is used in many skin-lightening creams and gels to remove freckles, age spots and other hyperpigmented areas of skin. It is also found in some pesticide formulations. It is a severe skin, eye and respiratory tract irritant and allergen as well as a suspected carcinogen.

HYDROXYCAPRILIC ACID
See Alpha-hydroxy acids

HYDROXYCITRONELLOL

A synthetic floral fragrance, it is also a contact allergen, and skin, eye and lung irritant.

IMIDAZOLIDINYL UREA

A broad-spectrum antibacterial preservative with particularly good activity against *Pseudomonas* species, this, after *Parabens*, is the most commonly used cosmetic preservative. It is found in baby shampoos, personal-care products and fragrances, and is a sensitising agent and a primary cause of contact dermatitis. It can release *Formaldehyde* into the formulation and is most dangerous when used in combination with ethanolamines (any ingredient names containing the acronyms DEA, MEA or TEA).

IODOFENPHOS

An organophosphate insecticide found in a variety of commercial products used to control cockroaches, lice, flies and mosquitoes, fleas, mites and ticks, the data on toxicity in humans are lacking. However, in common with other organophosphates, exposure may cause headache, nausea, sweating, altered heart rate, salivation, fatigue and anxiety.

ISO E SUPER

This synthetic floral, woody fragrance is similar in structure to synthetic musk compounds and may have similarly devastating, hormone-disrupting health effects. It has been poorly studied for safety. For that reason, the US National Toxicology Program has recently called for more and better data to be provided for this chemical.

ISOBUTANE

E943b

A propellant used in cosmetics, household and garden products, and foods, chronic exposure can produce a range of central nervous system symptoms such as headache, breathing difficulties, mood swings, nausea, vomiting, dizziness and symptoms mimicking drunkenness.

Isobutane is a highly inflammable volatile organic chemical (VOC) popular with solvent abusers because it produces a quick 'high' – however, it can also result in convulsions, coma and rapid death. VOCs also accumulate in human breastmilk. While it doesn't damage the earth's ozone shield, it does contribute to the formation of ground-level ozone, or smog, which can cause serious breathing problems. See also *Butane* and *Propane.*

ISOBUTYLPARABEN

See Parabens

ISOCYANATES

Plasticisers found in paints and packaging materials, isocyanates can cause asthma and other lung problems, even with very low exposure levels. They can also irritate your eyes, nose, throat and skin.

ISOEUGENOL

See Eugenol

ISOMALT

See Sugar alcohols

ISOPENTANE

Methylbutane, 2-methylbutane

A solvent and propellant, and a major component of gasoline vapour, this chemical relative of **Isobutane** can produce symptoms such as breathing difficulties, dry skin, contact dermatitis, altered heart rhythms, dizziness and headaches. It also has an anaesthetic effect on the skin.

ISOPHORONE

An industrial solvent found in some printing inks, paints, lacquers and adhesives, this is also used in some herbicide and pesticide formulations. Fumes can cause irritation of the skin, eyes, nose and throat as well as dizziness and fatigue. Animal studies suggest that chronic exposure to isophorone vapours may cause kidney damage and birth defects, and slow the growth of offspring. Ingestion has been linked to an increase in tumours of the kidneys and liver as well as the lymph and reproductive glands.

ISOPROPANOL

See Isopropyl alcohol

ISOPROPILTHIOXANTONE

IXT

A food-packaging chemical found in aseptic or Tetra Paks, it can leach into fatty foods and beverages (such as milk). However, it is poorly studied in terms of how safe or otherwise it is for humans to consume or be exposed to. Sunlight appears to activate this chemical, and human data suggest that topical exposure plus sunlight can cause skin rashes.

ISOPROPYL ALCOHOL

A solvent found in glass cleaners and windscreen-wiper solutions, this chemical irritates eyes and mucous membranes, and causes central nervous system depression. Prolonged contact can cause eczema and sensitisation. Animal studies show that inhalation can damage the liver; ingestion results in drowsiness, unconsciousness and death.

ISOPROPYL PALMITATE

Palmitic acid, hexadecanoic acid

Used in cosmetics as a thickening agent and emollient, this can be synthetic or derived from the palmitic acid in coconut oil. It is often used in moisturisers, where it forms a thin layer and easily penetrates the skin. It can clog pores.

ISOTRIDECYL SALICYLATE

See Salicylates

ISOXABEN

A broad-spectrum herbicide found in garden weed-control products, its fumes can cause eye and respiratory irritation. Based on animal data, it is a potential carcinogen and reproductive toxin, and able to cause detrimental changes in blood chemistry if ingested.

KATHON CG

A preservative compound widely used in cosmetics, this is a mixture of two synthetic chemicals: **Methylchloroisothiazolinone** and **Methylisothiazolinone**. It is a contact allergen and sensitiser. Methylisothiazolinone has recently been identified as a neurotoxin that can damage nerve endings with repeated exposure.

KEROSENE

Mineral spirits

This is a neurotoxic solvent found in all-purpose cleaners, furniture polishes and waxes. An eye and skin irritant, it can damage lung tissues, and may contain the carcinogen **Benzene**.

LACTIC ACID

E270, butyl lactate, ethyl lactate

Used in a variety of food products as an acidity regulator and flavouring, this is generally considered safe to consume. In cosmetics, it can often be found in anti-ageing products, where it is used as an **Alpha-hydroxy acid**.

LAMBDA CYHALOTHRIN

A synthetic pyrethroid insecticide used to control cockroaches, mosquitoes, ticks, flies and aphids, this agent is a powerful neurotoxin that can provoke tingling, burning or numbness (particularly at the point of skin contact), tremors, muscle incoordination, paralysis or other disrupted motor functions, and confusion or loss of consciousness. It is also highly toxic to many fish, aquatic invertebrate species and bees.

LANOLIN

Derived from wool fat, and used as an emollient and thickener in a wide range of cosmetics, hair products, ointments and lotions, lanolin itself is non-toxic and unlikely to cause adverse effects, but impurities mixed in with it can cause allergic skin rashes in some people. Cosmetic-grade lanolin can be contaminated with toxic pesticides such as **DDT**, **Dieldrin** and **Lindane**, which are carcinogenic, and **Diazinon**, which is neurotoxic. These chemicals can enter the bloodstream through the skin. Labels do not disclose which lanolin-based ingredients are pure.

LAURAMIDE DEA

See Diethanolamine

LAURETH COMPOUNDS

Ingredients such as laureth-7, laureth-10 and laureth-23 are commonly used as emulsifiers in cosmetic products. These compounds are known as 'ethoxylated alcohols' and, due to the way they are processed, they can be contaminated with the carcinogen 1,4-**dioxane**.

LAURIC ACID

Dodecanoic acid

The major fatty acid found in coconut oil or palm-kernel oil, lauric acid is a common ingredient in many cosmetics, soaps and detergents. In foods, it is used in the manufacture of various flavourings for beverages, desserts, baked goods and puddings, and is generally regarded as safe.

LILIAL

A synthetic fragrance known to cause sensitisation when applied topically, this can cause immune suppression after inhalation.

LIMONENE

This synthetic citrus fragrance is found in perfumes, colognes, personal-care products, household cleaners and air fresheners, and is a common pesticide in flea-control products. It can cause skin and eye irritation, and may trigger asthma attacks. It is a powerful sensitiser, and can produce tumours, reproductive abnormalities and delayed growth in some animals.

LINALOOL

A synthetic herbal/woody fragrance found in perfumes, colognes, personal-care products, household cleaners and air fresheners, it is also a common pesticide in flea-control products. Able to cause skin, eye and respiratory irritation, it has a narcotic effect in high doses, and has been shown to cause central nervous system disorders in animals. Symptoms include altered mood, poor muscle coordination and reduced spontaneous motor activity. Exposure can cause fatal respiratory disturbances. It attracts bees (and thus poses a threat to people who are allergic to bee stings).

LINDANE

An organochlorine insecticide and fumigant used to control a wide range of soil-dwelling and plant-eating insects, this is also used in some lotions, creams and shampoos for the control of lice and mites in humans. Readily absorbed through the skin, its toxic effects include central nervous system stimulation (usually developing within an hour), mental/motor impairment, excitation, clonic (intermittent) and tonic (continuous) convulsions, increased respiratory rate and/or failure, pulmonary oedema and dermatitis. In animals, it has been shown to damage the liver, kidneys, pancreas, testes and immune system, and to produce a variety of tumours.

LYE

See Sodium hydroxide

MAGNESIUM OXIDE

E530

An anticaking and firming agent, and pH adjuster in foods, inhalation of this agent can cause fevers in humans. In animals, ingestion of magnesium oxide has produced tumours.

MALATHION

An organophosphate insecticide used for the control of garden pests as well as mosquitoes, flies, animal parasites, and head and body lice, this is easily absorbed through the skin. Acute exposure can produce symptoms of numbness, tingling sensations, incoordination, headache, dizziness, tremor, nausea, abdominal cramps, sweating, blurred vision, difficulty breathing or respiratory depression and slow heartbeat. Very high doses may result in unconsciousness or incontinence. In test animals, malathion has caused reproductive abnormalities, and damaging effects to the central nervous and immune systems, adrenal glands, liver and blood.

MALTITOL
See Sugar alcohols

MANEB
An ethylene(bis)dithiocarbamate (EBDC) fungicide used in a variety of garden products, this is irritating to the skin, eyes and respiratory tract. Acute exposure to it may result in effects such as hyperactivity and incoordination, loss of muscle tone, nausea, vomiting, diarrhoea, loss of appetite, weight loss, headache, confusion and drowsiness. In the body, it targets the thyroid, kidneys and heart and, in animals, has been shown to cause increased rates of stillbirth.

MANNITOL
See Sugar alcohols

MCPP
Mecoprop

A phenoxy herbicide found in weed and feed products, mecoprop is irritating to skin and eyes. It causes redness and swelling, and can cause cloudy vision. Human studies suggest exposure can cause cancer of soft tissues and non-Hodgkin's lymphoma. Animal data show it may increase the risk of miscarriage.

METHANOL
Methyl alcohol, wood alcohol

A solvent and denaturant, this is a systemic poison easily absorbed through all routes of exposure, and a neurotoxin that can produce symptoms of headache, dizziness, confusion, abdominal pain and weakness. Ingestion can damage the eyes and cause blindness. Methanol is one of the toxic breakdown products of the artificial sweetener *Aspartame*.

METHOPRENE
This hormone-disrupting insecticide is used to control mosquitoes and several types of ants, flies, lice, moths, beetles and fleas. It is also used in animal feeds or mineral blocks for cattle. Data on its toxicity are incomplete. In the body, it primarily targets the liver.

METHYL ALCOHOL
See Methanol

METHYL ANTHRANILATE
Derived from *Coal tar* and used as a synthetic grape flavouring agent in foods and beverages, this is also found in perfumes and fruit-essence aromas and, occasionally, as a sunscreening agent in cosmetics. It can irritate the skin. Used in agriculture to repel animals, it may be present as a coating on fruit and vegetables. Toxicity data in humans are almost non-existent. In animals, it targets the kidneys and liver.

METHYL BROMIDE
Used primarily as a pesticide to fumigate soil and buildings, inhalation causes dizziness, headache, vomiting, abdominal pain, confusion and convulsions. Chronic exposure can cause central nervous system depression and kidney injury.

METHYL CELLULOSE

Used as a thickener in sauces and salad dressings, and as a thickener and stabiliser in ice creams, where it prevents ice crystals from forming during freezing, this is a bulk laxative and eating large amounts can cause flatulence, distention of the abdomen or intestinal obstruction. It may also affect the absorption of minerals. Methyl cellulose is used in cosmetics as a viscosity adjuster and in laundry detergents as an anti-redisposition agent (in other words, it keeps dirt from being redeposited on clothes during the wash). It is generally regarded as safe when used topically.

METHYL HEPTINE CARBONATE

A synthetic fragrance used in perfumes and air fresheners to impart a fresh, sweet, green, fruity scent, it is a cause of skin sensitisation and may trigger breathing difficulties.

METHYLCHLOROISOTHIAZOLINONE

This cosmetic preservative is usually combined with *Methylisothiazolinone* (a combination also known as *Kathon CG*). It is a strong allergen that binds quickly to the skin, remaining there long after use. Laboratory studies suggest it is a potential mutagen, and a suspected carcinogen due to its corrosive action.

METHYLENE CHLORIDE

Used as an industrial solvent and a paint-stripper, this may also be found in some aerosol and pesticide products. Harmful if swallowed, inhaled or absorbed through skin, it is a potential carcinogen that affects the central nervous system, liver, cardiovascular system and blood, and causes irritation to skin, eyes and respiratory tract.

METHYLISOTHIAZOLINONE

This cosmetic preservative is usually combined with *Methylchloroisothiazolinone* (in a combination known as *Kathon CG*). It is a strong allergen that binds quickly to the skin and remains there long after use. Laboratory studies suggest this substance causes nerve damage. It is also a potential mutagen, and a suspected carcinogen due to its corrosive action on the skin.

METHYLPARABEN

See Parabens

MICROBAN

See Triclosan

MINERAL OIL

See Parafinnum liquidum

MONOETHANOLAMINE

2-aminoethanol

A surfactant found in wash-off toiletries, it is a relative of **Diethanolamine**. Often denoted by the prefix or suffix MEA, as in cocamide MEA, linoleamide MEA or stearamide MEA, it is a skin and eye irritant. Inhaling MEA can irritate the lungs and trigger asthma attacks. It is also a gastrointestinal and liver nervous system toxin.

MONOSODIUM GLUTAMATE
E621, MSG

This controversial flavour enhancer is contained in gelatin, textured protein, autolysed yeast, monopotassium glutamate, yeast extract and any kind of hydrolysed protein. MSG is a neurotoxin with adverse reactions, including migraine headache, asthma, nausea and vomiting, fatigue, tightness in the chest, a burning sensation in the forearms and back of the neck, disorientation and depression. Recent studies suggest long-term eye damage as a result of its use including retinal lesions, thinning of the retina itself and macular degeneration.

MORPHOLINE

A contaminant found in the waxy coatings used to preserve fruit and vegetables, this is toxic on inhalation, ingestion and skin contact. The World Health Organization reports the morpholine can turn into the carcinogen N-nitrosomorpholine during storage.

MURIATIC ACID
See Hydrochloric acid

MYRISTAMINDE DEA
See Diethanolamine

N-BUTANE
See Butane

NAPHTHAS

A collective term for solvents derived from both petroleum distillation and **Coal tar**, these can normally be found in dry cleaning fluids and industrial-strength cleaners. Petroleum naphtha has a lower order of toxicity than coal-tar naphtha; however, overexposure to either type may cause central nervous system depression, with symptoms of inebriation followed by headache and nausea. Naphthas can enter into your system through inhalation of their vapours, ingestion, and eye and skin contact. They are irritating to the skin, eyes and upper respiratory tract. Skin-chapping and sensitivity to light may develop after repeated contact.

NAPHTHALENE

A **coal-tar** derivative that is poisonous to humans and a potential carcinogen, this is one of a number of possible petroleum distillates that may be present in air fresheners. It is also a solvent, and pesticide, insecticide and fungicide. It is used in the manufacture of lacquers and varnishes. Like all petroleum distillates, it is irritating to the skin, eyes, mucous membranes and upper respiratory tract. Exposure can cause nausea, vomiting and profuse sweating. Prolonged exposure is known to cause damage to the kidneys, liver and red blood cells, and is thought to possibly cause cancer.

NEOTAME

A close chemical relative of **Aspartame**, this artificial sweetener is a staggering 7000 to 13,000 times sweeter than ordinary sugar. Since it is made from the same chemicals as aspartame, there is no reason, and no independent evidence, to suggest that it is any safer, though the manufacturers say it is more heat stable than its predecessor. In animal studies, neotame ingestion increased weight gain beyond what would normally be expected from the given amount of food, suggesting an effect on the body that is potentially dangerous.

NITRATE

This is a naturally occurring form of nitrogen found in soil. Nitrogen is essential to all life. Most crop plants require large quantities to sustain high yields and, in moderate amounts, nitrate is a harmless constituent of food and water. In children and adults who have insufficient stomach acid, excessive nitrate ingestion can cause methaemoglobinaemia, the most obvious symptom of which is a bluish colour of the skin, especially around the eyes and mouth. Nitrate in food and drinking water can be converted into toxic **Nitrites** in the body.

NITRITES

The collective term for potassium and sodium nitrite used in smoked and cured meats such as bacon, salami, frankfurters and sausages, nitrite preservatives greatly delay the development of botulinum toxin (causing botulism, a fatal food poisoning) in meat. It is used to develop a cured meat flavour and colour, retards rancidity during storage, and preserves the flavour of spices and smoke. Nitrites are also used as preservatives in other foods such as beer, fish and fish byproducts, and some cheeses. Nitrites combine with chemicals naturally present in foods and in the gastrointestinal tract to form powerful carcinogens known as nitrosamines (the same carcinogens can also form in cosmetics; see Chapter 6). There is no 'safe' dose of nitrosamines.

NITROBENZENE

A highly toxic solvent used in metal and shoe polishes, and many other products, this can enter your body through inhalation, skin and eye contact, and ingestion, and lead to spleen and liver damage. It also affects the central nervous system, producing headache, fatigue, weakness, vertigo and, in some cases, severe depression, unconsciousness and coma. Drinking alcohol increases toxic effects. Nitrobenzene quickly crosses the placenta and can cause birth defects.

2-NITRO-p-PHENYLENEDIAMINE

See Phenylenediamines

NITROPHENYLENEDIAMINE

See Phenylenediamines

OCTAFLUOROCYCLOBUTANE

946

A refrigerant and propellant used in sprayed food products, it can irritate the skin, eyes, nose and throat, and cause respiratory distress.

OCTOCRYLENE

See Cinnamates

OCTYL METHOXYCINNAMATE

See Cinnamates

OCTYL SALICYLATE

See Salicylates

OLEAMIDE DEA

See Diethanolamine

OLEIC ACID

Derived from various animal and vegetable fats, this is used in the food industry to make synthetic butters and cheeses. It is also used to flavour baked goods, sweets, ice creams and sodas. In cosmetics, it is an emollient and emulsifier. Although generally regarded as safe to ingest, because of its film-forming ability, it can clog pores when applied topically.

OLESTRA

A synthetic fat substitute used in snack and convenience foods, it has no calories and cannot be digested. However, it is not healthy because it attaches to valuable nutrients known as carotenoids and flushes them out of the body. Carotenoids protect against diseases such as lung cancer, prostate cancer, heart disease and macular degeneration. The Harvard School of Public Health states that 'the long-term consumption of olestra snack foods might therefore result in several thousand unnecessary deaths each year from lung and prostate cancers and heart disease and hundreds of additional cases of blindness in the elderly due to macular degeneration. Besides contributing to disease, olestra causes diarrhoea and other serious gastrointestinal problems, even at low doses.'

Olestra is banned in Canada.

OLETH

Cosmetic emulsifiers and surfactants denoted by names such as oleth-5 and oleth-2, they can produce allergic skin reactions and, because they are in the same family as **PEG** compounds, they may also contain impurities linked to breast cancer (e.g. 1,4-**Dioxane**, **Ethylene oxide**). They are toxic to aquatic organisms.

OPTICAL BRIGHTENERS

Used in laundry detergents, and carpet and upholstery cleaners, these compounds put a thin chemical film on your clothes that converts ultraviolet light to visible blue light, making clothes look brighter. Like thousands of minuscule mirrors, they reflect light back to the eye, giving the impression that the cleaning product has worked better than it has. Optical brighteners belong to a family of agents that were once used in food products like flour and sugar to make them look whiter. They have long since been banned for this purpose. As they are used today, they can cause skin sensitisation and allergic reactions.

ORTHO-AMINOPHENOL

Found in hair dyes, it imparts a light-brown colour to hair. This is a derivative of p-phenylenediamine (see **Phenylenediamines**).

ORTHO-PHENYLENEDIAMINE

See Phenylenediamines

OXALIC ACID

A poisonous organic compound commonly used in household cleaners, this is also used for cleaning car radiators and other metals. Oxalic acid can damage the kidneys and liver, irritate the eyes and respiratory tract, and is corrosive to the mouth and stomach.

OXYBENZONE
See Benzophenones

PABA
Para-aminobenzoic acid

PABA and its related compounds, which include ethyl dihydroxypropyl PABA, padimate-O (ocyl dimethyl PABA), padimate-A and glyceryl PABA, are used as sunscreening agents. Applied topically, they can cause skin irritation and sensitisation as well as leading to light sensitivity (with blistering and peeling skin) in some individuals. PABAs are *Formaldehyde*-forming chemicals that can form carcinogenic nitrosamines when combined with amines such as DEA, TEA and MEA. PABAs can cause skin irritation, and are relatives of the cosmetic preservatives *Parabens*. In addition to being irritating to the skin, they are also thought to be oestrogenic.

PADIMATE-A
Amyl dimethylaminobenzoate
See PABA

PADIMATE-O
Octyl dimethyl PABA
See PABA

PALMITIC ACID
An emollient, moisturiser and emulsifier found in a wide range of cosmetics, this can cause contact dermatitis in some individuals.

PARA-AMINOBENZOIC ACID
See PABA

PARA-AMINOPHENOL
This reddish-brown colour found in hair dyes must be mixed with an oxidising agent (e.g. *hydrogen peroxide, resorcinol*) to produce the required colour. It can trigger moderate-to-severe skin reactions in some individuals. Once in the body, it can cause kidney damage.

PARABENS
Butylparaben, ethylparaben, isobutylparaben, methylparaben, propylparaben

The most widely used group of preservatives found in cosmetics, it is estimated that more than 90 per cent of all cosmetic products contain some form of parabens. They are also used in foods as a preservative such as in dried meats, cereals and snack foods.

Applied topically, they can cause skin irritation, contact dermatitis and contact allergies. Animal and laboratory studies have long shown that parabens have a weak oestrogenic activity. Butylparaben and isobutylparaben have the strongest hormonal effects, followed by propylparaben, ethylparaben and methylparaben. Whether that poses any health risk for humans is still unclear. In animal studies, ingested parabens can induce cell proliferation (often a precursor of cancer) in the fore-stomach, and birth defects in mice and rats. Recently, when scientists conducted an analysis of breast-cancer tissue, they found accumulated parabens in every sample examined. The researchers suggested that parabens in deodorants and antiperspirants could be the cause.

Our bodies are exposed to oestrogens from many sources, and it is possible that regularly ingesting or absorbing weak oestrogens from a number of different sources may add up to a strong oestrogenic effect in the body. Too much oestrogen in the body is a trigger for oestrogen-dependent cancers of the breast, ovary, uterus and testicles, and may even have effects on foetal development. Although parabens are used in small amounts in individual products, they are widely used in all toiletries and cosmetics – usually in products that are left on for long periods of time. It is likely that we absorb parabens from each of the products we use. Thus, parabens need to be viewed in the light of the larger problem of exposure to environmental oestrogens.

PARADICHLOROBENZENES
PDCBs

Paradichlorobenzenes are neurotoxic solvents commonly found in toilet fresheners, mothballs, room deodorants, and industrial-strength odour controllers and moth-repellents as well as in general insecticides and mildew-control agents. They replaced the older chemical **Naphthalene**, a suspected carcinogen. Symptoms of exposure to PDCB fumes include eye and nose irritation, drowsiness, weakness, headache, swollen eyes, stuffy head, loss of appetite, nausea, vomiting, and throat and eye irritation. They are particularly toxic to small children and infants who have experienced severe toxic reactions on being dressed in clothing stored in mothballs.

PARAFFINUM LIQUIDUM
905a, mineral oil, baby oil

A transparent, odourless and colourless oil derived from petroleum, this is used in foods as a glazing agent, release agent and sealing agent. In cosmetics, it is an emollient and film-former. Ingested, it can inhibit the absorption of essential fats and have a mild laxative effect. This is also a human carcinogen and reproductive toxin if inhaled.

In cosmetics, it is used as an emollient to produce a temporary moisturising effect. However, prolonged use destroys the natural oily barrier of the skin, leading to more persistent dryness. By destroying the protective oily barrier of the skin, mineral oil also acts like a penetration enhancer, allowing other chemicals to be more easily absorbed into the skin and bloodstream. In addition, mineral oil can be contaminated with **Polycyclic aromatic hydrocarbons** (PAHs). The US National Toxicology Program recognises some PAHs as potential human carcinogens. Studies link them with an increased risk of breast cancer. If inhaled, it can cause fatal pneumonia and, in the US, products containing mineral oil are obliged to carry a warning and have childproof caps.

Manufacturers have slowly been replacing the mineral oil in their products with other synthetics such as **Silicones**.

PARA-PHENYLENEDIAMINE
p-Phenylenediamine

The black colour found in hair dyes, this must be mixed with an oxidising agent (e.g. **Hydrogen peroxide**, **Resorcinol**) to produce the required colour. It can trigger moderate-to-severe skin reactions in some individuals. Once in the body, it can cause kidney damage. See also *Phenylenediamines*.

PARA-TOLUENEDIAMINE

p-Toluenediamine

The brown colour found in hair dyes, this must be mixed with an oxidising agent (e.g. *Hydrogen peroxide*, *Resorcinol*) to produce the required colour, and can trigger moderate-to-severe skin reactions in some individuals. Once in the body, it can cause liver damage. It belongs to a family of dyes and intermediaries known as *Diaminotoluenes*.

PARETH

This surfactant belongs to the same family as *Polyethylene glycol*.

PARFUM

Perfume, fragrance

'Parfum' is the collective name given to hundreds of different chemicals used to produce a fragrance in cosmetics and toiletries, pesticides, household cleaners, air fresheners, foods and cigarettes (where it is called an *Aroma*). Perfumes contain every kind of poison known to man, which is why many perfume ingredients double up as pesticides. Most, for instance, are solvents and, as such, are neurotoxic. Many are persistent (i.e. they don't break down in the environment, and they accumulate in human tissue and breastmilk) and can cause birth defects. Artificial musks, a common ingredient in fragrances and toiletries, are hormone-disrupting and cancer-causing. Immediate reactions to parfum include headache, mood swings, depression, forgetfulness and irritation. It is also a major trigger of attacks in asthmatics

Of the 20 most common perfume ingredients, four – *acetone*, ethanol, *ethyl acetate* and *methylene chloride* – are classified as hazardous waste by the US Environmental Protection Agency.

Other commonly used chemicals in perfume include *Propylene glycol*; cyclohexanol, a central nervous system depressant; *Linalool*, which can provoke depression, loss of equilibrium and respiratory disturbances; methyl ethyl ketone, which is toxic to liver and kidneys, and irritating to the eye, nose and throat; and *Formaldehyde*, a known carcinogen. Spray formulations mean you inhale more of these toxic chemicals.

PARTIALLY HYDROGENATED VEGETABLE OIL

See Hydrogenated vegetable oil

PEG

Polyethylene glycol

Polyethylene glycol (PEG) compounds are derived from natural gas, and have numerous functions in toiletries, including: moisturisers, emulsifiers, emollients and antioxidants as well as plasticisers, solvents and softeners. Adding PEG to a product will also prevent moisture loss during storage.

On the ingredients label, PEGs are usually listed followed by a number (e.g. PEG-4 or PEG-350) that refers to its molecular weight. These numbers represent the liquidity of the compound: the higher the number, the more solid it is. PEG compounds can be contaminated with the carcinogen 1,4-*dioxane*. They can also form carcinogens when mixed with DEA and TEA compounds (see also Chapter 6).

PENDIMETHALIN

A herbicide used to control grasses and weeds, this can be irritating to the skin and lungs; it is toxic to the liver with long-term use.

PENTACHLORONITROBENZENE

PCNB, quintozene

An organochlorine fungicide, very high doses can induce fatigue, possible dizziness and lethargy. Long-term exposure is toxic to the liver.

PENTACHLOROPHENOL

PCP

A reproductive toxin found in products like laundry starch, it is associated with foetal abnormalities and birth defects.

PENTANE

Often found in dryer sheets and fabric softeners, this is irritating to the eyes and can cause skin rashes. Its vapours may cause headache, nausea, vomiting, dizziness, drowsiness, irritation of the respiratory tract and loss of consciousness. Prolonged and repeated inhalation of vapours may cause central nervous system depression.

PENTASODIUM DISODIUM EDTA

See Disodium EDTA

PERCHLOROETHYLENE

PERC, tetrachloroethylene, ethylene tetrachloride

A solvent commonly found in dry-cleaning fluids and spot removers, PERC is fat-soluble and so collects in the tissues of living organisms and accumulates in the environment. Its vapours are irritating to skin, eyes and upper respiratory tract, and can produce giddiness, headache, inebriation, nausea, vomiting and sinus inflammation. Chronic inhalation can cause serious depression of the central nervous system as well as kidney and liver damage.

The coin-operated dry-cleaning machines that can be found in laundrettes have been associated with acute PERC poisonings. Long-term exposure can cause liver and central nervous system damage. It is a proven carcinogen in animals and suspected human carcinogen.

PERMETHRIN

A synthetic pyrethroid insecticide used against a variety of pests, including flies and cockroaches, this compound can cause irritation to the skin and eyes. Human studies are lacking, but animal studies suggest it can suppress the immune system and is toxic to the liver.

PETROLATUM

Petroleum jelly, Vaseline

This chemical lubricant derived from petroleum is used to make skin creams feel smoother. It can provoke allergic skin reactions and, over time, will destroy the natural oily barrier on the skin, leaving it more prone to drying, flaking and cracking.

PHENOL
Carbolic acid

The largest single use of phenol is in resins used in the plywood, adhesive, construction, automotive and appliance industries. It is also used as an intermediate in the production of caprolactam, which is used to made nylon and other synthetic fibres, and ***Bisphenol-A***, which is used to make epoxy and other resins. In household products, phenol is used as a disinfectant, for instance, in bathroom and toilet cleaners, and as an anaesthetic in medicinal preparations, including ointments, ear- and nosedrops, cold-sore lotions, throat lozenges and antiseptic lotions. Exposure to its fumes can irritate the eyes, nose and throat, and cause sweating, pallor, weakness, headache, dizziness, muscle ache and pain, tremors and twitches, ringing in the ears, shock and, in extreme cases, a profound fall in body temperature.

PHENOXYETHANOL

This is a cosmetic preservative that can cause skin irritation, contact dermatitis and contact allergies.

PHENOXYISOPROPANOL

A preservative and solvent found in acne treatments, shampoos and facial cleansers, this is a strong irritant that can only be used in wash-off products. Skin reactions are likely.

PHENYLENEDIAMINES

A family of dyes commonly found in permanent and semi-permanent hair colours, they can damage skin, cause allergic reactions (sometimes fatal ones) and are irritating to the eyes. Phenylenediamines are also carcinogenic, and can cause immune system dysregulation as well as kidney and liver damage. They are toxic to wildlife and soil. The type of phenylenediamine used depends on the end colour, thus:

- para-phenylenediamine (black)
- para-toluenediamine (brown)
- ortho-phenylenediamine (brown)
- para-aminophenol (reddish-brown)
- ortho-aminophenol (light brown).

PHENYLMERCURIC ACETATE
PMA

An organomercury compound used as a fungicide and herbicide, mercury is a neurotoxin and there is no safe dose. It is corrosive to the skin and eyes, and animal studies suggest it is a reproductive and developmental toxin.

2-PHENYLPHENOL
o-Phenylphenol, 2-biphenylol, o-hydroxybiphenyl

A fungicide and disinfectant of the phenol family, this is found in household disinfectant sprays and timber treatments. It's also used as a post-harvest fungicide for vegetables and fruits, especially citrus, and as an antimicrobial preservative in cosmetics and a flavouring in food. A recognised carcinogen, and suspected hormone disrupter, neurotoxin and reproductive toxin implicated in liver and kidney damage, exposure can cause skin and respiratory irritation. Common symptoms include headache, giddiness, nervousness, blurred vision, weakness, nausea, cramps, diarrhoea and discomfort in the chest. Rarely, when used in cosmetics, it can cause skin depigmentation and photoallergy (light sensitivity).

PHENYL-p-PHENYLENEDIAMINE
See Phenylenediamines

PHOSPHOLIPIDS
Fat substances found in all living cells, phospholipids are critical building blocks for all body cells. Lecithin, found in soya beans and other seeds as well as in eggs, contains several phospholipids, such as phosphatidylcholine, phosphatidylethanolamine, phosphatidylinositol or phosphatidylserine. In cosmetics, they are extracted from natural sources or synthesised in the lab to be used as emollients, moisturisers, emulsifiers, dispersants, wetting agents and stabilisers. They are generally regarded as safe.

PHOSPHORIC ACID
A common ingredient in metal cleaners and rust removers, this is irritating to the skin and lungs. Phosphoric acid is also used to acidify foods and beverages such as various colas. Ingesting high levels of this leaches essential calcium from the bones, and raises the risk of brittle bones and fractures. Children consuming at least six glasses (1.5 litres) of phosphoric acid-containing soft drinks daily have more than five times the risk of developing low blood levels of calcium compared with children who don't drink sodas.

PHTHALATES
Phthalates are a class of widely used industrial compounds that have become ubiquitous, not just in the products in which they are intentionally used, but also as contaminants in almost everything. They can be used as softeners in plastics, oily substances in perfumes and additives to hairsprays, lubricants and wood finishers. Phthalates are oestrogen mimics that can easily leach out of products in our homes. Animal studies show that exposure to very low levels of the phthalates dibutyl phthalate (DBP) and diethylhexyl phthalate (DEHP) in the womb caused demasculinisation of male foetuses and increased the rate of reproductive disorders such as hypospadias (where the urethra opens on the underside of the penis). Phthalate exposure is also linked to reduction in sperm quality.

PINE OIL
A common antimicrobial component of household cleaning solutions, its fumes are irritating to the mucous membranes and gastrointestinal tract. Large exposures can cause severe respiratory distress, cardiovascular collapse, severe central nervous system effects and kidney failure.

PIPERONYL BUTOXIDE
This is a synergist that is used in a wide variety of insecticides. Synergists are chemicals which, while lacking killing properties of their own, enhance the pesticidal properties of other active ingredients. Piperonyl butoxide is used in conjunction with insecticides such as **Pyrethrins**, pyrethroids, **Rotenone** and carbamates.

PIRIMIPHOSMETHYL
An organophosphate insecticide that is irritating to the eyes, respiratory system and skin,

high exposure can result in headache, nausea, vomiting, abdominal cramps, diarrhoea, dizziness, sweating, extreme weakness, blurred vision, muscle tremors and tightness in the chest.

POLYCHLORINATED BIPHENYLS

PCBs

Related to **DDT** and **dioxins**, PCBs were once used extensively in transformers, for insulating cooling equipment, and in hydraulic fluids, lubricants and other electrical components. Banned since the 1970s, they are still present in many older electrical installations. PCBs resist biodegradation, are fat-soluble and tend to accumulate in animals higher up the food chain. PCBs are both antioestrogens and antiandrogens (in other words, they disrupt signalling from both female and male hormones). Exposure to PCBs in food has been linked to delayed brain development and reduced IQ in children. PCBs can still be found as contaminants in plastics, dyes, inks, older types of carbonless copy paper, adhesives, wood treatments and pesticides. It has also been detected as contaminants in foods such as meat and fish, waterfowl, poultry, eggs and milk.

POLYCYCLIC AROMATIC HYDROCARBONS

Polycyclic aromatic hydrocarbons (PAHs) are a group of over 100 different chemicals created by incineration of plastic waste such as polyvinyl chloride (PVC), high-density polyethylene (HDPE) and polypropylene as well as other industrial waste; large quantities are released during natural events such as volcanic eruptions and forest fires, but also by many human activities such as burning coal, oil and wood for heat, smoking cigarettes, frying food and gas-powered motor travel. They are found in asphalt, creosote, coal-tar pitch, roofing tar, coal and crude oil. A few PAHs are used in products such as medicines, plastics, dyes and pesticides.

Animal studies have also shown that PAHs can have harmful effects on the skin, body fluids and immune system after both short- and long-term exposure. Mice exposed to high levels of PAHs during pregnancy had difficulty reproducing, as did their offspring. These offspring also had higher rates of birth defects and lower body weights. In laboratory animals, PAHs produced a variety of cancers.

POLYETHYLENE GLYCOL

See PEGs

POLYOXYETHYLENE ALKYL ETHERS

This family of detergents, surfactants and wetting agents is found in household cleaning products and cosmetics. Lauryl alcohol and cetyl alcohol as well as sorbitan are polyoxyethylene compounds found in cosmetics and in toiletries as emulsifying agents. In household cleaning compounds like nonyl phenol, these are used because of their strong degreasing effects. Some polyoxyethylene compounds are also used as fabric softeners and antistatic agents. They are mostly non-irritating, but can be contaminated with the carcinogen 1,4-**dioxane**.

POLYSORBATES

Emulsifiers and surfactants used in foods and cosmetics, these belong to a large group of chemicals known as **Polyoxyethylene alkyl ethers**, and can be contaminated with the carcinogen 1,4-**dioxane**.

POLYTETREFLUOROETHYLENE
PTFE, Teflon
> See *Teflon*

POLYVINYLPYRROLIDONE
E1201
> A clarifying additive in wine, beer and vinegar, and used in the production of dietary supplements, PVP compounds can also be found in some hair-styling products, especially hairsprays. Inhalation of PVP damages the lungs; when ingested, animal studies suggest it is associated with damage to the kidneys and liver as well as an increased risk of cancer.

POTASSIUM BENZOATE
> See *Benzoates, sodium benzoate*

POTASSIUM HYDROXIDE
E525, caustic potash, lye
> A harsh alkali used as an intermediate in soap production and as a neutraliser in food production, this is also found in nail-cuticle softeners and depilatories. It is corrosive to the eyes, mucous membranes and skin, and can cause dermatitis and burns even in dilute solutions.

POTASSIUM NITRITE
E249
> See *Nitrites*

PPG-3 METHYL ETHER
> See *Propylene glycol*

PPG-14 BUTYL ETHER
> Used primarily in cosmetics as a preservative, solvent PPG-14 butyl ether is a relative of **Propylene glycol**. In addition to being a skin irritant and neurotoxin, it is potentially toxic to the kidneys and liver. In the US, it is a pesticide component used in sprays to protect animals from flies, gnats and mosquitoes. It is poisonous in high concentrations and can enhance the skin penetration of other, more toxic chemicals.

PRONAMIDE
> A herbicide used either before weeds emerge (pre-emergence) and/or after weeds come up, it controls a wide range of annual and perennial grasses, as well as certain annual broadleaf weeds.
>
> Pronamide has caused liver tumours in mice after two years at high doses, suggesting that it could be carcinogenic in humans exposed to sufficient quantities. Target organs identified in animal studies include the liver, and thyroid, adrenal and pituitary glands. It is poorly studied in humans.

PROPANE
> A petroleum-derived propellant for aerosol sprays, especially after the ban of **Chlorofluorocarbons** (CFCs), skin contact may result in frostbite and burns. A central nervous

system toxicant, it can produce symptoms such as rapid breathing, incoordination, rapid fatigue, excessive salivation, disorientation, headache, nausea and vomiting.

PROPOXUR

Used to control a variety of insect pests, including ants, cockroaches, crickets, flies and mosquitoes, signs of propoxur intoxication over the short or long term include nausea, vomiting, abdominal cramps, sweating, diarrhoea, excessive salivation, weakness, imbalance, blurring of vision, breathing difficulty, increased blood pressure, incontinence and death. Animal studies suggest it can reduce birth weight, retard the development of some reflexes and impair the central nervous system.

PROPYL GALLATE

E310

An antioxidant used in foods such as fats, oils, mayonnaise, shortening, baked goods, sweets, dried meat, fresh pork sausage and dried milk to keep oils and fats in products from turning rancid, it is usually found in combination with another antioxidant, ascorbyl palmitate, as each enhances the effect of the other. It is also used in cosmetics, hair products, adhesives and lubricants. It has low toxicity, but can cause contact dermatitis in those who are exposed to it regularly.

PROPYLENE GLYCOL

PPG, 1,2-propanediol

This is a solvent, humectant and wetting agent found in foods, cosmetics and household products. In foods, it is used as an emulsifier and viscosity adjuster for confectionery, chocolate products, ice creams, beverages and baked goods. Irritating to the eyes, skin and respiratory tract, applied topically, it acts as a penetration enhancer, altering skin structure, thereby allowing other, more toxic chemicals to penetrate deeply into the skin and eventually the bloodstream.

PVP

See Polyvinylpyrrolidone

PYRETHRINS

Pyrethrins are natural insecticides produced by certain species of the chrysanthemum plant. The flowers of the plant are harvested shortly after blooming, and are either dried and powdered, or the oils within the flowers are extracted with solvents. The active insecticidal components in these dusts and extracts are collectively known as pyrethrins. Synthetic pyrethrins are usually referred to as 'pyrethroids', and the term 'pyrethrum' is a general name covering both compounds.

Pyrethrums have been used primarily to control human lice, mosquitoes, cockroaches, beetles and flies. They are contact poisons that quickly penetrate the nerve system of the insect. Synthetic pyrethroids are considered more powerful toxins than their natural counterparts. Inhaling high levels of pyrethrum may bring about asthmatic breathing, sneezing, nasal stuffiness, headache, nausea, incoordination, tremors, convulsions, facial flushing, and swelling, burning and itching sensations. At high doses, pyrethrum can be damaging to the central nervous system and the immune system. When the immune system is attacked by pyrethrum, allergies can be worsened. Animals fed large doses of pyrethrins may experience liver damage.

QUATERNARY AMMONIUM COMPOUNDS

This large family of strong disinfectants and surfactants is found in household cleaners, but also in medications such as ophthalmic preparations and in cosmetics. Highly toxic and implicated in the rise of drug-resistant bacteria in homes and hospitals, in eyedrops, they can damage eyes on contact. Examples of quaternary ammonium compounds include **Benzalkonium chloride,** alkyl triethanol ammonium chloride, benzethonium chloride and cetrimide (cetyltrimethylammonium bromide).

In cosmetics, they are used as preservatives, examples of which include quaternium-15, quaternium-18 and quaternium-80. Applied to the skin, they can be irritating and, because they are **Formaldehyde**-forming compounds, they can produce carcinogenic nitrosamines when mixed with DEA and TEA (see also Chapter 6).

RED PETROLATUM

A reddish-brown, grease-like petroleum jelly, its natural pigments are effective in blocking the sun's ultraviolet rays. During World War II, red petrolatum was extensively used by the military. It has largely fallen out of fashion, but is still used as a sunblocker in some products.

RESMETHRIN

A synthetic pyrethroid used to control flying and crawling insects in homes and greenhouses, this is also used for fabric protection, pet sprays and shampoos. Symptoms of exposure by any route may include incoordination, twitching, loss of bladder control and seizures. Dermal exposure may lead to local numbness, itching, burning and tingling sensations near the site of exposure. In animal studies, it damaged the liver, decreased blood glucose levels and increased the rate of stillbirth. It is also highly toxic to bees and fish.

RESORCINOL

1,3-benzenediol, m-dihydroxybenzene, resorcin

An oxidising agent commonly found in permanent and semi-permanent hair dyes, this is also used as an antidandruff agent in shampoo and in sunscreen products as well as in pesticide formulations. Resorcinol fights fungal and bacterial organisms, and promotes softening, dissolution and peeling of the skin; it is sometimes used to treat acne, eczema, psoriasis, corns, calluses, warts and other skin conditions. Irritating to eyes and skin, it can cause contact allergies. Resorcinol may be absorbed into the body through the skin and into the bloodstream, where it acts like a hormone disruptor. It has been linked to reproductive effects, thyroid damage, and central nervous system effects such as dizziness, nausea, altered heart beat and restlessness.

ROTENONE

Rotenone is used in home gardens for insect control, lice and tick control on pets. Local effects on the body include conjunctivitis, dermatitis, sore throat and congestion. Ingestion produces effects ranging from mild irritation to nausea and vomiting. Growth retardation and vomiting in rats and dogs resulted from chronic exposures. In female rats, it reduced fertility. Chronic exposure may produce changes in the liver and kidneys as also indicated by the animal studies cited above.

S-BIOALLETHRIN

See Bioallethrin

S-METHOPRENE
See Methoprene

SACCHARIN
Hermesetas, Sweetex (EU), Sweet 'N Low (US), Sucaryl, Sugar Twin and Sweet Magic

The grandfather of artificial sweeteners, saccharin was discovered in 1879 and was widely used during both world wars, compensating for sugar shortages. It is 200 to 300 times sweeter than sugar, but tends to have a bitter or metallic aftertaste. Saccharin is still ubiquitous today, as it is cheap, has a long shelf-life and is heat-resistant. It is thus often added to baked goods, jams and processed fruits, but it also crops up in salad dressings and sauces.

In the 1970s, it was found to cause bladder cancer in rats. The US Food and Drug Administration (FDA) all but banned it outright, but reprieved it in 1991, although requiring the label to declare it to be potentially carcinogenic. The Canadian authorities banned it outright until 1997. In the UK, it has never been prohibited.

Although it is still widely used, the US government's National Toxicology Program classifies saccharin as an 'anticipated carcinogen', in 2002, a group of Canadian scientists concluded that there was 'ample evidence' that it can cause bladder cancer in laboratory animals and possibly in humans at high doses.

SALICYLATES

This is a vast range of chemicals that can be used as flavourings and aromas in foods (e.g. amyl, phenyl, menthyl and glyceryl salicylate), and as perfume ingredients in fragranced cosmetics and household products (e.g. benzyl salicylate, CIS-3-hexenyl salicylate). One of their most widespread uses is in cosmetics as sunscreening agents (e.g. homosalate, ethylhexyl salicylate, octyl salicylate, isotridecyl salicylate and trolamine salicylate). People who are sensitive to aspirin may develop allergic-type reactions after ingesting salicylates or applying them to the skin. In addition, salicylates are penetration enhancers that allow other chemicals in the product to get deeper into the bloodstream; research also shows that some salicylates used in suncreams are oestrogenic.

SALICYLIC ACID

Used as a preservative in food products and cosmetics, this is also a common dandruff treatment in shampoos. In anti-ageing creams, salicylic acid is a **Beta-hydroxy acid**, used as a chemical peel to dissolve and remove the outermost layer of skin. Because of its exfoliating action, salicylic acid can increase photosensitivity of the skin and cause contact dermatitis (see also *Salicylates*).

SELENIUM SULPHIDE

An antidandruff agent that is irritating to the skin and eyes, it is best to avoid contact of this agent with broken skin.

SEMICARBAZIDE
SEM

A breakdown product of azodicarbonamide, a chemical used in the plastic seals for jars and other types of food packaging, this is a contaminant that leaches into foods from the plastic gaskets used to seal glass jars with metal twist-off lids. SEM has been detected at low levels in a number of such food products, including baby foods. It has also been detected in seaweed-derived products (e.g. *Carrageenan*), used widely in food production. In addition, azodicarbonamide is also approved as a food additive in a number of countries for use as a bleaching agent in cereal flour and as a dough conditioner. Azodicarbonamide is also used in certain pesticide formulations and industrial applications. Animal studies show that semicarbazide is carcinogenic.

SIDURON

A herbicide used in weed-control products, this is moderately irritating to skin, eyes and mucous membranes.

SILICA

A natural mineral (silicon dioxide) used as an anticaking agent in salts and salt substitutes and other dry food items; in cosmetics, it is used as an abrasive, absorbent and viscosity adjuster. Inhaling silica dust is a risk factor in developing lung cancer (see *Crystalline silica*, *Hydrated silica*).

SILICATES

This is a family of naturally occurring, quartz-containing minerals (e.g. *silica*). In dry form, they are used in powder bases for cosmetics such as face powder, eyeshadow or blusher.

Magnesium silicate, or *Talc*, is a good example of a silicate used for this purpose. Other types of powdered silicates are used as abrasives in toothpastes and household cleaners. Inhaling silica dust is a risk factor in developing lung cancer.

SILICONES

A group of semisynthetic fluid oils, rubbers and resins derived from silica (e.g. *Dimethicone*, *Simethicone*), these are widely used in cosmetics as film-formers, skin-conditioning agents and water repellents. They are generally considered safe, though poorly studied with regard to toxicity in humans.

SIMETHICONE

This synthetic silicone-based moisturiser and film-former is used in cosmetics. Film-formers trap other substances (including other ingredients in the product) beneath them. Because they do not allow the skin to breathe, they may exacerbate skin irritation caused by sweat or other substances.

SODIUM BENZOATE

This preservative is used in food such as margarines, soft drinks, pickles, jellies and jams. Ingestion has caused birth defects in experimental animals. Currently, there is concern that sodium benzoate and its salts react with ascorbic acid (vitamin C) in soft drinks to form the carcinogen *Benzene*.

SODIUM BICARBONATE
Baking soda

Often used as a flour treatment agent and baking aid in bakery goods and in toothpastes as a whitening/bleaching agent, this can be a harsh abrasive if used in concentrated form. However, it is generally regarded as safe.

SODIUM BISULPHATE

Sulphuric acid

A strong deodoriser that is corrosive and irritating to the skin and eyes, if ingested, it can damage body tissues. Its fumes are a trigger of asthma attacks.

SODIUM CARBONATE

E500, soda ash, washing soda

A strong alkali used as a neutraliser in dairy products, cocoa products and in the canning of olives, ingesting large amounts can cause gastrointestinal upset and even damage. Sodium carbonate can be found in more concentrated forms in household cleaners as a disinfectant and bleaching agent. It can be irritating to the skin and may produce sensitivity reactions.

SODIUM COCOATE

A detergent derived from coconut oil, this is generally considered mild and safe.

SODIUM COCOYL ISETHIONATE

This detergent/surfactant made from entirely synthetic sources can be irritating to the skin.

SODIUM CHLORIDE

Salt

Simple table salt can be added as a water softener to help the product rinse better in hard water. It is used in cosmetics and household cleaners as a viscosity adjuster (thickener).

SODIUM DODECYLBENZENESULPHONATE

A harsh detergent commonly found in car and wheel shampoos, metal polishes, dish and laundry detergents, and even foaming bath products, sodium dodecylbenzenesulphonate can produce skin irritation.

SODIUM FLUORIDE

See Fluoride

SODIUM HYDROXYMETHYLGLYCINATE

A broad-spectrum antimicrobial that is active against a variety of bacteria, yeasts and moulds, this is used as a preservative in toiletries and household cleaners. It is a **Formaldehyde**-forming ingredient that can mix with other ingredients to form carcinogenic nitrosamines (see **Diethanolamine**; see also Chapter 6).

SODIUM HYDROXIDE

Lye, caustic soda

This caustic bleaching/cleaning agent, commonly found in bathroom cleaners, toilet-bowl cleaners, oven cleaners and drain cleaners, is also used in the manufacture of soaps.

In its pure form, lye will quickly eat through skin and body tissue. Mixed with acids, it will release harmful vapours. It is also corrosive, alkaline and poisonous. If accidentally splashed in the eyes, it will cause blindness.

SODIUM HYPOCHLORITE

Bleach

An effective disinfectant and bleaching agent commonly found in cleaners, disinfectants, laundry products, toilet bowl cleaners, tub and tile cleaners, bleach is one of the household cleaners most frequently implicated in household poisonings. It can irritate the skin and respiratory tract and if ingested can damage the mouth, oesophagus and stomach.

SODIUM ISETHIONATE

A detergent made from entirely synthetic sources, this can be irritating to the skin.

SODIUM LAURETH SULPHATE

SLES

A detergent and foaming agent found in bath foams, bubble baths and shampoos, this can be irritating to eyes and skin. Laureth compounds can be contaminated with the carcinogen 1,4-**dioxane**.

SODIUM LAURYL SULPHATE

SLS

A detergent and foaming agent found in bath foams, bubble baths, shampoos and toothpastes, SLS is not carcinogenic, but can nevertheless be damaging. It is so harsh that it is used in medical research to induce a kind of benchmark skin irritation against which all other potential skin irritants are measured. Used in toothpastes, it can damage the delicate mucosal lining of the mouth and, if it gets into the eyes during shampooing, it can damage the cornea. Because it strips the protective oily layer from the skin, it can also act as a penetration enhancer, making it easier for other toxic chemicals to be absorbed into the body.

As new detergents have been invented, the popularity of SLS among manufacturers has waned, but it is still found in many products. Often, its presence is a good indicator of other undesirable ingredients, including **Formaldehyde**-containing preservatives (e.g. **Imidazolidinyl urea**) and nitrosamine-forming agents (e.g. **cocamide DEA, Triethanolamine**) as well as a long list of skin and hair conditioners necessary to repair some of the initial damage it causes.

SODIUM LAUROAMPHOACETATE

This detergent/surfactant is found in body washes and shampoos. It is comparatively mild, so is often found in sensitive or 'no tears' baby shampoos.

SODIUM METABISULPHITE

E223

A preservative and bleaching agent found in alcoholic beverages, juices and dried fruits, ingestion can trigger asthma attacks. It is also used in cosmetics as a preservative where it can cause skin irritation (see **Sulphites**).

SODIUM MONOFLUOROPHOSPHATE

See Fluoride

SODIUM PALM KERNELATE

A detergent synthesised from the oil of palm kernels, it is usually found in soap and bath bars, and is generally thought to be non-toxic.

SODIUM PALMATE
A detergent synthesised from the oil of palm kernels, this is usually found in soap and bath bars, and is generally considered to be non-toxic.

SODIUM SILICATE
A commonly used corrosion inhibitor found in laundry detergents, it is a strong alkali; inhalation is irritating to the lungs and mucous membranes.

SODIUM STEARATE
Found in shampoos and facial washes, this is a fatty acid added as a skin softener to replace the oils that are stripped away from the skin by detergents in these products.

SODIUM SULPHITE
See Sulphites

SODIUM TALLOWATE
A detergent synthesised from animal fats found in facial and bath soaps, this is generally non-toxic.

SODIUM TRIPOLYPHOSPHATE
With various applications such as a preservative for seafood, meats, poultry and pet foods, this agent is also used in toothpaste, and as a builder and water softener in household cleaners and laundry detergents, improving their cleansing ability. It is a caustic that can be irritating to the skin.

SOLVENTS
The solvents used in household products are called 'organic' – not because they are free from harmful chemicals, but because they contain the carbon atoms common to all life on earth.

All organic solvents are hazardous. They are easily absorbed through the skin and via their fumes. Solvents have been associated with liver and kidney problems, birth defects and nervous system disorders. Most recently, solvent exposure has been linked to an increased risk of developing Parkinson's disease. Many of these problems develop slowly over time and are thought to be the result of chronic low-level exposure to solvents such as *Isopropanol*, *Propylene glycol* and *Ethanol*.

SORBITAN LAURATE
An emulsifier and surfactant used in cosmetics, this is generally mild, but it can cause skin irritation in some.

SORBITAN OLEATE
Used in cosmetics as an emulsifier and surfactant, this is synthesised from olive oil. Generally mild, it can nevertheless cause skin irritation in some.

SORBITAN STEARATE
A modified fatty acid derived from beef tallow, it is used as an emulsifier, stabiliser and surfactant in cosmetics. Generally mild, it can cause blackheads in some individuals.

SORBITOL

Used in foods and some toiletries as a sweetener and tartar-control agent, as well as a humectant (keeps the product moist), sorbitol is an alcohol-derived sugar that tastes sweet, but only breaks down in the gut. If swallowed, sorbitol can cause gastrointestinal cramps and bloating. Because of its laxative effects, the use of gel toothpastes (which can contain up to 70 per cent sorbitol) by small children should be supervised and possibly even discouraged, by parents. See also *Sugar alcohols*.

SOYTRIMONIUM CHLORIDE

A *Quaternary ammonium compound* used as a surfactant and detergent in foaming bath products and shampoos, this is toxic by all routes of exposure. Skin and airways irritation are common. Depending on the concentration, quaternary compounds may also produce nausea, vomiting, abdominal pain, anxiety, restlessness, coma, convulsions and respiratory muscle paralysis.

STANNOUS CHLORIDE

Tin dichloride

An antioxidant found in sodas and tinned asparagus, this may be irritating to the skin and mucous membranes.

STEARALKONIUM CHLORIDE

Originally developed by the fabric industry as a softener, it is commonly found in hair conditioners and creams, and may cause allergic reactions.

STEARAMIDE MEA

See *Monoethanolamine*

STEARAMIDOPROPYL DIMETHYLAMINE

Part of a larger group of *Glycol ethers* (the same family as *Propylene glycol* and *Polyethylene glycol* compounds), glycol ethers are solvents and wetting agents that are quickly absorbed into the skin. In the body, they are reproductive toxins.

STEARETH

Waxy compounds (e.g. steareth-2, steareth-21) used as emulsifiers, they are part of a larger group of ethoxylated alcohols that are toxic and potentially carcinogenic, and may also be contaminated by the carcinogen 1,4-*dioxane*.

STEARIC ACID

A lubricant and emulsifier derived from both animal and vegetable sources, this is a fatty acid added as a skin softener. Found in shampoos and facial washes, it replaces the oils stripped away from the skin by the mix of detergents. It can be irritating to the skin, eyes and respiratory tract.

STEARYL ALCOHOL

An emollient, moisturiser and stabiliser derived from animal fats, this is also used as a lubricating agent to help the product go on more smoothly. It is thought to be non-toxic, but can cause mild skin irritation and even contact dermatitis.

STEVIA

A natural sweetener derived from the shrub *Stevia rebaudiana*, stevia has been used for centuries in South America, Japan, China and Korea. However, it is not a permitted food additive in either the EU or the US on the basis of insufficient safety data.

Fears have been raised that stevia may be carcinogenic, damage DNA and affect fertility, but a 2003 review of all the evidence concluded that the plant is, in fact, of 'very low toxicity' and that it is 'safe when used as a sweetener'. It also has the added advantage of reducing blood pressure in people with hypertension.

The main concern is that the plant is a source of phytosterols that may cause reproductive abnormalities in men. However, official concern as to the toxicity of plant sterols seems to be a moveable feast. All over the Western world, men and women gulp down plant oestrogens and sterols in the form of soya supplements that have been approved as 'safe'. Likewise, we are encouraged to eat sterol-containing spreads and yoghurt drinks to lower cholesterol on the basis that these are 'healthy'. The concern is legitimate, and better research is needed to show to what extent sterols in all these foods may have an oestrogenic effect in humans.

Stevia, which can have a slight liquorice flavour and a bitter aftertaste if not processed correctly, is available as a nutritional supplement in the US, but not in Europe.

STRONTIUM CHLORIDE

Added to some toothpastes to reduce periodontal disease, this is also found in some treatment shampoos and facial washes. Considered toxic, it can be irritating to skin and mucous membranes.

SUCRALOSE

Splenda

One of the few sweeteners to be derived from sugar itself, sucralose tastes more like sugar than other artificial sweeteners and contains about one-eighth the calories and carbohydrates of sugar. However, it is produced by chlorinating sugar.

Animal studies, conducted by the manufacturers, have found a range of problems at high doses, including shrunken thyroid glands, and kidney and liver problems. Human studies suggest that a dose at half the current approved level for six months could raise blood-glucose levels. It is widely used in soft drinks, desserts and confectionery, and as a table-top sweetener; consumer reports suggest a wide range of adverse effects from regular ingestion of sucralose including gastrointestinal upsets, cramping and bladder problems.

SUGAR ALCOHOLS

Sorbitol, xylitol, lactitol, mannitol, maltitol, isomalt, hydrogenated starch hydrolysates (HSH)

Though not technically artificial sweeteners, these are lower-calorie sweeteners derived from sugar alcohol. Sugar alcohols have fewer calories than sugar and are claimed not to promote tooth decay or cause sudden increases in glucose in diabetics. They have a pleasant sweet taste similar to sucrose, and are often used in sweets, biscuits and chewing gum.

The regulatory authorities classify sugar alcohols as GRAS (generally recognised as safe), but they may cause diarrhoea, bloating and stomach pain in high doses over 1 gram. This is because they are more slowly digested and remain longer in the intestinal tract, rather than being absorbed into the blood. The non-absorbed carbohydrates create an osmotic effect that pulls water into the intestines. Also, when the non-absorbed carbohydrates reach the colon, normal bacteria metabolise them into gases and short-chain fatty acids.

SULISOBENZONE

This is a sunscreening agent. See **Benzophenones**.

SULPHITES

A class of chemical preservatives used widely in food production, they can keep cut fruit and vegetables looking fresh, preventing discoloration in apricots, raisins and other dried fruits. They can also control 'black spot' in freshly caught shrimp, and prevent discoloration, bacterial growth and fermentation in wine. Until the early 1980s, they were considered safe, but research now shows they can provoke sometimes severe allergic reactions, especially in asthmatics. In 1995, the US Food and Drug Administration banned sulphites from most (but not all) commercially prepared fruit and vegetables. They are still widely used elsewhere, however.

SULPHUR DIOXIDE

Used to bleach vegetable colours, and preserve fruits and vegetables, this is an antioxidant and preservative found in a wide variety of foods, including wines, beverages, soups and condiments. Poisonous and highly irritating, it also destroys the vitamin content of foods. This is on the US Environmental Protection Agency's list of extremely hazardous substances.

SULPHURIC ACID

A cleaner and disinfectant used in toilet-bowl cleaners and metal polishes, this can produce severe skin burns even when diluted. Also, it is very dangerous when splashed in the eyes, and has been known to cause blindness.

TALC

Magnesium silicate

Talc is made up of finely ground particles of stone. It is used widely in powdered cosmetics and is an absorbent on its own. As it originates in the ground and is a mined product, it can be contaminated with other substances. Asbestos is a good example, and recent reports of the talc used in crayon manufacture being contaminated with this poisonous substance have caused alarm to every parent whose child has ever sucked a crayon.

Regular use is also associated with respiratory problems in adults and children. Because it comprises finely ground stone, it can lodge in the lungs and never leave. In women, its use in the genital area has been linked to ovarian cancer; it is now estimated that women who frequently use talc have three times the risk of developing ovarian cancer compared with non-users.

TEA LAURYL SULPHATE

See Triethanolamine

TEA SODIUM LAURYL SULPHATE

See Triethanolamine

TEFLON

Polytetrafluoroethylene, PTFE

This is the non-stick coating found on cookware, and in the packaging of fast and microwaveable foods such as french fries, popcorn and pizza, as well as in sweet wrappers and other products. As a waterproof coating on fabrics, it is known as Stainmaster, Gore-tex and Scotchgard. It's also frequently used as a film-former in cosmetics.

According to the US Environmental Protection Agency, one of the breakdown products of Teflon, known as PFOA (perfluorooctanoic acid), is an expected human carcinogen. PFOA can be released when Teflon is heated and can cause severe respiratory distress (and is deadly to pet birds). It is a persistent chemical pollutant found in almost every animal on the planet, including humans. As evidence of PFOA's toxicity continues to accumulate, some observers believe that its effect on humans may yet make **DDT** look almost safe by comparison.

TETRAMETHRIN

A synthetic pyrethroid insecticide used to control wasps, ants and other garden insects, this is a skin, eye and respiratory irritant, neurotoxin and suspected carcinogen.

TETRASODIUM EDTA

Tetrasodium ethylenediaminetetraacetic acid

A cosmetic preservative used in soaps and other toiletries, it helps to isolate impurities such as metals that cause the mixture to degrade. It can cause skin, mucous membrane and eye irritation, as well as contact dermatitis and contact allergies, and also acts as a penetration enhancer. Environmentally persistent, it binds with heavy metals in lakes and streams, aiding their re-entry into the food chain.

TETRASODIUM ETIDRONATE

A synthetic preservative used to stop impurities such as metals from making the product deteriorate, it can be irritating to the skin.

THIMEROSAL

This mercury-containing preservative is found in certain cosmetics such as mascara as well as in ophthalmic preparations. Highly toxic and damaging to the eyes, it may add to the body's burden of the neurotoxin mercury.

TITANIUM DIOXIDE

E171

Titanium dioxide is extracted from the naturally occurring mineral ilmenite. It is used in foods such as cottage and mozzarella cheese, horseradish cream and sauces, lemon curd, in sweets, where it is often used to provide a barrier between different colours, and in sauces to increase their opacity. It is also found in tablets and capsules, and is used as a colouring, opacifier and sunscreening agent in cosmetics. Thought not to be easily absorbed and generally considered safe when used in topical formulations, ingestion can produce detectable amounts in the blood, brain and glands, with the highest concentrations being in the lymph nodes and lungs. It is banned in Germany.

TOLUENE

Toluol, methylbenzene

This and its chemical cousin **Xylene** are **Aromatic hydrocarbons** used primarily as **Solvents**. Commonly found in dry cleaning solutions and perfume, toluene easily enters the body through inhalation and ingestion, but is poorly absorbed via the skin. Irritating to the skin and respiratory tract, it can cause damage to several organs, including eyes, liver, kidneys and the central nervous system (where it acts like a narcotic). Symptoms of chronic exposure include fatigue, weakness, confusion, headache, watery eyes, muscular fatigue, insomnia, dermatitis and photosensitivity.

2,4-TOLUENEDIAMINE
4-methyl-m-phenylenediamine
  See Phenylenediamines

TRIADIMEFON
A triazole fungicide used to control powdery mildews, rusts and other fungal pests in turf, shrubs and trees, it is irritating to the lungs. Long-term exposure can produce pathological changes in red blood cell counts, increase blood cholesterol levels and damage the liver. Animal studies indicate that it may have reproductive effects such as causing more neonatal deaths and lower birth weights in offspring.

TRIBUTYLTIN OXIDE
TBT

A fungicide used as a wood treatment and preservative, it can cause irritation of the skin, eyes and respiratory tract. It is a central nervous system toxin that can produce headache, nausea, vomiting, dizziness, breathing difficulties and flu-like symptoms. It is also a suspected reproductive toxin and carcinogen, based on limited animal data.

1,1,2-TRICHLOROETHANE
A solvent for chlorinated rubbers, fats, oils, waxes and resins, this is common in household products such as typewriter correction fluid, paint removers, adhesives and spot removers, and can cause stinging and burning sensations on the skin. It is poorly studied for its potential capacity to cause cancer, reproductive defects and central nervous system damage.

TRICHLOROETHANE
TCA

A solvent and cleaning agent commonly found in spot removers, metal polishes and fabric cleaners, film cleaner, insecticides, paint and varnish removers, and degreasers, it is also used as an aerosol propellant.

It is absorbed into the body by inhalation and ingestion, is an irritant to the eyes and nose, and can result in central nervous system depression, and liver and kidney damage, if ingested.

TRICHLOROETHYLENE
TCE

Found in spot cleaners and dry cleaning fluids, TCE is another commonly used solvent. It is a suspected carcinogen. When inhaled, it can cause dizziness and sleepiness and, in some cases, memory loss. Irritating to the eyes and nose, it can cause skin to become dry and flaky, and may produce rashes. It is associated with central nervous system disorders and damage to vital organs such as the kidneys and liver. It can also cause cardiac failure.

Trichloroethylene can persist on fabrics long after its application. It is also a common groundwater contaminant that easily works its way back into the food chain and water supply.

TRICHLORPHON

An organophosphate insecticide used to control cockroaches, crickets, silverfish, bedbugs and fleas, long-term exposure can provoke impaired memory and concentration, disorientation, severe depression, irritability, confusion, speech difficulties, delayed reaction times, nightmares, sleepwalking and drowsiness or insomnia. This is a highly toxic substance that is a reproductive toxin, carcinogen and mutagen, and toxic to birds and fish.

TRICLOPYR

A herbicide that is irritating to skin and eyes, and that may damage the liver and kidneys.

TRICLOSAN

2,4,4'-trichloro-2'-hydroxy diphenyl ether

An antibacterial agent found in household cleaners, toothpastes, mouthwashes, face washes and bath products, it is used as a coating on plastics (e.g. cutting boards and storage containers), and it is known as Microban. Applied to the skin, it can cause allergic reactions and ulceration. In the mouth, it kills both 'good' and 'bad' bacteria, and makes users more vulnerable to infection. It can also cause premature cell death in the gingival tissues, resulting in gum damage. It's easily absorbed into the body via the mouth, and has been associated with liver damage and eye irritation. A chlorinated aromatic compound, Triclosan is molecularly similar to **Dioxins**, **PCBs** and Agent Orange. Indeed, the manufacturing process of Triclosan can release dioxins – powerful hormone disrupters – into the environment. It is also a chlorophenol, a class of chemicals that can cause cancer in animals. Commonly used as a pesticide, the widespread use of Triclosan in commercial products is also implicated in our increasing rates of bacterial resistance.

TRIETHANOLAMINE

TEA

A surfactant, emulsifier, dispersant and pH adjuster commonly used in shampoos and foaming bath products, this can be irritating to the skin and eyes. More worryingly, it may, during storage, on the skin or in the body after absorption, mix with **Formaldehyde**-forming chemicals in the product to form carcinogenic compounds called nitrosamines (see also Chapter 6). TEA is a suspected endocrine disrupter. Animal studies have demonstrated liver and kidney damage due to chronic exposure.

TRIETHANOLAMINE LAURYL SULPHATE

See Triethanolamine

TRIFLURALIN

A herbicide used to control many annual grasses and weeds, ingestion of this agent can cause nausea and severe gastrointestinal discomfort. Inhalation may cause irritation of the lining of the mouth, throat, or lungs. Animal studies suggest that long-term exposure can reduce red blood cell counts and raise cholesterol levels as well as lead to malignant tumours in the kidneys, bladder and thyroid.

TRIISOPROPANOLAMINE

TIPA

This alkanolamine (the same family as **Diethanolamine**, **Triethanolamine** and **Monoethanolamine**) is a hormone-disrupting solvent and surfactant.

TRIPOLYPHOSPHATE

Used as a water softener and emulsifier, it may cause oesophageal stricture and violent vomiting if swallowed.

TRISODIUM EDTA

See Tetrasodium EDTA

UREA

E927b, carbamide

Naturally found in urine and other body fluids, today it is synthesised from ammonia and carbon dioxide and used as a fertiliser; in foods, it can be used as a texturiser in chewing gum and, in skincare products, it is used to moisturise hardened skin. Generally regarded as safe, although regular topical applications can cause thinning of the skin.

VA/VINYL BUTYL BENZOATE/CROTONATES COPOLYMER

A petroleum-based vinyl acetate that forms a thin plastic-like film on the hair that aids styling, it can cause mild skin irritation.

VINYL ACETATE/ACRYLIC COPOLYMER

A petroleum-based checmical that forms a thin plastic-like film on the hair that aids styling, it can cause mild skin irritation.

XYLENE

Xylol, dimethylbenzene

A chemical cousin of **Toluene** and one of the **Aromatic hydrocarbons** used primarily as a **Solvent**, this is commonly found in dry cleaning solutions and perfume. Xylene easily enters the body through inhalation and ingestion, but is poorly absorbed via the skin. It is irritating to the skin and respiratory tract, and can cause damage to the eyes, liver, kidneys and central nervous system. Symptoms of chronic exposure include fatigue, weakness, confusion, headache, watery eyes, insomnia, dermatitis and photosensitivity.

XYLITOL

See Sugar alcohols

ZINC OXIDE

This popular mineral-based sunblocker is generally considered safe and effective although, in some individuals, it can cause skin irritation.

ZINC STEARATE

Found in shampoos and facial washes, it is a fatty acid added as a skin softener to replace the oils stripped away from the skin by detergents.

ZIRAM

A carbamate fungicide, also used as a bird and rodent repellent, it is irritating to the skin, eyes and mucous membranes. Animal studies indicate it can reduce fertility, delay development in offspring, and cause chromosomal damage and cancer. In humans it can cause nerve and visual disturbances, chromosomal damage and enlarged thyroid glands.

afterword
Pick your poison

WE ARE BOTH PASSIVE AND DIRECT recipients of pollution. Reading through this book, you may find yourself becoming dismayed at the overwhelming number of ways in which the products you use every day can affect your health, but don't give up and don't get discouraged.

In an ideal world, the absolute best way to stay healthy is to avoid being exposed to chemical toxins altogether. But this is not realistic. Given how badly we have polluted our planet and our home environments, none of us can avoid all the known poisons that are threatening our day-to-day health and wellbeing. But you do have more power than you think and you can, to a very large and influential extent, learn to pick your poisons.

One way to do this is to be aware of what your particular weak spots are. These may be genetic vulnerabilities, or weak spots developed in your own lifetime. For instance, if you have a family history of cancer, it makes sense to avoid carcinogenic chemicals and metals as far as is possible. If your family has a history of neurological disorders (for instance, multiple sclerosis) or autoimmune diseases (such as arthritis), you should be on the lookout for neurotoxic and immunotoxic chemicals. If you suffer from menstrual problems, chemicals that disrupt your hormones may play a part. Get to know what these chemicals are and learn to avoid them.

It may also mean making the occasional compromise. If there is something that you absolutely can't live without, then keep using it. But try to make 'chemical savings' elsewhere in your life by, for instance, saving perfume or makeup for special occasions only, using a fluoride-free tooth-paste, cutting down on the number of other largely unnecessary toiletries you use, getting rid of toxic air fresheners, making use of some of the sug-gestions in this book for chemical-free cleaning or pest control, or seeking out paints and other home decoration supplies that are low in toxic ingre-dients.

By doing this, you are protecting yourself as well as your children – who are the most vulnerable to the effects of chemical exposures – and ensuring that they have a healthy future to look forward to.

You are in control, you do have the power and it is your responsibility.

appendices

A complete guide to E numbers

Foods sold in the European Union (EU) have had full ingredient labelling since the mid-1980s. For ease of reference and to help avoid the problems of translating them into the wide range of languages used in Europe, many of these ingredients are abbreviated as 'E numbers'. In Australia and New Zealand, these same numbers are used but without the E prefix.

This simple numbering system for food additives is now being adapted for international use by the Codex Alimentarius Commission, an organisation created in 1963 by the Food and Agriculture Organization (FAO) of the United Nations and the WHO (World Health Organization). When this system is finally adopted, it will be known as the International Numbering System (INS), and will use mostly the same numbers (but without the E prefix).

As the table below shows, the list of food additives is simply staggeringly long. Many of these E numbers began life as naturally derived substances. However, most are now prepared/produced in the lab as synthetically produced compounds are often less expensive than the natural product.

While the E-numbering system may seem dense and impenetrable, there is a logic to it. Each group of numbers represents a particular type or group of additive:

▓ E100s are colours

▓ E200 to E282 are preservatives and acids

▓ E300 to E341 are antioxidants and acid regulators

- E400s include emulsifiers, stabilisers, thickeners, anticaking agents, release agents and bulking agents

- E500s are mineral salts and anticaking agents

- E620 to E640 are flavour enhancers

- E900 and upwards are additives that don't fall into any of the above categories.

The list is constantly being updated and changed, which makes it hard for conscientious shoppers to keep track of it. The list below gives an overview of the additives currently permitted in the EU. Most of these are permitted elsewhere but, in the US for instance, they are known by their chemical names. Those additives in the table without an E prefix are unique to Australia and New Zealand. Remember, not all E numbers have been fully tested for safety, so it is impossible to say categorically which ones are safe and which ones are not. Likewise, some individuals may be more sensitive than others to the effects of certain additives such as colours and sulphites.

COLOURS

E100   Curcumin
Derived from the root of the curcuma plant, but can be artificially produced. No known adverse effects.

E101   Riboflavin, riboflavin- 5'-phosphate
Doubles as colour and added nutrient. Synonyms: Vitamin B2

E102   Tartrazine
Known to provoke asthma attacks and skin rashes, altered states of perception and behaviour, and hyperactivity. Suspected carcinogen. Inhibits zinc metabolism and interferes with digestive enzymes. Banned in Norway, Austria and Finland. Restricted use in Sweden and Germany. Synonyms: FD&C Yellow 5; CI Acid Yellow 23, CI Food Yellow 4

103   Alkanet
Natural 'port-wine' colour from A. tinctoria plant. Banned in US; not approved in Europe.

E104   Quinoline Yellow
May cause asthma, rashes and hyperactivity. Aspirin-sensitive people must avoid it. Banned in Japan, US, Norway and Australia. Synonyms: D&C Yellow 10

E105   Fast Yellow AB
Effects unknown.

E106   Riboflavin-5'-[sodium phosphate]
Doubles as a colour and added nutrient. Synonyms: Vitamin B5

E107   Yellow 2G
May cause asthma, rashes and hyperactivity. People sensitive to aspirin should avoid it. Banned in Australia, Austria, Belgium, Denmark, France, Germany, Japan, Norway, Sweden, Switzerland and the US. Synonyms: Acid Yellow 17, CI Food Yellow 5

E110   Sunset Yellow FCF, Orange Yellow S
Can provoke allergic reactions, abdominal pain, hyperactivity, hives, nasal congestion, bronchoconstriction. Suspected carcinogen. Has been linked to growth retardation, severe weight loss and increased incidence of tumours in animals. Banned in Finland, Norway and the UK. Synonyms: FD&C Yellow 6, CI Food Yellow 3

E120   Cochineal
Can promote hyperactivity, rhinitis, urticaria (hives) and asthma. Banned in the US.

E122   Carmoisine
Can trigger asthmatic reactions and hyperactivity, urticaria and oedema. Suspected carcinogen. Banned in Austria, Japan, Norway, Sweden and the US. Synonym: Azo rubine

E123   Amaranth
Associated with birth defects and foetal deaths. Can cause urticaria and liver problems. Suspected carcinogen. Banned in Austria, Japan, Norway, Russia, Sweden and the US. Synonyms: FD&C Red 2, CI Acid Red 27, CI Food Red 9

E124   Ponceau 4R
Carcinogenic in animals, can trigger asthma and allergic reactions. Banned in Canada, Norway and the US (in 1976 for cancer-causing agents). Restricted in Sweden. Synonym: Cochineal Red A

E127   Erythrosine
Linked with sensitivity to light and learning difficulties; can increase thyroid hormone levels and lead to hyperthyroidism; was shown to cause thyroid cancer in rats. As a pesticide, kills maggot larvae and flies. Banned in Norway. Synonym: FD&C Red 3

E128   Red 2G
Should be avoided by hyperactive people, asthmatics and aspirin-sensitive people. Suspected carcinogen. Banned in Australia, Austria, Belgium, Denmark, Germany, Japan, Switzerland, New Zealand and the US.

E129   Allura Red AC
Suspected carcinogen. Prohibited throughout the EU. Synonyms: FD&C Red 40

E131   Patent Blue V
May cause dermatitis and purpura. Banned in Australia, Norway, Japan, New Zealand and the US.

E132   Indigotine, Indigo Carmine
Can cause nausea, vomiting, high blood pressure, skin rashes, breathing problems and allergic reactions. Suspected carcinogen. Banned in Norway. Synonyms: FD&C Blue 2

E133   Brilliant Blue FCF

Can cause hyperactivity, skin rashes, bronchoconstriction (when combined with E127 and E132). Linked with chromosomal damage. Banned in Austria, Belgium, France, Germany, Norway, Switzerland and Sweden. Synonyms: FD&C Blue 1, CI Acid Blue 9, CI Food Blue 2, CI Pigment Blue 24

E140   Chlorophylis, chlorophyllins

Generally harmless, although an excess can cause sensitivity to light.

E141   Copper complexes of chlorophyll and chlorophyllins; copper phaeophytins

No adverse effects are known.

E142   Green S

May cause asthma, rashes and hyperactivity. Mutagenic in animal tests. Banned in Canada, Japan, Sweden, the US and Norway. Synonyms: CI Acid Green 50, CI Food Green 4

E150(a)   Plain caramel

Plain caramel is mostly naturally derived. Other forms such as those made with ammonia are toxic and can provoke hyperactivity. Some caramels may damage genes, slow down growth, cause enlargement of the intestines and kidneys, and may destroy vitamin B.

E150(b)   Caustic sulphite caramel

See 150(a)

E150(c)   Ammonia caramel

See 150(a)

E150(d)   Sulphite ammonia caramel

See 150(a)

E151   Brilliant Black BN

Can trigger asthma attacks and hyperactivity in asthmatics, as well as urticaria and rhinitis. Also known to interfere with some digestive enzymes. Banned in Denmark, Australia, Belgium, France, Germany, Switzerland, Austria, the US and Norway, and greatly restricted in Sweden. Synonyms: Black PN, CI Food Black 1

E153   Vegetable carbon

Suspected carcinogen due to impurities. Banned in the US.

E154   Brown FK

Potential carcinogen. Banned in Austria, Australia, Japan, New Zealand, Switzerland, the US and all EU countries except the UK. Synonyms: Kipper Brown, Food Brown

E155   (Chocolate) Brown HT

Can provoke asthmatic reactions, hyperactivity and skin sensitivity. Suspected carcinogen. Banned in Austria, Belgium, Denmark, France, Germany, Norway, Switzerland, Sweden and the US.

E160(a) Carotene (alpha-, beta-, gamma-)
Natural orange/yellow colour; human body converts it to vitamin A in the liver; found in carrots and other yellow or orange fruit and vegetables.

E160(b) Annatto
Can cause urticaria and flare-ups of angioneurotic oedema, asthma and hyperactivity. Synonyms: bixin, norbixin

E160(c) Paprika extract, capsanthin, capsorubin
Natural colours derived from fruit pods of the red pepper. No known adverse effects.

E160(d) Lycopene
Can be derived from GM sources. Banned in some countries, including Australia.

E160(e) Beta-apo-8'-carotenal (C 30)
Natural orange colour. No known adverse effects.

E160(f) Ethyl ester of beta-apo-8'-carotenic acid (C 30)
Natural orange colour. No known adverse effects.

E161 Xanthophylls
Natural yellow colour derived from plants and animals, naturally found in green leaves, marigolds and egg yolk. No known adverse effects.

E161(b) Xanthophylls (lutein)
See E161

E161(g) Xanthophylls (canthaxanthin)
Yellow colour possibly derived from animal sources such as shellfish, fish and flamingo feathers. No known adverse effects.

E162 Beetroot Red, Betanin
Purple colour derived from beets. No known adverse effects.

E163 Anthocyanins
Violet, red, blue colour matter of flowers, buds and plants. No known adverse effects.

E170 Calcium carbonate
Mineral salt; may be derived from rock mineral or animal bones. High doses create mineral imbalance and many other physical problems such as haemorrhoids, kidney stones, abdominal pain and confused behaviour.

E171 Titanium dioxide
No known adverse effects.

E172 Iron oxides and hydroxides
High doses can create mineral imbalances.

E173 Aluminium
Suspected neurotoxin, linked to osteoporosis.

E174   Silver
No adverse effects known, but high doses can lead to bluish-grey skin (cyanosis). Banned in Australia.

E175   Gold
Rarely used. Adverse effects unknown.

E180   Latolrubine BK
Probable cause of rashes and hyperactivity, and potentially dangerous to asthmatics. Banned in Australia and New Zealand.

E181   Tannic acid, tannins
Clarifying agent in alcoholic drinks; derived from the nutgalls and twigs of oak trees; occurs naturally in tea. May cause gastric irritation.

PRESERVATIVES

E200   Sorbic acid
Either obtained from berries or synthesised from ketene; possible skin irritant, and may cause rashes, asthma and hyperactivity. Inhibits yeast and bacteria growth.

E201   Sodium sorbate
See E200

E202   Potassium sorbate
See E200

E203   Calcium sorbate
See E200

E210   Benzoic acid
Obtained from benzoin, a resin exuded by trees native to Asia. Can cause hyperactivity and asthma, especially in those using steroid asthma medications. Also reputed to cause neurological disorders and to react with sulphur bisulphite (E222). Synonyms: flowers of benzoin, phenlycarboxylic acid, carboxybenzene.

E211   Sodium benzoate
Causes nettle rash and aggravates asthma. Suspected neurotoxin.

E212   Potassium benzoate
Can provoke allergic reactions.

E213   Calcium benzoate
See E212

E214   Ethyl p-hydroxybenzoate
See E210. Banned in France and Australia.

E215   Sodium ethyl p-hydroxybenzoate
See E210. Banned in Australia.

E216   Propylparaben
Suspected hormone disrupter, allergen. Synonym: Propyl p-hydroxybenzoate

E217   Sodium propyl p-hydroxybenzoate
See E210. Banned in France and Australia.

E218   Methylparaben
Suspected hormone disrupter; allergen. Synonym: Methyl p-hydroxybenzoate

E219   Sodium methyl p-hydroxybenzoate
See E210. Banned in France and Australia.

E220   Sulphur dioxide
Can provoke gastric irritation, nausea, diarrhoea, skin rash, asthma attacks; difficult to metabolise for those with impaired kidney function. Also destroys vitamin B1, and should be avoided by anyone suffering from conjunctivitis, bronchitis, emphysema, bronchial asthma or cardiovascular disease.

E221   Sodium sulphite
See E220.

E222   Sodium hydrogen sulphite
See E220. Synonym: Sodium bisulphite.

E223   Sodium metabisulphite
See E220

E224   Potassium metabisulphite
See E220

E225   Potassium sulphite
See E220

E226   Calcium sulphite
May cause asthma. A gastric irritant. Destroys vitamins B and E. Banned in Australia.

E227   Calcium hydrogen sulphite
May cause an allergic reaction. Banned in Australia.

E228   Potassium hydrogen sulphite
See E220. Synonym: Potassium bisulphite

E230   Biphenyl, diphenyl
A constituent of the wood preservative creosote. Banned in Australia.

E231   Orthophenyl phenol
Toxic antifungal; not recommended for consumption by children. Banned in Australia.

E232   Sodium orthophenyl phenol
See E231

E233   Thiabendazole
High regular doses associated with anorexia, nausea, vomiting and vertigo.

E234   Nisin
Antibiotic derived from bacteria. Effects unknown.

E235   Natamycin
Can cause nausea, vomiting, anorexia, diarrhoea and skin irritation.

E236   Formic acid
Cumulative tissue poison with risk of acidosis (disturbance in the body's acid-base balance). Banned in Australia.

E237   Sodium formate
See E236. Banned in Australia.

E238   Calcium formate
See E236. Banned in Australia.

E239   Hexamethylene tetramine
Obtained by reacting ammonia with formaldehyde. Not recommended for children. Banned in Australia.

E242   Dimethyl dicarbonate
Effects unknown.

E249   Potassium nitrite
Nitrites can affect oxygen-carrying capacity, resulting in shortness of breath, dizziness and headaches; potential carcinogen; not permitted in foods for infants and young children.

E250   Sodium nitrite
May provoke hyperactivity and other adverse reactions. Suspected carcinogen

E251   Sodium nitrate
See E250

E252   Potassium nitrate
May provoke hyperactivity and other adverse reactions. Suspected carcinogen. Restricted in many countries. See E249.

E260   Acetic acid
No known adverse effects.

E261   Potassium acetate
Should be avoided by people with impaired kidney function.

E262   Sodium acetate and anhydrous, sodium diacetate
No known adverse effects.

E263   Calcium acetate
No known adverse effects.

E264   Ammonium acetate
Can cause nausea and vomiting.

E270   Lactic acid

No known adverse effects.

E280   Propionic acid

Propionates are linked with migraine headaches.

E281   Sodium propionate

See E280

E282   Calcium propionate

Can cause symptoms similar to a gallbladder attack. See also E280.

E283   Potassium propionate

See E280

E284   Boric acid

Suspected neurotoxin often used as a pesticide.

E290   Carbon dioxide

Suspected neurotoxin.

ACIDS, ANTIOXIDANTS, MINERAL SALTS

E296 Malic acid, D,L-malic acid

No known adverse effects.

E297   Fumaric acid

No known adverse effects.

E300   Ascorbic acid

Very large doses can cause dental erosion, vomiting, diarrhoea and dizziness. Take under medical advice if you have kidney stones, gout or anaemia. Synonym: Vitamin C

E301   Sodium ascorbate

See E300

E301   Calcium ascorbate

See E300

E301   Potassium ascorbate

See E300

E301   Ascorbyl palmitate, ascorbyl stearate

See E300

E306   Tocopherols (concentrate, mix)

No known adverse effects. Synonym: Vitamin E

E307   alpha-Tocopherol

See E306

E308   gamma-Tocopherol

See E306

E309   delta-Tocopherol
See E306

E310   Propyl gallate
May cause gastric or skin irritation; not permitted in foods for infants and small children because it is known to cause the blood disorder methaemoglobinaemia.

E311   Octyl gallate
See E310

E312   Dodecyl gallate
See E310

E315   Erythorbic acid
No known adverse effects.

E316   Sodium erythorbate
See E315

E318   Sodium erythorbin
See E315

E319   tert-Butylhydroquinone
May cause nausea, vomiting, delirium.

E320   Butylated hydroxyanisole (BHA)
Not permitted in infant foods; can provoke an allergic reaction, hyperactivity. Suspected carcinogen and hormone disrupter.

E321   Butylated hydroxytoluene (BHT)
See E320

E322   Lecithin
No adverse effects known.

E325   Sodium lactate
No known adverse effects. See E270.

E326   Potassium lactate
See E325

E327   Calcium lactate
See E325

E328   Ammonium lactate
See E325

E329   Magnesium lactate
See E325

E330   Citric acid
No known adverse effects.

E331   Sodium citrates
No known adverse effects.

E332   Potassium citrates (monopotassium, tripotassium)

No known adverse effects.

E333   Calcium citrates

No known adverse effects.

E334   Tartaric acid

No known adverse effects.

E335   Sodium tartrates

People with cardiac failure, high blood pressure, damaged liver or kidneys, and fluid retention may wish to avoid this additive.

E336   Potassium tartrates

See E335

E337   Sodium potassium tartrate

See E335

E338   Phosphoric acid

Too much leads to the loss of calcium in bones and the onset of osteoporosis.

E339   Sodium phosphates

See E338

340   Ammonium phosphates

No known adverse effects.

E340   Potassium phosphates

See E338

E341   Calcium phosphates

No known adverse effects.

E343   Magnesium phosphates

No known adverse effects.

E350   Sodium malates (sodium hydrogen malate)

No known adverse effects.

E351   Potassium malate

No known adverse effects.

E352   Calcium malates

No known adverse effects. Synonym: D,L-Calcium malate

E353   Metatartaric acid

No known adverse effects.

E354   Calcium tartrate

No known adverse effects.

E355   Adipic acid

Only a small amount can be metabolised by humans. Possible teratogen (foetal toxin).

E357   **Potassium adipose**
No known adverse effects.

E363   **Succinic acid**
Large doses associated with stomach upsets. Banned in Australia.

E365   **Sodium fumarate**
No known adverse effects.

E366   **Potassium fumarate**
No known adverse effects.

E367   **Calcium fumarate**
No known adverse effects.

E370   **1,4-Heptonolactone**
Poorly studied. Banned in Australia.

E375   **Niacin**
No known adverse effects. Synonym: Vitamin B3

E380   **Tri-ammonium citrate**
May interfere with liver and pancreas function.

E381   **Ammonium ferric citrates**
Unsafe in large amounts

E385   **Calcium disodium, ethylenediamine tetraacetic acid (EDTA)**
Causes mineral imbalance. Known enzyme and blood-coagulant inhibitor.
Gastrointestinal disturbances, blood in urine, kidney damage and muscle cramps are side-effects. Banned in Australia.

VEGETABLE GUMS, EMULSIFIERS, STABILISERS AND OTHERS

E400   **Alginic acid**
No known adverse effects.

E401   **Sodium alginate**
See E400

E402   **Potassium alginate**
See E400

E403   **Ammonium alginate**
See E400

E404   **Calcium alginate**
See E400

E405   **Propylene glycol alginate**
No known adverse effects.

E406   Agar
No known adverse effects.

E407   Carrageenan
Known adverse effects include gastrointestinal ulcers (but it is also used to treat ulcers in humans), liver damage and effects on the immune system; it is suspected to cause cancer.

E410   Locust bean gum
Mild laxative effect.

E412   Guar gum
Derived from the seeds of Cyamopsis tetragonolobus; can cause nausea, flatulence and cramps.

E413   Tragacanth
Resin form the tree Astragalus gummifer; possible allergen.

E414   Acacia
Derived from the sap of Acacia senegal; possible allergen.

E415   Xanthan gum
No known adverse effects.

E416   Karaya gum
Derived from the tree Sterculia urens; possible allergen.

E417   Tara gum
Derived from the tara bush, Caesalpinia spinosa; no known adverse effects.

E420   Sorbitol
Can cause stomach upset.

E421   Mannitol
Possible allergen; not permitted in infant foods due to its ability to cause diarrhoea and kidney dysfunction; also may cause nausea and vomiting.

E422*   Glycerol
Large quantities can cause headaches, thirst, nausea and high blood sugar.

E432*   Polysorbate 20
Banned in some countries.

E433*   Polysorbate 80
May increase the absorption of fat-soluble substances.

E434*   Polysorbate 40
Avoid it; banned in some countries.

E435*   Polysorbate 60
See E433

E436*   Polysorbate 120
See E433

E440(a)   Pectin

Large quantities may cause temporary flatulence or intestinal discomfort.

E440(b)   Amidated pectin

No known adverse effects.

E441*   Gelatine

Possible allergen.

E442   Ammonium phosphatides

No known adverse effects.

E450   Diphosphates

High intakes may upset the calcium/phosphate balance.

E460   Cellulose

No known adverse effects.

E461   Methyl cellulose

Can cause flatulence, distention, intestinal obstruction.

E463   Hydroxypropyl cellulose

Effects unknown. Banned in some countries.

E464   Hydroxypropyl methyl cellulose

Effects unknown.

E4120   Ethyl methyl cellulose

Effects unknown.

E466   Carboxy methyl cellulose, sodium carboxy methyl cellulose

No known adverse effects.

E469   Sodium caseinate

No known adverse effects.

E470*   Sodium, potassium and calcium salts of fatty acids

In large amounts can interfere with intestinal function. Banned in some countries.

E471*   Mono and diglycerides of fatty acids

No known adverse effects.

E472*   Esters of glycerides of fatty acids

No known adverse effects.

E473*   Sucrose esters of fatty acids

No known adverse effects.

E474*   Sucroglycerides

Effects unknown. Banned in some countries.

E475*   Polyglycerol esters of fatty acids

No known adverse effects.

E476* Polyglycerol polyricinoleate
No known adverse effects.

E477* Propylene glycol esters of fatty acids
No known adverse effects.

E479(b)* Thermally oxidised soya bean oil interacted with mono- and diglycerides of fatty acids
In laboratory tests, oxidised and heated (modified) fats fed in very large amounts to test animals can produce toxic symptoms, including liver and thyroid changes, and the development of tumours. May be GM-derived.

E480 Dioctyl sodium sulphosuccinate
No known adverse effects.

E481* Sodium stearoyl-2-lactylate
No known adverse effects.

E482* Calcium stearoyl-2-lactylate
No known adverse effects.

E483* Stearyl tartrate
Suspected carcinogen. Banned in some countries.

E491* Sorbitan monostearate
No known adverse effects.

E492* Sorbitan tristearate
May increase the absorption of fat-soluble substances.

E493* Sorbitan monolaurate
May be harmful or act as an irritant; effects largely uninvestigated. Banned in some countries.

E494* Sorbitan monooleate
No known adverse effects.

E495* Sorbitan monopalmitate
Effects unknown.

MINERAL SALTS AND ANTICAKING AGENTS

E500 Sodium carbonates
No known adverse effects.

E501 Potassium carbonates
No known adverse effects.

503 Ammonium carbonates
Irritant to mucous membranes, alters pH of urine and may cause loss of calcium and magnesium.

E504   Magnesium carbonate
No known adverse effects.

E507   Hydrochloric acid
Suspected teratogen (foetal toxin) and co-carcinogen when mixed with formaldehyde.
Safe in small quantities.

E508   Potassium chloride
Large quantities can cause gastric ulceration.

E509   Calcium chloride
No known adverse effects.

E510   Ammonium chloride
Should be avoided by people with impaired liver or kidney function.

E511   Magnesium chloride
No known adverse effects.

E513   Sulphuric acid
Teratogenic (foetal-toxic) properties. Banned in Australia.

E514   Sodium sulphates
May upset water balance.

E515   Potassium sulphates
No adverse effects known, but large doses can cause severe gastrointestinal bleeding

E516   Calcium sulphate
No known adverse effects

E517   Ammonium sulphate
White solid; used in water purification

E518   Magnesium sulphate
Dangerous to people with kidney problems and possible teratogen (foetal toxin).
Synonym: Epsom salts

E519   Copper sulphate
High doses of copper can act as a cumulative poison.

E524   Sodium hydroxide
Caustic. Banned in Australia. Synonym: Lye

E525   Potassium hydroxide
Caustic. Banned in Australia.

E526   Calcium hydroxide
No known adverse effects.

E527   Ammonium hydroxide
Dilute household ammonia. Banned in Australia.

E528   Magnesium hydroxide
Laxative effects. Banned in Australia.

E529   Calcium oxide
No known adverse effects.

E530   Magnesium oxide
Laxative effects. Banned in Australia.

E535   Sodium ferrocyanide
No known adverse effects.

E536   Potassium ferrocyanide
Reduces oxygen transport in the blood, which may cause breathing difficulties, dizziness or headache. Banned in the US.

E540   Dicalcium diphosphate
Unknown effects. Banned in Australia.

E541(i)   Sodium aluminium phosphate, acidic
A risk to babies, the elderly and people suffering from kidney and heart complaints. Possible links with osteoporosis, Parkinson's and Alzheimer's disease.

E541(ii)   Sodium aluminium phosphate, alkaline
Aluminium compounds are potentially neurotoxic. Banned in Australia.

E542   Bone phosphate, edible bone phosphate
No known adverse effects.

544   Calcium polyphosphates
May cause enzyme-blocking in the digestive system and cause calcium phosphorus imbalance. Banned in Australia.

545   Ammonium polyphosphates
Banned in Australia. See E544

E551   Silicon dioxide
No known adverse effects.

E552   Calcium silicate
No known adverse effects.

E553(i)   Magnesium silicate (synthetic)
No known adverse effects.

E553 (ii) Magnesium trisilicate
No known adverse effects.

E553(iii) Talc
No known adverse effects.

E554   Sodium aluminium silicate
Aluminium is known to cause placental problems in pregnancy and has been linked with Alzheimer's, Parkinson's and bone loss.

E556   Calcium aluminium silicate
See E554

E558   **Bentonite**
No known adverse effects.

E559   **Aluminium silicate**
See E554. Synonym: Kaolin

E570   **Stearic acid**
No known adverse effects.

572   **Magnesium stearate**
No known adverse effects.

E575   **Glucono delta-lactone**
No known adverse effects.

E576   **Sodium gluconate**
Concentrated traces of heavy metals in the product. Banned in Australia.

E577   **Potassium gluconate**
See E576

E578   **Calcium gluconate**
See E576

579   **Ferrous gluconate**
In small amounts, it is safe but may cause gastrointestinal stress.

E585   **Ferrous lactate**
Effects unknown.

FLAVOUR ENHANCERS

E620   **Glutamic acid**
Can cause similar problems to E621.

E621   **Monosodium L-glutamate (MSG)**
Neurotoxin linked with headaches and migraines, and also diseases such as
Huntington's, Alzheimer's and Parkinson's. Children, pregnant women,
hypoglycaemics, asthmatics, the elderly and those with heart disease may be
particularly sensitive.

E622   **Monopotassium L-glutamate**
Can cause nausea, vomiting, diarrhoea and abdominal cramps. Not for babies under
12 months old or for people with impaired kidneys. See E621.

E623   **Calcium di-L-glutamate**
Possible problems for asthmatics and aspirin-sensitive people. See E621.

E624   **Monoammonium L-glutamate**
See E621

E625   Magnesium di-L-glutamate.
See E621

E626   Guanylic acid
No known adverse effects.

E627   Disodium guanylate
Not permitted in foods for infants and young children. Those with gout, hyperactivity, asthma and aspirin sensitivity should avoid it.

E629   Calcium guanylate
Effects unknown.

E630   Inosinic acid
Effects unknown.

E631   Disodium inosinate
Frequently contains E621.

E635   Disodium 5'-ribonucleotide
Made from E627 and E631. Associated with itchy skin rashes for up to 30 hours after ingestion.

E636   Maltol
In large quantities, it can help aluminium pass into the brain, so is potentially linked to Alzheimer's disease. Some countries ban it for babies and young children.

637   Ethyl maltol
See E636

E640   Glycine (and its sodium salts), glycol, amino acetic acid
Mildly toxic if ingested.

MISCELLANEOUS

E900   Dimethyl polysiloxane
No known adverse effects.

E901   Beeswax (white and yellow)
No known adverse effects.

E902   Candelilla wax
No known adverse effects.

E903   Carnauba wax
Occasionally causes allergic reactions and is a possible carcinogen.

E904   Shellac
Derived from the lac insect of India; occasionally causes skin irritation.

905(a)   Mineral oil (white)
Listed as having teratogenic (foetal-toxic) properties; linked with bowel cancer.

905(b)   Petrolatum (petroleum jelly)
May inhibit absorption of fats and fat-soluble vitamins. Is a mild laxative. Suspected teratogen (foetal toxin).

E905   Paraffins, microcrystalline wax
Possible link with bowel cancer.

E907   Refined microcrystalline wax
Effects unknown.

E912   Montanic acid esters
Effects unknown.

E913   Lanolin
No known adverse effects. Synonym: Hydrous wool fat.

E914   Oxidised polyethylene wax
Effects unknown.

E920   L-Cysteine monohydrochloride
A known neurotoxin.

E921   L-Cysteine
See E920

E924   Potassium bromate
Large quantities can cause nausea, vomiting, diarrhoea, abdominal pain, kidney damage and failure. The WHO classifies it as a possible carcinogen.

E925   Chlorine
Destroys nutrients, known carcinogen.

E926   Chlorine dioxide
See E925

E927   Azodicarbonamide
Effects unknown. Banned in Australia.

E927(b)   Carbamide
Potential allergen.

E928   Benzoyl peroxide
Similar effects to E210.

E931   Nitrogen
Effects unknown.

E932   Nitrous oxide
Safe in small quantities. Long exposure has been linked to liver and kidney disease and cancer.

E938   Argon
Effects unknown.

E939   Helium
Effects unknown.

E941   Nitrogen
Effects unknown.

E948   Oxygen
No known adverse effects.

E950   Acesulfame potassium
Possible carcinogen in humans (caused cancer in test animals). Synonym: Acesulfame K

E951   Aspartame
Carcinogenic neurotoxin; linked to reproductive disorders.

E952   Cyclamic acid
Known to cause migraines and other reactions; can be carcinogenic; found to be a reproductive toxin in animal tests. Banned in the US and UK.

E953   Isomalt, isomaltitol
Can cause softer than normal stools and intestinal gas. Not permitted in infant foods.

E954   Saccharine
Interferes with normal blood coagulation, blood-sugar levels and digestive function. Potential carcinogen. Banned in France, Germany, Hungary, Portugal and Spain. Banned as food additive in Malaysia and Zimbabwe. Banned as a beverage additive in Fiji, Israel, Peru and Taiwan.

955   Sucralose
Can cause bloating, gas, nausea. In animal tests before being accepted in Australia, this showed detrimental effects to the thalamus glands, liver and kidney enlargement, and renal mineralisation. Synonym: Trichlorogalactosucrose

956   Alitame
Unknown effects, but possibly similar to E951.

E957   Thaumatin
Effects unknown.

E959   Neohesperidine DC
Effects unknown.

E965   Maltitol, hydrogenated glucose syrup
Stomach upsets; laxative in high concentrations.

E966   Lactitol
Stomach upsets; laxative in high concentrations.

E967   Xylitol
Stomach upsets; laxative in high concentrations.

E999   Quillaia extract
Effects unknown.

1001 Choline salts and esters

Effects unknown.

1100 Amylase

Effects unknown.

1101 Proteases (papain, bromelain, ficin)

Effects unknown.

1102 Glucose oxidase

Effects unknown.

E1103 Invertase

Effects unknown.

1104 Lipases

Effects unknown.

E1105 Lysozyme

Effects unknown.

E1200 Polydextrose

E1201 Polyvinylpyrrolidone

Made from formaldehyde. Excess may cause damage to the lungs or kidneys, gas and faecal impaction. Suspected carcinogen.

E1202 Polyvinylpolypyrrolidone (PPVP)

May cause damage to kidneys and stay in the system for up to a year.

1400 Dextrin roasted starch

Effects unknown.

1401 Acid-treated starch

No known adverse effects.

1402 Alkaline-treated starch

No known adverse effects.

1403 Bleached starch

Effects unknown.

E1404 Oxidised starch

Effects unknown.

1405 Enzyme-treated starch

No known adverse effects.

E1410 Monostarch phosphate

No known adverse effects.

E1412 Distarch phosphate

No known adverse effects.

E1413   Phosphated distarch phosphate

No known adverse effects.

E1414   Acetylated distarch phosphate

No known adverse effects.

E1420   Acetylated starch

No known adverse effects.

1421   Starch acetate esterified with vinyl acetate

No known adverse effects.

E1422   Acetylated distarch adipate

No known adverse effects.

E1440   Hydroxypropyl starch

No known adverse effects.

E1442   Hydroxy propyl distarch phosphate

No known adverse effects.

E1450   Starch sodium octenyl succinate

No known adverse effects.

E1451   Acetylated oxidised starch

No known adverse effects.

E1505   Triethyl acetate or citrate

No known adverse effects

E1510   Ethanol, ethyl alcohol

Suspected neurotoxic hazard; may provoke symptoms in people with Candida and allergies.

E1517   Glycerol diacetate

May cause headaches, nausea, vomiting, dehydration, diarrhoea, thirst, dizziness and mental confusion.

E1518   Glycerol triacetate, triacetin

Binder for solid rocket fuels. Fungicide, humectant and solvent. Effects unknown.

E1519   Benzyl alcohol

Consumption of large doses may cause vomiting, diarrhoea and central nervous system depression.

E1520   Propylene glycol

Large doses can cause central nervous system depression and kidney damage.

1521   Polyethylene glycerol 8000

Effects unknown.

* Additives which probably or definitely are of animal (mostly pig) derivation

Foods that fight toxic damage

A good diet can go a long way towards keeping you healthy. Along with essential nutrients, many foods also contain important cofactors, enzymes and fibre that turn them into what are known as 'functional foods' – that is, foods that bring extra bonuses that go beyond basic nutrition, such as helping the body to eliminate chemical toxins. Consider these simple kitchen-cupboard solutions to keeping your body free from chemical toxins:

- **Garlic and onions** contain powerful antioxidants that aid the body's natural day-to-day efforts to detox. Use these liberally in cooking. Other sulphur-rich foods such as broccoli, and bile stimulants such as lemon and bitter greens, also assist in detoxification.

- **Peas, beans and lentils** also contain unique antioxidants, and are high in fibre, which can bind to toxins and aid their removal from the body. Pulses are a good alternative source of protein, so consider substituting a couple of meat meals each week with one based on (organic) pulses.

- **A high-fibre diet** in general is useful for trapping toxins and assisting in the elimination of heavy metals. Fibre helps reduce intestinal permeability, sometimes known as a 'leaky gut' – a condition that can sometimes lead to allergies and toxic buildup in the bloodstream. It also prevents deactivated oestrogens from being reactivated and reabsorbed. Consider adding water-soluble mucilaginous fibres such as psyllium seeds and flaxseeds to your diet. These can be ground up, and sprinkled onto cereals, soups and baked foods.

- **Pectin**, found in apple and pear seeds, can protect your body from damage by toxic metals. It works by blocking the absorption of toxins while aiding detoxification. Try making apples or pears stewed with their seeds a regular feature of your diet.

- **Bananas** have antioxidant qualities that help to fight chemical damage.

- **Eggs** protect against lead and mercury contamination.

- **All leafy dark-green vegetables**, especially cruciferous vegetables (belonging to the cabbage family), can inhibit the carcinogenic effects of chemicals. Try to include plenty of kale, spinach, broccoli and brussels sprouts in your diet. Other green foods that contain chlorophyll are also natural chelators that can draw heavy metals out of the system. Herbs like coriander (cilantro) are a good choice. A good way to take your greens is to buy a juicer and use it to make vegetable juices – they are not as sweet as fruit juices, but they pack more punch in the detox stakes.

- **Consider seaweeds**. Seaweeds and alginates can also bind to heavy metals. There is evidence, for instance, that the freshwater green algae Chlorella can draw persistent chemicals, such as PCBs, out of the system. Similarly, research stretching back several decades shows that Arctic seaweeds are an aid to detoxification. These can be taken as supplements or added to your diet.

- **Black and green teas** are packed with antioxidants that may provide some protection from heavy-metal toxicity.

- **Forget your fat phobia**. Increasing your intake of healthy fats is important to maintaining good health. Good fats such as omega-3 and -6 can help leach toxins out of your system, prevent inflammation and protect the gut from toxic damage. Modern diets are particularly low in omega-3 fatty acids. The best natural sources of these are flaxseed, hempseed, canola, soybean and walnut oils, dark-green leaves, and coldwater fish, such as salmon, mackerel and sardines. The best natural sources of omega-6 are safflower, sunflower, hemp, soybean, walnut, pumpkin, sesame and flax oils as well as borage seed, blackcurrant seed and evening primrose oil. To get your daily dose of good fats, include more of the following foods in your diet:

  For omega-3 fats:
  Hempseed oil, 1 tablespoon; Flaxseed oil, 1 tablespoon; Flaxseeds, 2 tablespoons; Pumpkinseeds, 4 tablespoons; EPA/DHA supplement, 1000 mg.

  For omega-6 fats:
  Hempseed, 1 tablespoon ; Sunflowerseeds, 1 tablespoon; Pumpkinseeds, 2 tablespoons; Sesame seeds, 1½ tablespoons; Evening primrose oil, 1000 mg; Borage oil, 500 mg.

  Choose one source of omega-3 and omega-6 from each list to achieve a good intake of essential fatty acids (EFAs). Another good source of both types of fatty acids is dried beans such as kidney, haricot and soya. Regularly including these in your diet will ensure your 'good fat' needs are met.

- **Juice**. Fruit juices – even freshly squeezed ones – are tasty, but full of sugar; when it comes to detoxing, they cannot compare with the powerful effect of vegetable juices. Having said that, you need to be choosey about which vegetables you select. Veggie juices made from carrots and beetroot taste good, but are as full of sugar as most fruit juices. Mild detox drinks can be made from greens such as celery, fennel (anise) and cucumber. This is a good way to introduce yourself to the taste and effects of veggie juices if you've never had them before.

However, it is the dark-green leafy vegetable juices, though sometimes less palatable, that will benefit you the most. This is partly because of their chlorophyll content and partly because of their high antioxidant content. Once you get used to the milder juices, you can introduce more powerful mixtures made from lettuces such as red leaf, green leaf, romaine and endive, as well as other greens like escarole, spinach, cabbage, and Chinese cabbage or pak choi (bok choy).

Adding herbs like parsley and coriander (cilantro) to the juices will add flavour as well as further detoxification benefits. Start with small amounts and monitor your body's responses.

Other types of greens you can use (but sparingly, as they are very bitter) include kale, collard greens, dandelion greens and mustard greens.

Make sure you wash all your greens thoroughly before juicing and, where possible, buy organic for even more health benefits.

Better buying

Below is a brief list of companies that specialise in producing less-toxic products. However, with a rare few exceptions, it is impossible to unreservedly recommend every product that each of these companies produces. Instead, it is advised that consumers ask questions, read labels and choose for themselves those products with which they feel safe.

FOOD

General stores

Goodness Direct
www.goodnessdirect.co.uk

Hider
www.hider-foods.co.uk

Naturally Good Food Ltd
www.goodfooddelivery.co.uk

Real Food Direct
www.realfooddirect.co.uk

Traidcraft
www.traidcraft.co.uk

Australian Organic Food Directory
www.organicfooddirectory.com.au

Food-buying groups

Clearspring
www.clearspring.co.uk

Community Foods
www.communityfoods.co.uk

Eostre Organics
www.eostreorganics.co.uk

Essential Trading
www.essential-trading.coop

Organico
www.organico.co.uk

Suma
www.suma.co.uk

Organic beef, lamb, pork & poultry

Graig Farm Organics
www.graigfarm.co.uk

Higher Hacknell Farm
www.higherhacknell.co.uk

Sheepdrove Organic Farm
www.sheepdrove.com

The Real Meat Company
www.realmeat.co.uk

Well Hung Meat
www.wellhungmeat.com

Fresh fish

Inverawe Smokehouses
www.smokedsalmon.co.uk

The Organic Smokehouse
www.organicsmokehouse.com

Oeverill Trout Farm
www.purelyorganic.co.uk

Beers, ales & cider

Beers in a Box
www.beersinabox.com

Black Isle Organic Beers
www.blackislebrewery.com

Broughton Ales
www.broughtonales.co.uk

Mountain Goat Beer
www.goatbeer.com.au

Wine

Festival Wines
www.festivalwines.co.uk

Pure Wine
www.purewine.co.uk

Vinceremos
www.vinceremos.co.uk

Vintage Roots
www.vintageroots.co.uk

Organic Wine
www.organicwine.com.au

Spirits

Juniper Green Organic Gin
www.junipergreen.org

Stonelink Farm (organic sloe gin)
www.stonelinkfarm.co.uk

Coffee & tea

A Lot of Coffee
www.alotofcoffee.co.uk

Cafe Direct
www.cafedirect.co.uk

Clipper Teas
www.clipper-teas.com

Dragonfly Tea
www.dragonflyteas.com

Equal Exchange
www.equalexchange.com

Origin
www.origincoffee.co.uk

The Bean Shop
www.thebeanshop.com

Tobys Estate
www.tobysestate.com.au

BEAUTY

Bodycare essentials

The Organic Pharmacy
www.theorganicpharmacy.com

Pure Skin Care
www.pureskincare.co.uk

Barefoot Botanicals
www.barefoot-botanicals.com

Dr Bronner's
www.21stcenturyhealth.co.uk

Duchy Originals
www.duchyoriginals.com

Earthbound Organics
www.earthbound.co.uk

Green People
www.greenpeople.co.uk

My Being Well
www.mybeingwell.com

Neal's Yard Remedies
www.nealsyardremedies.com

REN
www.renskincare.com

Weleda
www.weleda.co.uk

Jurlique
www.jurlique.com.au

Sanitary products

Natracare
www.natracare.com

Nature Women Care
www.naty.com

Menses
www.menses.co.uk

The Mooncup
www.mooncup.co.uk

Make-your-own cosmetics

Aromantic
www.aromantic.co.uk

Bay House Aromatics
www.bay-house.co.uk

Cosmetics at Home
www.cosmeticsathome.co.uk

New Directions
www.newdirectionsuk.com

The Soap Tub
www.meltsandpoursupplies.com

BABY & CHILD

Baby basics

Born
www.borndirect.com

Green Baby
www.greenbaby.co.uk

Greenfibres
www.greenfibres.co.uk

Hejhog
www.hejhog.co.uk

Nature's Child
www.natureschild.com.au

Baby toiletries

Burt's Bees
www.myburtsbees.co.uk

Earth Friendly Baby
www.earth-friendly-baby.co.uk

Earth Mama Angel Baby
www.earthmamaangelbaby.com

Weleda
www.weleda.co.uk

Clothing

Baby Organics
www.babyorganics.co.uk

Bishopston Trading Company
www.bishopstontrading.co.uk

Gossypium
www.gossypium.co.uk

Huggababy
www.huggababy.co.uk

Little Earthlings
www.littleearthlings.com

Natural Child
www.naturalchild.com

Organics for Kids
www.organicsforkids.com

Schmidt Natural Clothing
www.naturalclothing.co.uk

Cloth nappies

See Saw
www.seesawnappies.co.uk

Snazzy pants
www.snazzypants.co.uk

The Nappy Lady
www.thenappylady.co.uk

HOUSEHOLD

Cleaning products

Bio D
www.biodegradable.biz

Ecotopia
www.ecotopia.co.uk

Ecover
www.ecover.com

Energy Wipe
www.energywipe.com

Enjo
www.enjo.net

Faith in Nature
www.faithproducts.com

Greenlands
www.greenlands-env.co.uk

Natural Collection
www.naturalcollection.com

Vertue
www.vertue.com

My Organic
www.myorganic.com.au

Paints

Auro Organic Paints
www.auro.co.uk

Earth Born Paints
www.earthbornpaints.co.uk

Ecomerchant
www.ecomerchant.co.uk

Ecopaints
www.ecopaints.co.uk

Decorating basics

Construction Resources
www.constructionresources.com

Ecomerchant
www.ecomerchant.co.uk

Green Building Store
www.greenbuildingstore.co.uk

The Green Shop
www.thegreenshop.co.uk

The Healthy House
www.healthy-house.co.uk

Nigel's Eco Store
www.theinsightecostore.com

Garden supplies

British Eco
www.britisheco.com

Green Gardener
www.greengardener.co.uk

The Organic Gardening Catalogue
www.organiccatalogue.com

Fertilisers

Enviromulch
www.wbpenviromulch.com

Fertile Fibre
www.fertilefibre.co.uk

Rooster Pelleted Manure
www.rooster.uk.com

Selected bibliography

An enormous amount of research has formed the background to this book, so these pages represent only a selection of the papers and books that readers may find of interest.

PAPERS & REPORTS

General

Abou-Donia MB et al. 'Neurotoxicity resulting from coexposure to pyridostigmine bromide, DEET, and permethrin: implications of Gulf War chemical exposures', *J Toxicol Environ Health*, 1996; 48 (1): 35–56

Arnold SF et al. 'Synergistic activation of estrogen receptors with combinations of environmental chemicals', *Science*, 1996; 272: 1489–92

Bearer CF. 'How are children different from adults?', *Environ Health Perspect*, 1995; 103 (Suppl 6): 7–12

Brown SK. 'Exposure to volatile organic compounds in indoor air: A review, in *Proceedings of the International Clean Air Conference of the Clean Air*', *Society of Australia and New Zealand*, 1992; 1: 95–104

Brown SK. 'Volatile organic pollutants in new and established buildings in Melbourne, Australia', *Indoor Air*, 2002; 12: 55–63

Carpenter DO et al. 'Human health and chemical mixtures: an overview', *Environ Health Perspect*, 1998; 106 (Suppl 6):1263–70

'Chemical Hazard Data Availability Study', US Environmental Protection Agency, 1998

Colbin T et al. 'Our Stolen Future', Online at: *www.ourstolenfuture.org*

Cooper SD et al. 'Identification of polar organic compounds found in consumer products and their toxicological properties', *Anal Environ Epidemiol*, 1995; 5: 57–75

Crinnion WJ. 'Environmental medicine, Part 1: The human burden of environmental toxins and their common health effects', *Altern Med Rev*, 2000; 5: 52–63

'Crisis in Chemicals: The threat posed by the "biomedical revolution" to the profits, liabilities and regulation of industries making and using chemicals', Friends of the Earth, May 2000

'Draft risk assessment of the potential human health effects associated with exposure to perfluorooctanoic acid and its salts', Environmental Protection Agency, January 4, 2005 (online at *www.epa.gov/oppt/pfoa*)

'11th Report on Carcinogens, National Toxicology Program', US Department of Health and Human Services, Public Health Service

Eaton KK, Anthony HM. 'Multiple chemical sensitivity recognition and management: A document on the health effects of everyday chemical exposures and their implications', Third Scientific Report of the British Society for Allergy, Environmental and Nutritional Medicine (BSAENM), March 2000

'Environmental Diseases From A to Z.' Publication no. 96–4145. National Institutes of Health, US Department of Health and Human Services, 1997

Epstein S et al. 'Synergistic toxicity and carcinogenicity of "freons" and piperonyl butoxide', *Nature*, 1967; 214: 526–8

Fujii K, Epstein S. 'Effects of piperonyl butoxide on the toxicity and hepatocarcinogenicity of 2-acetylaminofluorene and 4acetylaminobiphenyl, and their N-hydroxylated derivatives, following administration to newborn mice', *Oncology*, 1979; 36: 105–12

Harris C et al. 'The estrogenic activity of phthalate esters in vitro', *Environ Health Perspect*, 1997; 105: 802–11

'Health-Hazard Information', US Environmental Protection Agency, 1991

'How Chemical Exposures Affect Reproductive Health: Patient Fact Sheet', Greater Boston Physicians for Social Responsibility (GBPSR), 1996

'Identification of Polar Volatile Organic Compounds in Consumer Products and Common Microenvironments', US Environmental Protection Agency, 1991

Lichtenstein P et al. 'Environmental and heritable factors in the causation of cancer: Analyses of cohorts of twins from Sweden, Denmark, and Finland', *N Engl J Med*, 2000; 343: 78–85

Masters RD. 'Biology and politics: linking nature and nurture', *Ann Rev Polit Sci*, 2001; 4: 345–69

Meggs WJ. 'Neurogenic inflammation and sensitivity to environmental chemicals', *Environ Health Perspect*, 1993; 101: 234–8

Meggs WJ. 'Neurogenic switching: A hypothesis for a mechanism for shifting the site of inflammation in allergy and chemicals sensitivity', *Environ Health Perspect*, 1995; 103: 54–6

'National Report on Human Exposure to Environmental Chemicals', Centers for Disease Control and Prevention, Atlanta, GA: March 2001; online at: *www.cdc.gov/nceh/dls/report/*

'Neurotoxins: At home and the workplace', Report by the Committee on Science and Technology, US House of Representatives, September 15, 1986, No 99–827

Pearce N, Bethwait P. 'Increasing incidence of non-Hodgkin's lymphoma: occupational and environmental factors', *Cancer Res*, 1992; 52 (19 Suppl): 5496S–500S

'PFCs – A Family of Chemicals That Contaminate the Planet', Environmental Working Group, EWG, April 2003

'Second National Report on Human Exposure to Environmental Chemicals', Centers for Disease Control and Prevention, Atlanta, GA, March 2003. Online at: *www.cdc.gov/exposurereport/*

'Toxic Alert. A survey of high-street companies and their approach to suspect chemicals', Friends of the Earth, October 2000

'Toxic Nation: A report on pollution in Canadians', Environmental Defence, Canada Nov 2005; online at: *www.environmentaldefence.ca*

Warhurst M. 'Introduction to Hormone Disrupting Compounds', Online at: *http://website.lineone.net/~mwarhurst/*

Food

Brotons JA et al. 'Xenoestrogens released from lacquer coatings in food cans', *Environ Health Perspect*, 1995; 103: 608–12

'Children's drinks contain ingredients that can form benzene: FDA silent despite knowledge of the problem', Environmental Working Group press release, February 28, 2006

Cressey P et al. '1997/98 New Zealand Total Diet Survey, Part 1: Pesticide residues', Ministry of Health, 2000

'CSPI's Guide to Food Additives', Center for Science in the Public Interest. Online at: *www.cspinet.org/reports/chemcuisine.htm*

'Eating Oil: Food in a changing climate', Sustain, 2001

'Feeding Minds – The impact of food on mental health', Mental Health Foundation, Winter 2005; online at: *www.mentalhealth.org.uk*

Gunderson EL. 'FDA total diet study, April 1982–April 1984. Dietary intakes of pesticides, selected elements, and other chemicals', *J Assoc Off Anal Chem*, 1988; 71: 1200–9

Lau K et al. 'Synergistic interactions between commonly used food additives in a developmental neurotoxicity test', *Toxicol Sci*, 2006; 90 (1): 178–87

Lucas MEP, Hines C. 'Stopping the great food swap: Relocalising Europe's food supply', The Green Party, 2001

Mayer AM. 'Historical changes in the mineral content of fruits and vegetables: A cause for concern?', *Br Food J*, 1997; 99: 207–11

McCance RA, Widdowson EM. 'The Chemical Composition of Foods', 1st edn, Special Report Series no. 235. UK: Royal Society of Chemistry/MAFF, 1940

McCance RA, Widdowson EM. 'The Composition of Foods', 5th edn. UK: Royal Society of Chemistry/MAFF, 1991

'Pesticide residues monitoring: second quarter results April to June 2003', Pesticide Residues Committee 3 December 2003; online: *www.pesticides.gov.uk/prc_home.asp*

Pretty JN et al. 'Farm costs and food miles: an assessment of the full cost of the UK weekly food basket', *Food Policy*, 2005; 30: 1–19

'The 19th Australian Total Diet Survey', Australia New Zealand Food Authority, ANZFA, April 2001

'The Total Diet Study: summary of residues found ordered by food, Market baskets, 91-3–99-1', Food and Drug Administration, FDA, September 2000

Thomas D. 'Mineral depletion in foods over the period 1940 to 1991', *Nutr Pract*, 2001; 2: 27–9

Van der Weyer C. 'Changing diets, changing minds: How food affects mental well being and behaviour', Mental Health Foundation/Sustain, winter 2005; online at: *www.sustainweb.org*

'Vegetables without vitamins', Life Extension, March 2001; online at: *www.lef.org/magazine/mag2001/mar2001_report_vegetables.html*

'What's Wrong With Supermarkets?', 4th edn. Corporate Watch, April 2004; online at *www.corporateatch.org.uk*

White A. 'Pesticides in food: Why go organic?', Pesticide Action Network NZ/Safe Food Campaign NZ, New Zealand, 1999

Wiles R. Letter to Andrew C. von Eschenbach, MD, Acting Commissioner of Food and Drugs, U.S. Food and Drug Administration Environmental Working Group, February 28, 2006

'Working Party on Pesticide Residues – 1999 Report', London: MAFF Publications, 1999

Worthington V. 'Nutritional quality of organic versus conventional fruits, vegetables and grains', *J Alt Comp Med*, 2001; 7 (2): 161–73

Beauty

Anderson RC, Anderson JH. 'Acute toxic effects of fragrance products', *Arch Environ Health*, 1998; 53: 138–46

Brown LM et al. 'Hair dye use and multiple myeloma in white men', *Am J Public Health*, 1992; 82: 1673–4

Buchbauer G et al. 'Fragrance compounds and essential oils with sedative effects upon inhalation', *J Pharm Sci*, 1993; 82: 660–4

Cantor KP et al. 'Hair dye use and risk of leukemia and lymphoma', *Am J Publ Health*, 1988; 78: 570–1

Connor TH et al. 'Mutagenicity of cosmetic products containing Kathon', *Environ Mol Mutagen*, 1996; 28: 127–32

Cook LS et al. 'Hair product use and the risk of breast cancer in young women', *Cancer Causes Control*, 1999; 10: 551–9

Cramer DW et al. 'Genital talc exposure and risk of ovarian cancer', *Int J Cancer*, 1999; 81: 351–6

Darbre PD et al. 'Concentrations of parabens in human breast tumours', *J Appl Toxicol*, 2004 Jan–Feb; 24 (1): 5–13

Daughton C, Ternes T. 'Pharmaceuticals and personal care products in the environment: agents of subtle change?', *Environ Health Perspect*, 1999; 107 (suppl 6): 907–38

Eisenbrand G et al. 'N-Nitrosoalkanolamines in cosmetics in relevance to human cancer of N-nitroso compounds, tobacco smoke and mycotoxins', IARC (International Agency for Research on Cancer), 1991

Frosch PJ et al. 'Patch testing with fragrances: results of a multicentre study of the European environmental and contact dermatitis research group with 48 frequently used constituents of perfumes', *Contact Derm*, 1995; 33: 333–42

Gertig DM et al. 'Prospective study of talc use and ovarian cancer', *J Natl Cancer Inst*, 2000; 92: 249–52

Graves AB et al. 'The association between aluminum-containing products and Alzheimer's disease', *J Clin Epidemiol*, 1990; 43: 35–44

Grodstein F et al. 'A prospective study of permanent hair dye use and hematopoietic cancer', *J Natl Cancer Inst*, 1994; 86: 1466–70

Harlow BL, Weiss BS. 'A case-control study of borderline ovarian tumors: the influence of perineal exposure to talc', *Am J Epidemiol*, 1989; 130: 390–4

Hastings L et al. 'Olfactory primary neurons as a route of entry for toxic agents into the CNS', *Neurotoxicology*, 1991; 12: 707–14

Heller DS et al. 'The relationship between perineal cosmetic talc usage and ovarian talc particle burden', *Am J Obstet Gynecol*, 1996; 74: 1507–10

Holly EA et al. 'Hair-color products and risk for non-Hodgkin's lymphoma: a population-based study in the San Francisco bay area', *Am J Publ Health*, 1998; 88: 1767–73

Kumar P et al. 'Inhalation challenge effects of perfume scent strips in patients with asthma', *Ann Allergy Asthma Immunol*, 1995; 75: 429–33

Lawson R. 'Have you met this syndrome?', *Med Monit*, September 4, 1996: 66.

Mauller S et al. 'Occurrence of nitro and non-nitro benzenoid musk compounds in human adipose tissue', *Chemosphere*, 1996; 33: 17–28

Millqvist E, Lowhagen O. 'Placebo-controlled challenges with perfume in patients with asthma-like symptoms', *Allergy*, 1996; 51: 434–9

Nasca PC et al. 'Relationship of hair dye use, benign breast disease, and breast cancer', *J Natl Cancer Inst*, 1980; 64: 23–8

Routledge EJ et al. 'Some alkyl hydroxy benzoate preservatives (parabens) are estrogenic', *Toxicol Appl Pharmacol*, 1998; 153: 12–9

Schlumpf M et al. 'In vitro and in vivo estrogenicity of UV screens', *Environ Health Perspect*, 2001; 109: 239–44

Shafer N, Shafer RW. 'Potential of carcinogenic effects of hair dyes', *NY State J Med*, 1976; 76: 394–6

Shore RE et al. 'A case-control study of hair dye use and breast cancer', *J Natl Cancer Inst*, 1979; 62: 277–83

Shulman JD, Wells LM. 'Acute fluoride toxicity from ingesting home-use dental products in children, birth to 6 years of age', *J Publ Health Dent*, 1997; 57: 150–8

Spencer PS et al. 'Neurotoxic fragrance produces ceroid and myelin disease', *Science*, 1979; 204: 633–5

Spencer PS et al. 'Neurotoxic properties of musk ambrette', *Toxicol Appl Pharmacol*, 1984; 75: 571–5

Thun MJ et al. 'Hair dye use and risk of fatal cancers in US women', *J Natl Cancer Inst*, 1994; 86: 210–5

Weibel H et al. 'Penetration of the fragrance compounds, cinnamaldehyde and cinnamyl alcohol, through human skin in vitro', *Contact Derm*, 1996; 34: 423–6

Whitford GM. 'Fluoride in dental products: safety considerations', *J Dent Res*, 1987; 66: 1056–60

Household

Anderson RC, Anderson JH. 'Toxic effects of air freshener emissions', *Arch Environ Health*, 1997; 52: 433–41

Anderson RC. 'Toxic emissions from carpets', *J Nutr Environ Med*, 1995; 5: 375–86

'Exercise caution when using "nano-sealing sprays" containing a propellant!', Federal Institute for Risk Assessment, March 31, 2006 press release; online at: *www.bfr.bund.de/cms5w/sixcms/detail.php/7699*

Ott WR, Roberts JW. 'Everyday exposure to toxic pollutants', *Sci Am*, 1998; Feb: 86–91

Thomas P. 'Dawn of the domestic superbug', *Ecologist*, July/August 2005: 42–8

Wallace LA et al. 'Personal exposure, indoor-outdoor relationships, and breath levels of toxic air pollutants measured for 355 persons in New Jersey', *Environmental Protection Agency* 0589, presented at the Annual Meeting of Air Pollution Control Association, San Francisco, CA, 25 June 1984

Wallace LA et al. 'Personal exposure, indoor-outdoor relationships, and breath levels of toxic air pollutants exposures, outdoor concentrations, and breath levels of toxic air pollutants measured for 425 persons in urban, suburban and rural areas', *EPA 0589*, presented at the Annual Meeting of Air Pollution Control Association, San Francisco, CA, 25 June 1984

Warhurst AM. 'An environmental assessment of alkylphenol ethoxylates and alkylphenols', Friends of the Earth, London, 1995

White RF, Proctor SP. 'Solvents and neurotoxicity', *Lancet*, 1997; 349: 1239–43

Pesticides

'Chemical Trespass – A toxic legacy', World Wildlife Fund, WWF-UK, 1999

Davis JR et al. 'Family pesticide use and childhood brain cancer', *Arch Environ Contam Toxicol*, 1993; 24: 87–92

'European workshop on the impact of endocrine disrupters on human health and wildlife', 2–4 December 1996, Weybridge, UK. Proceedings, Report No. EUR 17549. Copenhagen, Denmark: European Commission DG XII, April 1997

Harrison PTC. 'Endocrine disrupters and human health', *BMJ*, 2001; 323: 1317–8

Harrison PTC et al. 'Reproductive health in humans and wildlife: are adverse trends associated with environmental chemical exposure?', *Sci Total Environ*, 1997; 205: 97–106

'Hormonally Active Agents in the Environment', Committee on Hormonally

Active Agents in the Environment, National Research Council, National Academy of Sciences, 2000

'Intolerance Risk: Pesticides in our children's food', Natural Resources Defences Council, Washington, DC: NRDC, 1989

Ritter L. 'Report of a panel on the relationship between public exposure to pesticides and cancer', Ad Hoc Panel on Pesticides and Cancer, National Cancer Institute of Canada. Cancer, 1997; 80: 2019–33

'The Secret Hazards of Pesticides: Inert ingredients', Attorney General of New York, New York State Office of the Attorney General, Environmental Protection Bureau, February 1996

Pets

Davenport GM. 'The impact of nutrition on skin and hair coat', Presented at the 4th World Congress of Veterinary Dermatology, in Current Research in Canine Dermatology, The IAMS Company, Dayton, Ohio, 2000: 4–9

Hawkins BJ. 'Periodontal disease in dogs and cats', Proceedings of the North American Veterinary Conference, Orlando, Fl, 1996: 137–9

Hayes KC et al. 'An ultrastructural study of nutritionally induced and reversed retinal degeneration in cats', Am J Pathol, 1975; 78: 505

Lewis RG et al. 'Evaluation of methods for monitoring the potential exposures of small children to pesticides in the residential environment', Arch Environ Contam Toxicol, 1994; 26: 37–46

Martin AN. '"Mad pet" disease: mad cow disease is killing Europe's pets', Nutrient Requirements of Cats. National Research Council, National Academy Press, Washington DC, 1986

Morris JG, Rogers QR. 'Assessment of the nutritional adequacy of pet foods through the life cycle', J Nutr, 1994; 124: S2520–34

Neff J. 'Dog eat dog & cats? Fur flies as charges of canine cannibalism and willful malnourishment roil pet industry', Food Processing, March 2002

'Nutrient Requirements of Dogs', National Research Council, National Academy Press, Washington DC, 1985

Pollak W. 'The effects of a natural vs. commercial pet food diet on wellness of common companion animals', Online at: www.healthyvet.com

Wallinga D, Greer L. 'Poisons on pets – health hazards from flea and tick products', Natural Resources Defense Council, November 2000

Williams R. 'Safe flea control and organic labelling', *Townsend Lett Docs*; 2003; April 1

'What Vets Don't Tell You: Special Report', London, UK: WDDTY, 2003. Available to order online at *www.wddty.co.uk*

BOOKS

Antczak S, Antczak G. *Cosmetics Unmasked*. Thorsons, 2001

Ashford N, Miller C. *Chemical Exposures: Low levels and high stakes*. Wiley & Sons, 1998

Blythman J. *Shopped! The shocking truth about British supermarkets*. Fourth Estate, 2004

Bowlby R. *Carried Away: The invention of modern shopping*. Faber & Faber, 2000

Bremner M. *Enquire Within*, 3rd ed. Helicon, 1994

Briggs SA and the Staff of the Rachel Carson Council. *Basic Guide to Pesticides*. USA & London: Hemisphere Publishing, 1992

Carson R. *Silent Spring*, reprint ed. Mariner Books, 1994

Cox P, Brusseau P. *Secret Ingredients*. Bantam Books, 1997

Engel C. *Wild Health: How animals keep themselves well and what we can learn from them*. Mariner Books, 2003

Epstein S et al. *The Breast Cancer Prevention Program*. Macmillan, 1997

Gosselin RE et al. *Clinical Toxicology of Commercial Products*, 5th edn. Williams & Wilkins, 1984

Harte J et al. *Toxics A to Z: A guide to everyday pollution hazards*. University of California Press, 1991

Lawrence F. *Not on the Label*. Penguin Books, 2004

Lijinsky W. *Chemistry and Biology of N-nitroso Compounds*. Cambridge University Press, 1990

Logan K. *Clean House, Clean Planet*. Pocket Books, 1997

Martin AN. *Foods Pets Die For: Shocking facts about pet food*, 2nd edn. New Sage Press, 2003

Monbiot G. *Captive State: The corporate takeover of Britain*. MacMillan, 2000

Mumby K. *The Complete Guide to Food Allergies and Environmental Illness*. Thorsons, 1993

Neal's Yard Remedies. *Make Your Own Cosmetics*. Aurum Press, 1997

Pagram B. *Natural Housekeeping*. Gaia, 1997

Palma RJ. *The Complete Guide to Household Chemicals*. Prometheus Books, 1995

Robbins C. *Poisoned Harvest: A consumer's guide to pesticide use and abuse*. Victor Gollancz, 1991

Roberts RJ. *Overview of similarities and differences between children and adults: implications for risk assessment*, in Guzelian PS et al. (eds). Similarities and Differences Between Children and Adults. Washington, DC: ILSI Press, 1992: 1–15

Ross Lewis G. *1001 Chemicals in Everyday Products*, 2nd edn. Wiley-Interscience, 1999

Sarjeant D, Evans K. *Hard to Swallow: The truth about food additives*. Alive Books, 1999

Schettler T et al. *Generations At Risk: Reproductive health and the environment*. MIT Press, 2000

Schlosser E. *Fast Food Nation: The dark side of the American meal*. Penguin Books, 2001

Seth A, Randall G. *The Grocers*. Kogan Page 1999

Steinman D, Epstein S. *The Safe Shopper's Bible: A consumers guide to nontoxic household products*. Macmillan, 1995

Steinman D, Wisner RM. *Living Healthy in a Toxic World*. Perigree, 1996

Thomas P. *Cleaning Yourself to Death*. New Leaf, 2001

Thomas P. *Living Dangerously*. New Leaf, 2003

Tickner J et al. *The Precautionary Principle in Action: A handbook.* Science and Environmental Health Network, 1998

Whitehead R, ed. *The UK Pesticide Guide 2000*. Wallingford, Oxon: CABI Publishing, CAB International

Winter R. *A Consumer's Dictionary of Food Additives*. Three Rivers Press, 2004

Wormwood VA. *The Fragrant Pharmacy*. Macmillan, 1990

Young W. *Sold Out: The true cost of supermarket shopping*. Vision, 2004

index

For more detailed information on individual chemicals see the A–Z listing on pages 289–354